STEROIDS – CLINICAL ASPECT

Edited by **Hassan Abduljabbar**

Steroids – Clinical Aspect
Edited by Hassan Abduljabbar

Published by InTech

Janeza Trdine 9, 51000 Rijeka, Croatia

Publishing Process Manager Bojan Rafaj

Technical Editor Teodora Smiljanic

Cover Designer InTech Design Team

Additional hard copies can be obtained from orders@intechopen.com

Steroids – Clinical Aspect, Edited by Hassan Abduljabbar
p. cm.
ISBN 978-953-307-705-5

For EU product safety concerns:
IN TECH d.o.o., Prolaz Marije Krucifikse Kozulić 3, 51000 Rijeka, Croatia,
info@intechopen.com or visit our website at intechopen.com.

Meet the editor

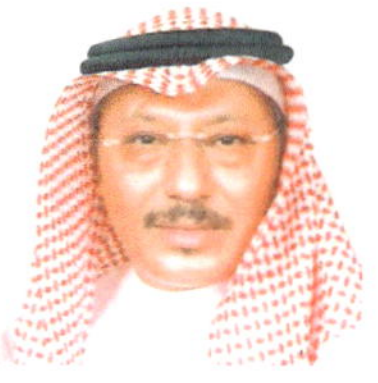

Professor Hassan Abduljabbar obtained his Medical degree from King Abdulaziz University, Jeddah, Saudi Arabia on June 1980. He then pursued his postgraduate training in Obstetrics and Gynecology at the University of Western Ontario, Canada. On Nov 1986 he became a Fellow of the Royal College of Physicians Surgeons of Canada. He obtained his American board in OBGYN on 1988. Currently he is a Professor and the chairman of the Department of Obstetrics and Gynecology at King Abdulaziz University Hospital, Jeddah, Saudi Arabia. He also is the Medical Director of United Doctors Hospital, Jeddah, Saudi Arabia from 1998 till present. He is a member of American Fertility Socitey, American Socitey of Gynecological laparscopy and The Saudi Obstetrics and Gynecology Society. His main interests are infertility, Stem Cells, and physiological and biochemical changes in the human body during pregnancy. He has a number of publications in different journals in Obstetrics and Gynecology.

Contents

Preface

The history of steroids is richly immersed and runs long and deep. The modern history of steroids started in the early 20th century, but its use has been traced back to ancient Greece where athletes ingested animal testicles to boost their energy and performance. This book covers the modern understanding and clinical use of steroids.

We divided the book into two sections. The first section contains information about steroids in the human body. The second section will cover the relationship of steroids.

Topics covered in the first section include the concentration of the steroids in various parts of the body, effects of steroids on body composition of athletes, the metabolic syndromes, and the effect of steroids on the development of the male reproductive system. The second section contains various clinical scenarios that involve steroids.

We hope that this book will contribute further to the literature available about steroids and enables the reader to further understand this interesting and rapidly evolving science.

Hassan Abduljabbar
Professor of Obstetrics and Gynecology,
King Abdulaziz University,
Kingdom of Saudi Arabia

Part 1

Steroid in the Body

1

The Concentration of Steroid Hormones in Blood and Peritoneal Fluid Depends on the Site of Sampling

N. Einer-Jensen[1], R.H.F. Hunter[2] and E. Cicinelli[3]
[1]*Institute of Molecular Medicine, University of Southern Denmark, Odense M,*
[2]*Institute for Reproductive Medicine, Hannover Veterinary University, Hannover,*
[3]*Dept Obstet Gynecol, University Hospital, Bari,*
[1]*Denmark*
[2]*Germany*
[3]*Italy*

1. Introduction

The concentration of steroid hormones in arteries varies according to the site of blood sampling. The hormone concentration is higher in the ovarian and testicular arteries than in the aorta resulting in a high impact on the target organs, opening a route for local hormonal regulation between organs. Local application of drugs may induce a potential method for semi-specific treatments. Vaginal application of hormones will therefore induce relatively higher concentrations in the uterus and urinary bladder area than a peripheral application. Likewise, nasal application will induce a higher relative concentration in brain arterial blood than peripheral application. This is due to local counter-current transfer between venous and arterial blood, and between the lymphatic and arterial vessels. Similarly, the concentration of steroids in peritoneal fluid varies according to the site of sampling.

2. The third way of humoral communication: local counter-current transfer

Humoral communication between cells can be either through local diffusion in the interstitial fluid between neighbouring cells or through the vascular system. The present paper will discuss a third possibility that is part of the vascular distribution. The paper will concentrate on local communication between organs belonging to the reproductive system and steroid hormones, but will also touch other organs (the adrenal, the brain and the peritoneal cavity) where local transfer of steroids seem to be involved in the physiological regulation.

McCracken et al. (1972) initiated the hormonal transfer investigations in the female. The anatomical structure had, however, been known for hundreds of years (Blancardi 1687, published in 1739). Ginther (1967) described the functional importance of a close connection between the ovarian artery and veins. The work involving steroid transfer in males was started by Jacks and Setchell (1973) and Einer-Jensen (1974). The documentation comes from investigations in several animal species as well as in man (see

Einer-Jensen et al., 1989; see Krzymowski, 1990; see Einer-Jensen and Hunter, 2005). Despite the anatomical differences between the species (one ovulation versus 10-20 ovulations, large uterine body and small uterine horns versus small uterine body and large horns), the picture of transfer is similar.

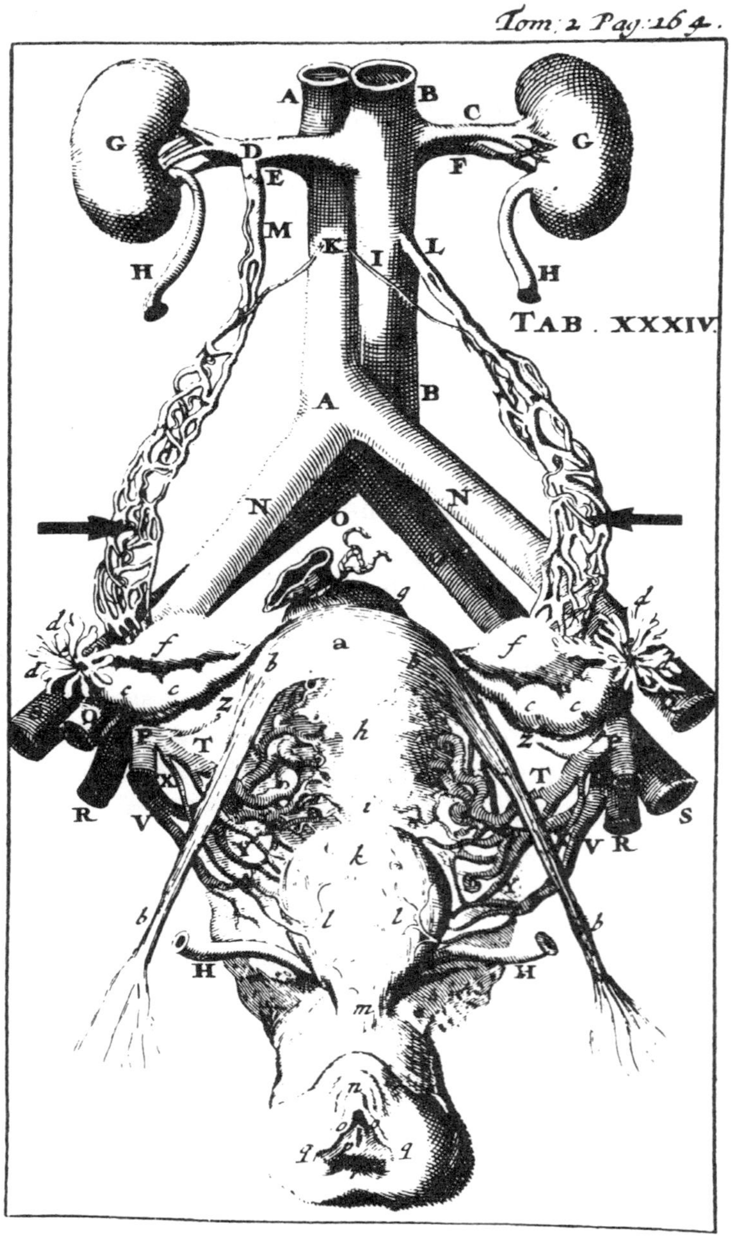

Fig. 1. The human genital organs and their vascular supply. The plexus formed by the ovarian artery and vein can be seen (arrows). (From Blancardi 1687).

Signal substances such as hormones produced in an organ will diffuse to the surrounding lymph and blood capillaries. Thus the signal substance will be present in the content of local lymph and blood vessels removing fluid and blood from the organ. The concentration will, of course, be high here compared to the peripheral fluids since no dilution has taken place (Einer-Jensen and Hunter, 2005).

In some hormone producing organs, the vessels removing the fluid from the organ are very intimately arranged with the artery supplying the organ. This is the case for steroid producing organs such as the gonads in both male and female. It is well known that the temperature in the extra-abdominal testis is a few degrees Centigrade lower than the general body temperature due to cooling through the scrotal wall and maintenance of the temperature gradient by counter-current transfer of heat energy. The transfer is expected to take place between the venous plexus (the Pampiniform plexus) and the convoluted testicular artery. The efficacy of the heat transfer is very high, close to 100% (Glad Sørensen et al., 1991), thus the cooling through the scrotal wall can be kept at a low level – which will diminish the waste of energy from the body. In most mammals, the testis is an organ positioned outside the abdomen, but even in animals with intra-abdominal testes the close apposition between the vessels is found, e.g. in small whales (Einer-Jensen, pers. com.). This strongly suggests that cooling is not the only reason for the vascular arrangement

The ovaries are always positioned in the abdomen and one would not expect temperature gradients within their tissues. The vessels to and from the ovary are closely apposed in a way similar to the male, indicating the potential for of a transfer system. However, the temperature of the pre-ovulatory follicles tends to be lower than deep body temperature (Hunter and Einer-Jensen, 2005; Hunter et al., 2006). Heat "consuming" proteins induce lower temperature and the temperature decrease is maintained by a very local heat-exchange mechanism in the vessels to and from the follicle.

3. Counter-current exchange

When blood or lymph flows through arteries, and veins and lymph vessels, and the vessels are in close contact, the flow can be described as counter-current flow.

Counter-current exchange along with Concurrent exchange comprise the mechanisms used to transfer some property of a fluid from one flowing current of fluid to another across a semipermeable membrane or thermally-conductive material between them. The property transferred could be heat, concentration of a chemical substance, or others. Counter-current exchange is a key concept in chemical engineering thermodynamics and manufacturing processes, for example in extracting sucrose from sugar beet roots. (Wikipedia, the figure below is also from Wikipedia).

The present authors expect the transfer to be passive; no active transfer mechanisms have been detected or proposed (to the best knowledge of the authors). The laws of physics, the respective rates of flow, the diffusion distance between the vessels, the chemical nature of the substances, especially the lipophility, will determine the rate of exchange. In general, a system will transfer heat at almost 100% (Glad Sørensen et al., 1991), whereas the exchange of tritiated water may be 20%, and the rate of steroid hormone transfer a few per cent.

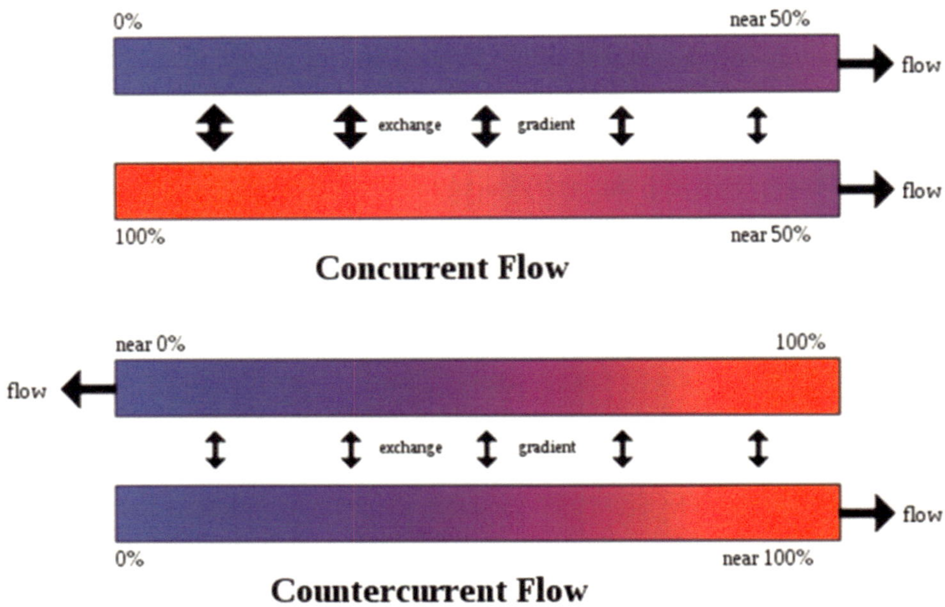

Fig. 2.

Many of the first experiments evaluating the transfer were performed with radioactive gases (^{133}Xenon and ^{85}Krypton). The efficacy of the transfer is similar to that of tritiated water. The advantage of using gas was the lack of recirculation since more than 95% of the gas is cleared during the first passage.

Even a limited transfer of steroids may have a marked physiological impact. Only non-protein bound steroids are biologically active. The hormone transferred will reach the arterial blood as free hormone and, because the binding takes some time (seconds), the steroid may reach the capillaries before it is bound to the plasma proteins (Einer-Jensen, 1984, 1989).

4. Steroid transferred from the gonads will reach the epididymis and the Fallopian tube

Like heat energy, substances may be transferred in areas with a close connection between lymph vessels, veins and arteries. The gonads are typical examples. The close connection between the winding testicular artery and the Pampiniform plexus is well known. It is not, however common knowledge that the blood supply to the first part of the epididymis also originates from the testicular artery. Thus, the epididymis is involved in the local transfer system and transfer of steroids will act to stimulate the epididymis more than indicated by the content of testosterone in peripheral blood. An intramuscular injection of testosterone may produce a high peripheral concentration of the hormone and produce a strong negative feedback on the pituitary gland. However, it will not produce the concentration difference between the blood in the testicular artery and any other arterial sample.

In the female, the arterial supply to the Fallopian tube and the proximal part of the uterus originates from the ovarian artery. Any hormone in or transferred to the ovarian artery will also reach the tube and part of uterus (Stefańczyk-Krzymowska et al., 1998; Einer-Jensen et al., 2002; Cicinelli et al., 2004a). The ovarian production of individual steroids is cyclic and the amount of hormone transferred will therefore fluctuate (Cicinelli et al., 2004c). The increased production of oestradiol shortly before ovulation and of progesterone in the days after ovulation may be especially important, since transfer to the blood supply of the Fallopian tube and proximal part of uterus will influence tissue function. The transfer has been documented in both experimental animals and in man. The border between the blood supply from the uterine and tubal arteries shifts during the ovulatory cycle in man, probably due to the local vasodilatory effect of oestrogens in the tubal artery (Cicinelli et al., 2004b; Cicinelli et al., 2005).

Cooling of the vagina induces a temperature fall in the vesica and corpus of uterus but not the tubal part, probably through a counter-current transfer mechanism (Einer-Jensen et al., 2001a). Application of steroids in the vagina will induce a semi-selective effect in the vesica and uterus (Cicinelli et al., 2001). Cycle dependent variations in transfer of ^{133}Xenon from vagina to uterus was found in rats (Zhao and Einer-Jensen, 1998).

5. Other organs may also have a local transfer mechanism

An important steroid producing gland, the adrenal, does not have the external artery-veins complex needed for a counter-current transfer. It is, however, known that glycogenic steroids potentiate the production of adrenalin. It is tempting to think that a local exchange mechanism exists within the adrenal gland. There is some anatomical evidence, but the hypothesis has not been documented sufficiently to exclude doubt (Einer-Jensen and Carter, 1995).

Local counter-current transfer between the brain blood vessels has been found in experimental animals (Krzymowski, 1992; Einer-Jensen and Larsen, 2000a and b; Einer-Jensen et al., 2001b; Einer-Jensen et al., 2002). The brain is (probably) not a steroid producing organ, but some neurons have steroid receptors. Nonetheless, the effect on the brain may be semi-selective when treated with nasal application of steroids as based on the following knowledge. When animals exercise intensively, the body temperature tends to increase. The brain is the first body organ to be damaged after a rather small increase of 3-5° Centigrade. Nature has developed a brain cooling mechanism. Large airflows through the nose will cool the nasal mucous membrane and the capillary blood. The venous blood will leave the head either through a superficial or a deep vein before reaching the jugular vein, the route being decided by an autoregulated mechanism. The higher the temperature, the more blood will reach the deeper vein. This vein is at one point in close connection with the carotid. In some animals, an arterial plexus (Rete Mirabile) is formed by the carotid creating a very effective transfer system which decreases the temperature of the carotid blood and therefore of the brain. Transfer of steroid hormones has been found in experiments involving nasal application in isolated, perfused heads from pigs (Skipor et al., 2003). The transfer mechanism may also be present in man.

6. The importance of high progesterone concentrations in peritoneal fluid

The peritoneal cavity, its lining membrane and fluids are active participants in local regulation of the reproductive processes. In women, peritoneal fluid was collected during abdominal surgery by means of cotton swaps in nine women all with an active corpus luteum. Several samples were collected during the same operation (over the active corpus luteum, over the opposite ovary, at the right left and right paracolic gutter and at the pouch of Douglas). Progesterone concentrations close to the corpus luteum were 4 times (range 1.4 - 9.2) higher than in the other peritoneal samples and, on average, 5 times higher than in the systemic blood (Cicinelli et al., 2009). Progesterone would be expected to enter the peritoneal cavity locally (close to the corpus luteum). The authors know of no similar investigations in farm or experimental animals. One may speculate on the physiological importance:

Nonetheless, female genital tissues and their mesenteries are bathed in fluid with an elevated concentration of steroid hormones and, in many species, peritoneal fluid also enters the Fallopian tube ostium around the time of ovulation. This is principally due to the ab-ovarian beat of the cilia on the inner surface of the fimbriated infundibulum. In addition, evidence from pigs indicates that vital dyes irrigated onto the mesometrium and mesosalpinx enter the lymphatic vessels bordering the genital tract of oestrous animals (Hunter, 2011). There is little doubt that steroid hormones would do likewise, eventually influencing the activity of the endosalpinx and its secretions at a time when gametes and/or embryos could be present in the lumen.

The contralateral ovary is bathed in the high progesterone-containing fluid, which may influence follicular development. Other steroids such as oestrogens may behave comparably. Although alternating ovulation between the two ovaries is far from obligatory, signal transfer via the peritoneal fluid may have an influence on such a phenomenon (Hunter et al., 2007).

7. References

Blancardi, S. *Anatomica Reformata*. Joannem ten Hoorn, 34, 1739. Amsterdami. Reproduced from Einer-Jensen's medical thesis: Counter current transfer between the blood vessels in the ovarian adnexa. (University of Southern Denmark, 1990).

Cicinelli E, Einer-Jensen N, Cignarelli M, Mangiacotti L, Luisi D, Schonauer S. *Preferential transfer of endogenous ovarian steroid hormones to the uterus during both the follicular and luteal phases.* Hum Reprod. 2004a Sep;19(9):2001-4. Epub 2004 Jul 8.

Cicinelli E, Einer-Jensen N, Galantino P, Alfonso R, Nicoletti R. *The vascular cast of the human uterus: from anatomy to physiology.* Ann N Y Acad Sci. 2004b Dec;1034:19-26.

Cicinelli E, Einer-Jensen N, Barba B, Luisi D, Alfonso R, Tartagni M. *Blood to the cornual area of the uterus is mainly supplied from the ovarian artery in the follicular phase and from the uterine artery in the luteal phase.* Hum Reprod. 2004c Apr;19(4):1003-8. Epub 2004 Feb 27.

Cicinelli E, Einer-Jensen N, Alfonso R, Marinaccio M, Nicoletti R, Colafiglio G, Bellavia M. *A dominant ovarian follicle induces unilateral changes in the origin of the blood supply to the tubal corner of the uterus.* Hum Reprod. 2005 Nov;20(11):3208-11. Epub 2005 Jul 8.

Cicinelli E, Einer-Jensen N, Hunter RH, Cignarelli M, Cignarelli A, Colafiglio G, Tinelli R, Pinto V. *Peritoneal fluid concentrations of progesterone in women are higher close to the corpus luteum compared with elsewhere in the abdominal cavity. Fertil Steril.* 2009 Jul;92(1):306-10. Epub 2008 Aug 9.

Einer-Jensen N. *Local recirculation of injected (^{3}H)testosterone from the testis to the epididymal fat pad and the corpus epididymidis in the rat.* J Reprod Fertil. 1974 Mar;37(1):145-8.

Einer-Jensen N. *Slow binding of progesterone to plasma proteins.* Acta Pharmacol Toxicol (Copenh). 1984 Jul;55(1):18-20.

Einer-Jensen N. *A new method for measurement of plasma protein steroid-binding kinetics in human plasma at 37° C.* Steroids. 1989 Aug;54(2):195-216.

Einer-Jensen N, McCracken JA, Schram W, Bendz A. *Counter-current transfer in the female adnex.* Acta Physiol Pol. 1989 Jan-Feb;40(1):3-11.

Einer-Jensen N, Carter AM. *Local transfer of hormones between blood vessels within the adrenal gland may explain the functional interaction between the adrenal cortex and medulla.* Med Hypotheses 1995 Jun;44(6):471-4.

Einer-Jensen N, Larsen L. *Transfer of tritiated water, tyrosine, and propanol from the nasal cavity to cranial arterial blood in rats.* Exp Brain Res. 2000a Jan;130(2):216-20.

Einer-Jensen N, Larsen L. *Local transfer of diazepam, but not of cocaine, from the nasal cavities to the brain arterial blood in rats.* Pharmacol Toxicol. 2000b Dec;87(6):276-8.

Einer-Jensen N, Cicinelli E, Galantino P, Pinto V, Barba B. *Preferential vascular-based transfer from vagina to the corpus but not to the tubal part of the uterus in postmenopausal women.* Hum Reprod. 2001a Jul;16(7):1329-33.

Einer-Jensen N, Khorooshi MH, Petersen MB, Svendsen P. *Rapid brain cooling in intubated pigs through nasal flushing with oxygen: prevention of brain hyperthermia.* Acta Vet Scand. 2001b;42(4):459-64.

Einer-Jensen N, Baptiste KE, Madsen F, Khorooshi MH. *Can intubation harm the brain in critical care situations? A new simple technique may provide a method for controlling brain temperature.* Med Hypotheses. 2002 Mar;58(3):229-31.

Einer-Jensen N, Cicinelli E, Galantino P, Pinto V, Barba B. *Uterine first pass effect in postmenopausal women.* Hum Reprod. 2002 Dec;17(12):3060-4.

Einer-Jensen N, Hunter RHF. *Counter-current transfer in reproductive biology.* Reproduction. 2005 Jan;129(1):9-18.

Ginther, OJ. *Local utero-ovarian relationships.* J. Anim. Sci. 1967; 26:1-17.

Glad Sørensen H, Lambrechtsen J, Einer-Jensen N. *Efficiency of the countercurrent transfer of heat and 133Xenon between the pampiniform plexus and testicular artery of the bull under in-vitro conditions.* Int J Androl. 1991 Jun;14(3):232-40.

Hunter RH, Einer-Jensen N. *Pre-ovulatory temperature gradients within mammalian ovaries: a review.* J Anim Physiol Anim Nutr (Berl). 2005 Aug;89(7-8):240-3.

Hunter RH, Einer-Jensen N, Greve T. *Presence and significance of temperature gradients among different ovarian tissues.* Microsc Res Tech. 2006 Jun;69(6):501-7.

Hunter RH, Cicinelli E, Einer-Jensen N. *Peritoneal fluid as an unrecognised vector between female reproductive tissues.* Acta Obstet Gynecol Scand. 2007;86(3):260-5.

Hunter RHF. *Components of oviduct physiology in Eutherian mammals.* Biological Reviews; 2011, in press.

Jacks F, Setchell BP. *A technique for studying the transfer of substances from venous to arterial blood in the spermatic cord of wallabies and rams.* J Physiol. 1973 Aug;233(1):17P-18P.

Krzymowski T, Kotwica J, Stefanczyk-Krzymowska S. *Uterine and ovarian countercurrent pathways in the control of ovarian function in the pig.* J Reprod Fertil Suppl. 1990;40:179-91

Krzymowski T. *New pathways in animal reproductive physiology frontiers and perspectives.* J Physiol Pharmacol. 1992 Dec;43(4 Suppl 1):5-19.

McCracken JA, Carlson JC, Glew ME, Goding JR, Baird DT, Gréen K, Samuelsson B. *Prostaglandin $F_{2\alpha}$ identified as a luteolytic hormone in sheep.* Nat New Biol. 1972 Aug 2;238(83):129-34.

Skipor J, Grzegorzewski W, Einer-Jensen N, Wasowska B. *Local vascular pathway for progesterone transfer to the brain after nasal administration in gilts.* Reprod Biol. 2003 Jul;3(2):143-59.

Stefańczyk-Krzymowska S, Grzegorzewski W, Wasowska B, Skipor J, Krzymowski T. *Local increase of ovarian steroid hormone concentration in blood supplying the oviduct and uterus during early pregnancy of sows.* Theriogenology. 1998 Nov;50(7):1071-80.

Zhao J, Einer-Jensen N. *Cycle dependent variations in transfer of 133xenon from vagina to uterus in rats.* Maturitas. 1998 Jan 12;28(3):267-70.

2

Steroid Prohormones: Effects on Body Composition in Athletes

Sergej M. Ostojic, Julio Calleja-Gonzalez and Marko Stojanovic
Center for Health, Exercise and Sport Sciences, Belgrade
Serbia

1. Introduction

Androgenic-anabolic steroid hormones (AAS) are synthetic derivatives of the male hormone testosterone and for many years have been popular among athletes both for performance enhancement, due to physiological and psychological effects, and for aesthetic reasons (Evans 2004; Hartgens & Kuipers 2004). The anabolic action of AAS is particularly interesting since its affects protein metabolism by stimulation of protein synthesis and inhibition of protein breakdown, which could induce muscle growth and enhance adaptation to resistance training (Yesalis & Bahrke 1995; Brown et al. 2006). Since the AAS use in sport is banned, different nutritional strategies have been developed in the past decades to circumvent this problem and administer other exogenous testosterone analogues (King et al. 1999).

In the past 2o years, different steroid prohormones or prosteroids (e.g. androstenedion, dehydroepiandrosterone, androstenediol, 19-nor androstenediol, 19-nor androstenedione, 1-testosterone) have been developed and aggressively marketed in athletic environment as legal nutritional supplements that are expected to convert to active anabolic steroid hormones in the body and enhance exercise performance (Brown et al. 1999; Brown et al. 2000; Earnest et al. 2000; Leder et al. 2000; Brown et al. 2001; Kanayama et al. 2001). The efficacy and safety of these prohormones are not well established but are highly promoted to have the same androgenic effects on building muscle mass and strength as AAS (Baulieu et al. 2000; Brown et al. 2006). A typical steroid prohormone is intended to be a precursor to both testosterone and estrogens, through different biochemical pathways (Figure 1), typically resulting in the action of dehydrogenases in skeletal muscle, adipose tissue, skin, prostate and adrenal gland (Griffin 2004).

Dehydroepiandrosterone (3β-hydrohy-5-androsten-17-one; DHEA) seems to be the master steroid prohormone due its precursor function and its conversion to other hormones (Brown et al. 2006). Although the mechanism of action of DHEA or other prosteroids is not completely understood, it could be hypothesized that DHEA could increase testosterone production (at least as an acute response) if supplemented in diet, and due to its anabolic action may affects nitrogen balance and protein synthesis (Morales et al. 1998).

Testosterone is synthesized through either the Δ-4 or Δ-5 pathway (Broeder 2003) with the effects of newly synthesized testosterone in humans occur by way of 2 main mechanisms: by activation of the androgen receptor (directly or as 5α-dihydrotestosterone), and by conversion to estradiol and activation of estrogen receptors (Wilson 1988). Free testosterone

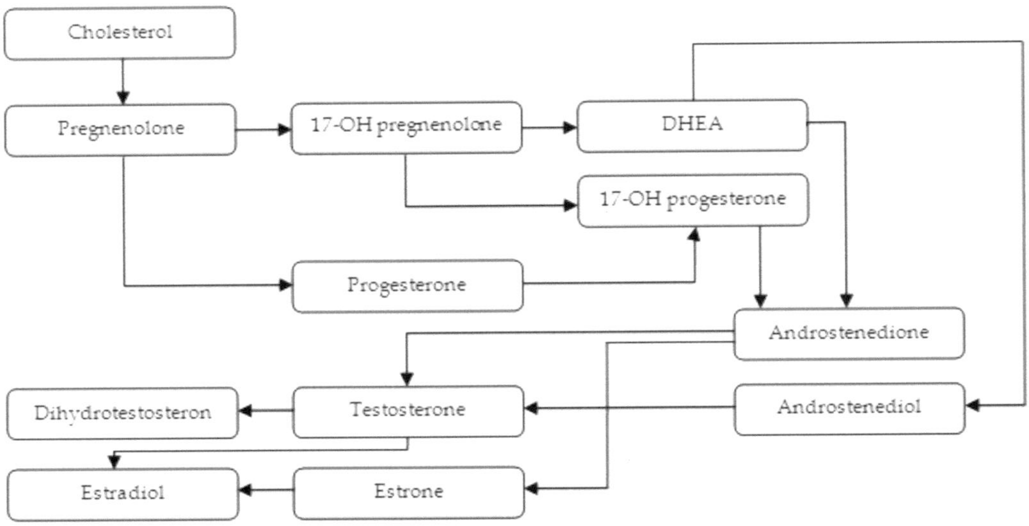

Fig. 1. Androgens biosynthesis from cholesterol to testosterone/dihydrotestosterone and estrogens (estrone and estradiol) via prohormone precursors (e.g. DHEA, androstenedione, androstenediol). *Abb.* DHEA – dehydroepiandrosterone.

is transported into the cytoplasm of target tissue cells, where it can bind to the androgen receptor, or can be reduced to 5α-dihydrotestosterone (DHT) by the cytoplasmic enzyme 5-alpha reductase (Hartgens & Kuipers 2004). DHT binds to the same androgen receptor even more strongly than testosterone, so that its androgenic potency is about 5 times that of testosterone (Breiner et al. 1986). The testosterone-receptor or DHT-receptor complex undergoes a structural change that allows it to move into the cell nucleus and bind directly to specific nucleotide sequences of the chromosomal desoxiribonucleic acid. The areas of binding are called hormone response elements, and influence transcriptional activity of certain genes, producing the anabolic effects (Saartok et al. 1984). Theoretically, the fewer interconversion steps a prohormone must complete in the syntheisis pathway to testosterone, the greater potential for enhancing active hormone production (Broeder 2003); for example, androstenedione converts to testosterone more rapidly than DHEA.

Existing data suggest that acute oral ingestion of DHEA, androstenediol or androstenedione modestly and transiently increase serum testosterone concentration; however, this is accompanied by greater increase in other steroids as well (i.e. estrogens, luteinizing hormone) (Ziegenfuss et al. 2002). Yet, it is questionable if this acute elevation in testosterone concentration induced by prosteroids necessarily result in enhanced transcriptional activity (Broeder 2003). Furthermore, research has shown that prosteroids may have significant biological activity by itself (Ostojic et al. 2009, Ostojic et al. 2010), affecting resting metabolic rate through futile cycling (Tagliaferro et al. 1986), increasing the flux of fatty acids through β-oxidation (Mohan et al. 1988), and alter the level of serotonin and dopamine (Cleary 1991; Ebeling et al. 1994; Kroboth 1999). Yet, the mechanism of action of prosteroids may differ between compounds because of variations in the steroid molecules (Hartgens & Kuipers 2004). These differences could be responsible for differences in the specificity of binding to receptor proteins or to interactions with various steroid-metabolizing enzymes (Wilson 1988; Creutzberg & Schols 1998) with future research needed to clarify the explaining physiological effects due to prosteroids use in humans.

2. History of steroid prohormones use in sport and exercise

Although the first documented reports of misuse of AAS by athletes stem from the 1950s (Yesalis 1999), the use of prosteroids in the athletic environment is rather new. Prosteroids were indirectly introduced with US Anabolic Steroid Control Act of 1990 (21 USCS Section 802), which defined anabolic steroids as *"...any drug or hormonal substance that promotes muscle growth in a manner physiologically similar to testosterone..."*, while steroid prohormones were not classified as anabolic steroids and could be purchased legally as dietary supplements (Broeder 2003; Brown et al. 2006). This document didn't appear to make a significant decrease in the use of anabolic steroids (Brainum 2008), but concern about the side effects linked to steroid use did lead to the development of another popular anabolic offering: prohormone nutritional supplements (Brown et al. 2003).

In December of 1996, androstenedione became available for over-the-counter sales in United States (Ziegenfuss et al. 2002), with subsequent availability of several other prohormones (e.g. androstenediol, DHEA, norandrostenedione). The non-critical promotion era of prosteroids in sport began with the disclosure of androstenedione use by Mark McGwire in 1998, who at the time was elite baseball player, which stimulated extensive media attention and dramatically increased the sales of prohormones among recreative and professional athletes (Brown et al. 2003, Brown et al. 2006).

In the past decades, prohormones have been highly marketed in the field of sport as lean body mass builders, fat reduction agents, and anticatabolic compounds. Recently, concerns over the safety of the prohormones use induced changes in US Anabolic Steroid Control Act in 2004 (21 USCS Section 802, amended), redefining anabolic steroids and classify prohormones as controlled substances. While the 2004 amendment specifically mentioned most of the current prohormones by name, that didn't stop some companies from marketing at least one anabolic steroid that the lawmakers had overlooked (Brainum 2008).

At the moment, it seems that legal status of prohormones is different throughout the world. In USA, Canada or Australia prosteroids are recognized as controlled substances and it is illegal to own or sell the product without prescription. On the other hand, no prescription is required for prosteroids purchase in several European countries, Russia or Japan, with products recognized as over-the-counter dietary supplements.

3. Epidemiology of steroids use among athletes: scope of the problem

Anabolic steroid usage has been recognized as a serious health and ethical problem among athletes for several decades (Foster & Housner 2004). Numerous examples of steroid usage rules violations have been highly publicized and have lead to the suspension and stripping of medals from international athletes, as well as many professional athletes (International Olympic Committee 1997; Wroble et al. 2002). Elite athletes are not the only population of individuals that use steroids. Recreational athletes also use steroids to enhance performance and to improve personal appearance (Wroble et al. 2002). Furthermore, evidence indicates that steroid usage often starts during high school (Yesalis et al, 1989; Kerr and Congeni 2007). Use of anabolic steroids is widespread in the athletic environment, particularly in power events and disciplines (e.g. football, track and field, body building, power lifting) (Foster & Housner 2004).

It seems that athletes have used AAS for more than 50 years, with first anecdotal evidence of use of animal testicular extracts even in 1890s (Yesalis 1999). Despite educational and preventive measures, steroid use increases (Windsor & Dumitru 1988). The prevalence of AAS abuse has been reported in several populations. The highest estimates have come from male bodybuilders with even more than 50% regularly using steroids (Tricker et al. 1989; Lindstrom et al. 1990). Lower rates have been reported among intercollegiate athletes, ranging from 15% to 20% (Dezelsky et al. 1985). Rates of steroids use vary greatly across individual sports and are used in higher frequency and higher doses by strength athletes (Sturmi & Diorio 1998). By contrast, only 1% of their nonathletic university student counterparts reported steroids use (Dezelsky et al. 1985). Perhaps the most surprising and alarming finding is the rather high rate of steroids abuse among high school students (Mulcahey et al. 2010). The typical rate reported in male students is between 5% and 6%, but rates as high as 11% have been reported (Johnson et al 1989). The most recent estimate reported a range of 5% to 15% for steroids use among high school boys. In female high school students, steroids abuse rates tend to be lower, but quite worrisome at 1% to 3% (Harmer 2010). Wroble and co-workers (2002) indicated that less than one percent (0.7%) of youth sports participants reported current or previous usage of anabolic steroids; the rate of usage was higher in males than females. Three percent of athletes had been offered steroids at some time with 22% of them admitted to using steroids. Of the reported anabolic steroid users, 27% admitted they used anabolic steroids for athletic performance; 18% used to improve personal appearance; 18% used for bodybuilding; and 18% took due to peer pressure. Twelve percent of all athletes said that they personally know someone who was using or had used steroids.

Although several prohormones are considered as AAS, and are banned by many sports governing bodies, including the International Olympic Committee (IOC), they are semi-legal substances available from many retail outlets, including internet health food stores. The overall prevalence of prohormones use is not known, although several reports indicated that prohormones are among the most popular dietary supplements especially in adolescent athletes (Smurawa & Congeni 2007). Even though usage has decreased by over 50% since 1989, steroid use in sport is still a serious problem. Insufficient knowledge and inappropriate attitudes regarding the benefits and risks of using anabolic steroids is also a major concern (Schwingel et al. 2011).

4. Testosterone production and musculotrophic effects of prosteroids

The most prevalent reason for athletes initiating AAS or prosteroids use is to promote muscle mass and strength (Yen et al. 1995). From long list of previous studies (for review see Hartgens & Kuipers 2004) it could be concluded that steroids administration may increase muscle mass. Exogenous testosterone administration (> 125 mg/week), with and without strength training program, may lead to increments of muscle volume and/or muscle fibre size. Yet, lower doses of testosterone (e.g. 25, 50 or 100 mg/week) had no effect on muscle fibre cross-sectional area. It seems that musculotrophic effect of steroids is dose-dependent. Therefore, the effects of prosteroids on muscle size and/or strength is highly influenced by its potential to increase serum testosterone after administration.

Existing data on testosterone-boosting effects of prosteroids are equivocal; it seems that age and basal serum testosterone concentration may influence the response to prosteroids intake (Brown et al. 2000). Several studies reported that serum sex steroid levels in both mature and young men were not significantly affected by prohormone supplementation, with only a minimal amount converted to testosterone and more to estrogen (Vogiatzi et al. 1996;

Morales et al. 1998; Kroboth et al. 1999; Yamada et al. 2007). No changes in levels of testosterone and estradiol were observed for men after supplementation with 50 mg of DHEA for 3, 6 and 12 months (Von Muhlen et al. 2008). In 19 young men (23 ± 1 yr old) participating in an 8-week resistance training, ingestion of 150 mg/day of DHEA did not affect serum testosterone and estrogen concentrations (Bowers 1999). On the other hand, ingesting 100 mg of androstenedione t.i.d. for 28 days increases serum-free testosterone concentration by 40% (Brown et al. 2000; Brown et al. 2001), while 200 mg of androstenediione increases testosterone area under the curve by approximately 15% during the 90 min post-administration (Earnest et al. 2000). In recent study (Ostojic et al. 2010) intake of DHEA resulted in significant increase of total testosterone in treated subjects after 28-days of supplementation. Accordingly, Wolf et al. (1997) reported 1.3-fold increase in testosterone levels after supplementation with 50 mg oral DHEA for 2 weeks in 25 men. Furthermore, serum estradiol levels were significantly elevated, indicating that a significant portion of the ingested prosteroids underwent aromatization. It seems that both the magnitude of the dose administered and the route of administration affect the extent of change in concentrations of sex hormones (Ziegenfuss et al. 2002). Furthermore, several studies confirm the importance of extraadrenal and extragonadal 3ß-hydroxysterodi dehydrogenase activity in the synthesis of androgens and estrogens after prohormones administration (Nestler et al. 1991; Kroboth et al. 1999).

Not all subjects respond to prohormones in same fashion, suggesting that additional factors (i.e. age, gender, diet, type and intensity of exercise) influence these responses. For example, research demonstrates that prohormone supplementation may acutely increase testosterone levels in women, thus producing a virilizing effect (Bahrke & Yesalis 2004). Furthermore, exercise could result in increased DHEA and DHEA-S concentrations (Bernton et al. 1995) and these elevated levels in athletes could influence response to supplementation, which requires further investigation. The recent study (Ostojic et al. 2010) reported an increase of total testosterone and estradiol while free testosterone is normal. These data can be consistent with an increase of sex hormone binding globulin (SHBG) by prosteroids administration (Nestler et al. 1991). Total testosterone was increased to keep normal free testosterone or in alternative free testosterone was normal due to an increase activation of 5-alpha reductase. Measuring SHBG luteinizing and folicle-stimulating hormone in future studies should prove these hypotheses. However, it is important to point out that simply producing an acute elevation in a particular hormone concentration (i.e. testosterone) does not necessarily result in increases in muscle mass or lean body mass. Prosteroids do not appear to have functional benefits when taken in daily concentrations up to 300 mg per day in young, middle-aged or older men (Wallace et akl. 1999; Ballantyne et al. 2000; Broeder 2003). Although oral DHEA intake enhanced testosterone production for 30%, Ostojic and co-workers (2010) did not found changes in total muscle mass or regional muscularity.

It seems that effect of prosteroids on serum hormones was not mediated by an effect on body composition. Increasing DHEA or other prohormones levels may not provide the optimal anabolic environment desired in spite of elevated total testosterone level, due to several possible mechanisms (i.e. genetic polymorphism of the androgen receptor, potential hormonal interconversions at the paracrine level) (Nestler et al. 1991). Whether the increase of testosterone after intake of prohormones translates into a meaningful change in body composition or rates of muscle protein synthesis is debatable. Studies must be evaluated in terms of the relative potency of various testosterone enhancers with varying effects on different tissues according to receptor-binding properties of the compound and its metabolites (Ebeling & Koivisto 1994). The relative potency of prosteroids seems to be small with inconsiderable advantageous anabolic properties. Several authors hypothesized that an important part of the musculotrophic effect of prosteroids may not be directly mediated through androgen receptors but instead involves interference with catabolic effects produced by glucocorticoid hormones binding to their specific receptors (Bernton et al. 1995; Morales et al. 1998). With an incomplete understanding of how prohormones exert their effects on skeletal muscle, further studies should analyze nitrogen balance indicators as noninvasive approximate index of muscle protein status.

5. Fat mass alteration and steroid prohormones intake

In the field of sports and exercise nutrition, prosteroids (DHEA in particular) are often promoted as fat-burning agent that could enhance body physique and estetize appearance (Kroboth et al. 1999). However, clear evidence supporting the use of prosteroids in athletic environment remains less clear. It is well known that age-related decreases in DHEA are associated with increases in obesity and a decline in fat free mass (Morales et al. 1998) yet the potential usefulness of DHEA as a slimming agent is mostly indicated by previous research in animals, particularly lower mammals (Cleary 1991). In the rat plasma concentration of DHEA ranges between 14 and 80 nM while in the plasma of humans DHEA-concentration ranges between 5 and 24 nM and DHEAS-concentration is up to 9 μM (Svec & Porter 1998). The anti-obesity effect of DHEA in animals could be due to several possible mechanisms (Cleary 1991; Ebeling & Koivisto 1994; Kroboth et al. 1999). However, studies that have investigated the effects of oral prosteroids supplementation on body composition in humans produced equivocal results, particularly in young men.
Nestler et al. (1988) reported that 28-day supplementation with DHEA (1600 mg/day) reduced body fat by 31% with no change in body mass in five normal men. Serum total testosterone, free testosterone, sex hormone-binding globulin, estradiol, and estrone levels did not change while serum DHEA-S and androstenedione rose 2.0- to 3.5-fold in DHEA group. Morales et al. (1998) founded that 100 mg of DHEA for 6 months induced decrease in body fat mass (6.1 ± 2.6%) in healthy non-obese men. On the other side, several investigators showed that body composition was not affected by prosteroids treatment in young and adult men, both obese and non-obese (Usiskin et al. 1990; Welle et al. 1990; Wallace et al. 1999). Vogiatzi et al. (1996) suggested that DHEA 40 mg administered sublingually twice daily for 8 weeks has no positive effects on body composition in obese young adults. In recent DAWN trial (Von Muhlen et al. 2008) no beneficial effects of 50 mg daily oral DHEA supplementation on body composition were found in 110 healthy mature men. In accordance with above research, the recent study (Ostojic et al. 2010) failed to show any beneficial effects of oral DHEA administration on body mass and body composition in non-obese young athletes. Authors did not found significant reduction in body fat of young soccer players after DHEA supplementation. Other indicators of body fatness (i.e. body mass index, waist-to-hip ratio) remained unchanged during the study in both DHEA and placebo group, indicating that treatment with DHEA does not result in significant changes to justify its use as an antiobesity or slimming agent. As in the case of cognition, negative results in healthy volunteers can be attributed either to a true lack of DHEA effect or to body composition too close to ideal at the study start to detect changes in the small numbers of subjects studied.

Although most studies found no beneficial effects of prosteroids supplementation on body composition in athletes, several investigators underlined possible beneficial effects of prosteroids supplementation for elderly. Hernandez-Morante et al. (2008) demonstrated for the first time in vitro that DHEA-S stimulates lipolysis in 85 obese patients, preferably in subcutaneous fat in women and in visceral fat in men. A study by Ho et al. (2008) suggested that low DHEA-S is associated with increased waist-to-hip ratio and reduced insulin sensitivity with aging while Hsu *et al.* (2008) had reported that body composition and insulin sensitivity can change with aging in early lifetime. Benefits of prosteroids supplementation in this regard for early middle-aged people requires more clinical investigation.

Although the body composition changes induced by steroids or prosteroids administration are rather small, after the drug withdrawal the alterations of body composition fade away in slow manner, but may be presented in part for period up to 3 months (Kuipers et al. 1991; Hartgens et al. 2001; Brown et al. 2006). Yet, the final net results of short-term steroids or prosteroids administration on body composition seems to be minute (Hartgens & Kuipers 2004). This is particularly true for all athletes who are not capable of maintaining the nutritional intake and training workload of the level required for significant body composition changes (Hartgens et al. 1996). It may be important that steroid cessation is followed by a period of hypogonadism, while testicular function gradually returns to normal, over a period of weeks or several months (Hartgens & Kuipers 2004). Although this has not been specifically studied, reduced circulating androgen during this period may help to accelerate the loss of any anabolic steroid-induced gains. How much of the gain can be sustained by physical training following drug cessation remains to be studied (Yesalis & Bahrke 2000).

6. Known and potential health risks of prosteroids administration

During the past 20 years, researches suggested that potential risk factors associated with prosteroids use were similar to those observed with anabolic steroids (Broeder 2002). The altered hormonal milieu caused by prohormone intake is similar to the hormonal milieu observed in men with gynecomastia, prostate cancer, testicular cancer and pancreatic cancer (Fyssas et al. 1997; Chang et al. 2005). Yet, no documented cases exist of these endocrine-related diseases caused by prohormone supplementation (Brown et al. 2006). Furthermore, it seems that athletes who regularly use prosteroids experienced several side effects (e.g. fatigue, headache, nasal congestion, acne, increased aggressiveness, increased blood pressure, masculinization in women, gynecomastia and testicular wasting in men) (Broeder et al. 2000). Although prohormones induces small decreases in high-density lipoprotein cholesterol (HDL-C), long-term implications of transient negative changes in blood lipids (e.g. 3-6 mg/dL reductions in HDL-C) have yet to be elucidated as the risk of sustaining a cardiac event (Ziegenfuss et al. 2002).

Regarding unfavourable body composition changes, it has been noted that prohormones could lead to changes in hydration of the fat free mass (via sodium and water retention), which could be interpreted as *hyperhydration* effect (Casaburi et al. 1996). Whether more prolonged (> 8-12 weeks) prohormones supplementation is safe or useful remains uncertain, but appears unlikely (Ziegenfuss et al. 2002). Although some health risks have been noted, thus far none of the prohormones tested appear to be overly toxic as no elevations in clinically relevant tissue enzymes (e.g. alanine aminotransferase, creatine kinase, aspartate aminotransferase, gamma-glutamyltransferase, lactate dehydrogenase) have been observed (Brown et al. 2000; Ziegenfuss et al. 2002). However, due to the lack of efficacy of oral prosteroids supplementation in athletes, its theoretical risks seem to fat outweight any potential benefits on body composition and should be discouraged (Earnest 2001).

7. Summary

In the past 2o years, different steroid prohormones or prosteroids have been aggressively marketed in athletic environment as legal nutritional supplements that are expected to convert to active anabolic steroid hormones in the body and enhance exercise performance. Although the mechanism of action of prosteroids is not completely understood it has been promoted that prosteroids increases testosterone production if supplemented in diet and due to its anabolic action may affects nitrogen balance and protein synthesis. Although popular among athletes, studies have demonstrated repeatedly that acute and long-term administration of these oral testosterone precursors does not effectively increase serum testosterone levels and fails to produce any significant changes in lean body mass, muscle strength, or performance improvement compared with placebo. It seems that increasing prohormone levels in athletes may not provide the optimal anabolic environment desired in spite of elevated total testosterone level (at least acutely), due to several possible mechanisms (i.e. genetic polymorphism of the androgen receptor, potential hormonal interconversions at the paracrine level). The relative potency of prosteroids seems to be small with inconsiderable advantageous anabolic properties. Furthermore, recent studies indicates that treatment with prosteroids does not result in significant changes to justify its use as an antiobesity or slimming agent. Not all subjects respond to prohormones in same fashion, suggesting that additional factors (i.e. gender, diet, type and intensity of exercise) influence these responses. Although some health risks have been noted, thus far none of the prohormones tested appear to be overly toxic. Yet, due to the lack of efficacy of oral prosteroids supplementation in athletes, its theoretical risks seem to far outweight any potential benefits on body composition and should be discouraged. Although the understanding of testosterone precursors as performance-enhancing drugs continues to advance, there are likely to be more revelations as scientific investigations continue.

8. References

Bahrke, M.S., & Yesalis, C.E. (2004). Abuse of Anabolic Androgenic Steroids and Related Substances in Sport and Exercise. *Current Opinion in Pharmacology*. Vol.4, No.6 (December 2004), pp. 614-620, ISSN 1471-4892.

Ballantyne, C.S., Phillips, S.M., MacDonald, J.R., Tarnopolsky, M.A. & MacDozgall, J.D. (2000). The Acute Effects of Androstenedione Supplementation in Health Young Men. *Canadian Journal of Applied Physiology*, Vol.25, No.1 (February 2000), pp. 68-78, ISSN 1066-7814.

Baulieu, E.E., Thomas, G., Legrain, S., Lahlou, N., Roger, M., Debuire, B., Faucounau, V., Girard, L., Hervy, M.P., Latour, F., Leaud, M.C., Mokrane, A., Pitti-Ferrandi, H., Trivalle, C., de Lacharrière, O., Nouveau, S., Rakoto-Arison, B., Souberbielle, J.C., Raison, J., Le Bouc, Y., Raynaud, A., Girerd, X., & Forette, F. (2000). Dehydroepiandrosterone (DHEA), DHEA Sulfate, and Aging: Contribution of the DHEAge Study to a Sociobiomedical Issue. *The Proceedings of the National Academy of Sciences of the United States of America*, Vol.97, No.8, (April 2000), pp. 4279-4284, ISSN 0027-8424.

Bernton, E., Hoover, D., Galloway, R., & Popp, K. Adaptation to Chronic Stress in Military Trainees: Adrenal Androgens, Testosterone, Glucocorticoids, IGF-1 and Immune Function (1995). *Annals of the New York Academy of Sciences*, Vol.774, (December 1995), pp. 217-231, ISSN 0077-8923.

Bowers, L.D. Oral Dehydroepiandrosterone Supplementation Can Increase the Testosterone / Epitestosterone Ratio. (1999). *Clinical Chemistry*, Vol.45, No.2, (February 1999), pp. 295-297, ISSN 0009-9147.

Branium, J. (2008). Bodybuilding Pharmacology. *Iron Man Magazine*, Vol.72, No.9, (September 2008), pp. 248-250, ISSN 0047-1496.

Breiner, M., Romalo, G. & Schweikert, H.U. (1986). Inhibition of Androgen Receptor Binding by Natural and Synthetic Steroids in Cultured Human Genital Skin Fibroblasts. *Klinische Wochenschrift*, Vol.64, No.16, (August 1986), pp. 732–737, ISSN 0023-2173.

Broeder, C.E:, Quindry, J., Brittingham, K., Panton, L., Thompson, J., Appakondu, S., Breuel, K., Byrd, R., Douglas, J., Earnest, C., Mitchell, C., Olson, M., Roy, T. & Yarlagadda, C. (2000). The Andro project: Physiological and Hormonal Influence of Androstenedione Supplementation in Men 35 to 65 Yeard Old Participating in High-Intensity Resistance Training Program. *Archives of Internal Medicine*, Vol.160, No.20, (November 2000), pp. 3093-3204, ISSN 0003-9926.

Broeder, C.E. (2003). Oral Andro-Related Prohormone Supplementation: Do the Potential Risks Outweight the Benefits? *Canadian Journal of Applied Physiology*, Vol.28, No.1, (February 2003), pp. 102-116, ISSN 1066-7814.

Brown, G.A., Vukovich, M.D., Sharp, R.L., Reifenrath, T.A, Parsons, K.A., & King, D.S. (1999). Effect of Oral DHEA on Serum Testosterone and Adaptations to Resistance Training in Young Men. *Journal of Applied Physiology*, Vol.87, No.6, (December 1999), pp. 2274-2283, ISSN 8750-7587.

Brown, G.A., Vukovich, M.D., Martini, E.R., et al. (2000). Endocrine Responses to Chronic Androstenedione Intake in 30- to 56-Year-Old Men. *Journal of Clinical Endocrinology and Metabolism*, Vol.85, No.11, (November 2000), pp. 4074-4080. ISSN 0021-972X.

Brown, G.A., Vukovich, M.D., Martini, E.R., Kohut, M,L,, Franke, W.D., Jackson, D.A. & King DS. (2001). Effects of Androstenedione-Herbal Supplementation on Serum Sex Hormone Concentration in 30- to 59-Year-Old Men. *International Journal for Vitamin and Nutrition Research*, Vol.71, No.5, (September 2001), pp. 293-301. ISSN 0373-0883.

Brown, W.J., Basil, M.D., & Bocarnea, M.C. (2003). The Influence of Famous Athletes on Health Beliefs and Practices: Mark McGwire, Child Abuse Prevention, and Androstenedione. *Journal of Health Communications*, Vol.8, No.1, (January-February 2003), pp. 41-57, ISSN 1081-0730.

Brown, G.A., Vukovich, M. & King, D.S. (2006). Testosterone Prohormone Supplements. *Medicine and Science in Sports and Exercise*, Vol.38, No.8, (August 2006), pp. 1451-1461. ISSN 0195-9131.

Casaburi, R, Storer, T. & Bhasin, S. (1996). Androgen Effects on Body Composition and Muscle Performance. In: *Pharmacology, Biology, and Clinical Applications of Androgens*, S. Bhasin, H. Gabelnick, J. Spieler, R. Swerdloff, C. Wang, & C. Kelly, (Eds.), pp. 487-491, Wiley-Liss, Inc., ISBN 978-047-1133-20-9, New York.

Chang, S.S., Ivey, B., Smith, A., Roth, B.J. & Cookson, M.S. (2005). Performance-Enhancing Supplement Use in Patients with Testicular Cancer. *Urology*, Vol.66, No2, (August 2006), pp. 242-245, ISSN 0834-6747.

Cleary, M.P. (1991). The Antiobesity Effect of Dehydroepiandrosterone in Rats. *Procceedings of the Society of Experimental Biology and Medicine*,Vo.196, No.1, (January 1991), pp. 8-16, ISSN 0037-9727.

Creutzberg, E.C., & Schols, A.M. (1998). Anabolic Steroids. *Current Oppinion in Clinical Nutrition and Metabiolic Care*, Vol.2, No.3, (May 1998), pp. 243-253, ISSN 1363-1950.

Dezelsky, T.L., Toohey, J.V. & Shaw, R.S. (1985). Non-Medical Drug Use Behaviour at Five United States Universities: A 15-year Study. *Bulletin on Narcotics*, Vol.37, N.2-3, (April-September 1985), pp. 49-53, ISSN 0007-523X.

Earnest, C.P. (2001). Dietary androgen 'supplements': separating substance from hype. *Physisian and Sportsmedicine*. Vol.29, No.5, (May 2001), pp. 63-79, ISSN 0091-3847.

Earnest, C.P., Olson, M.A., Broeder, C.E., Breuel, K.F. & Beckham, S.G. (2000). In Vivo 4-Androstene-3, 17-Dione and 4-Androstene-3 Beta, 16 Beta-Diol Supplementation in Young Men. *European Journal of Applied Physiology*, Vol.81, No.3, (February 2000), pp. 229-232. ISSN 1439-6319.

Ebeling, P., & Koivisto, V.A. (1994). Physiological Importance of Dehydroepiandrosterone. *Lancet*, Vol.343, No.8911, (June 1994), pp. 1479-1481, ISSN 0140-6736.

Evans, N.A. (2004). Current concepts in anabolic-androgenic steroids. *American Journal of Sports Medicine*, Vol.32, No.2, (March 2004), pp. 534-542, ISSN 0363-5465.

Foster, Z.J, & Housner, J.A. (2004). Anabolic-androgenic steroids and testosterone precursors: ergogenic aids and sport. *Curr Sports Medicine Reports*. Vol.3, No.4, (August 2004), pp. 234-241, ISSN 1537-890X.

Fyssas, I, Syrigos, K.N., Konstandoulakis, M.M., Papadopoulos, S., Milingos, N., Anapliotou, M., Waxman, J. & Golematis, B.C. (1997). Sex Hormone levels in the Serum of Patients with Pancreatic Adenocarcinoma. *Hormone and Metabolic Research*.Vol.29, No.3, (March 1997), pp. 115-118, ISSN 0018-5043.

Griffin, J.E., & Ojeda, S.R. (2004). *Textbook of Endocrine Physiology (5th ed)*, Oxford University Press, ISBN 978-019-5165-66-1, New York, USA.

Harmer, P.A. (2010). Anabolic-Androgenic Seroid Use Among Young Male and Female Athletes: Is the Game to Blame? *British Journal of Sports Medicine*, Vol.44, No.1, (January 2010), pp. 26-31, ISSN 0306-3674.

Hartgens, F., Kuipers, H., Wijnen, J.A. & Keizer, H.A. (1996). Body Composition, Cardiovascular Risk Factor and Liver Function in Long Term Androgenic-Anabolic Steroids Using Bodybuilders Three Months After Drug Withdrawal. *International Journal of Sports Medicine*, Vol.17, No.6, (August 1996), pp. 429-433, ISSN 0172-4622.

Hartgens, F., Van Marken Lichtenbelt, W.D., Ebbing, S., Vollaard, N., Rietjens, G. & Kuipers, H. (2001). Body Composition and Anthropometry in Bodybuilders: regional Changes Due to Nandrolone Decanoate Administration. *Intrenational Journal of Sports Medicine*, Vol.22, No.3, (April 2001), pp. 235-241, ISSN 0172-4622

Hartgens, F.& Kuipers, H. (2004). Effects of Androgenic-Anabolic Steroids in Athletes. *Sports Medicine*, Vol.34, No.8, (August 2004), pp. 513-554. ISSN 0112-1642.

Hernández-Morante, J.J., Pérez-de-Heredia, F., Luján, J.A., Zamora, S., & Garaulet, M. (2008). Role of DHEA-S on Body Fat Distribution: Gender- and Depot-Specific

Stimulation of Adipose Tissue Lipolysis. *Steroids*, Vol.73, No.2, (February 2008), pp. 209-215, ISSN 0039-128X.

Ho, C.T., Su, C.L., Chen, M.T., Liou, Y.F., Lee, S.D., Chien, K.Y., & Kuo, C.H. Aging Effects on Glycemic Control and Inflammation for Politicians in Taiwan. *Chininese Journal of Physiology*, Vol.51, No.6, (December 2008), pp. 402-407, ISSN 0304-4920.

Hsu, T.H., Liu, Y.F., Lee, S.D., Chen, S.M., Lee, J.P., Fang, C.L., Liu, T.C., & Kuo, C.H. (2008). Suppression of Age-Dependent Increase in Insulinemia in Early Middle-Aged Females with Exercise Habit. *Chinese Journal of Physioligy*, Vol.51, No.5, (October 2008), pp. 263-268, ISSN 0304-4920.

International Olympic Committee. (1999). *Statistics 1997 of the IOC Accredited Laboratories*, International Olympic Committee, Lausanne, Switzerland.

Johnson, M.D., Jay, M.S., Shoup, B. & Rickert, V.I. (1989). Anabolic Steroid Use by Male Adolescents. *Pediatrics*, Vol.83, No.6, (June 1989), pp. 921-924, ISSN 0031-4005.

Kanayama, G., Gruber, A.J., Pope Jr, H.G., Borowiecki, J.J. & Hudson, J.I. (2001). Over-the-Counter Drug Use in Gymnasiums: An Underrecognized Substance Abuse Problem? *Psychotherapy and Psychosomatics*, Vol.70, No.3, (May-June 2001), pp. 137-140, ISSN 0033-3190.

Kerr, J.M. & Congeni, J.A. (2007). Anabolic-Androgenic Steroids: Use and Abuse in Pediatric Patients. *Pediatric Clinics of North America*, Vol.54, No.4, (August 2007), pp. 771-785, ISSN 0031-3955.

King, D.S., Sharp, R.L., Vukovich, M.D., Brown, G.A., Reifenrath, T.A., Uhl, N.L. & Parsons, K.A. (1999). Effect of Oral Androstenedione on Serum Testosterone and Adaptations to Resistance Training in Youung Men; A Randomised Controlled Trial. *JAMA*, Vol.218, No.21, (June 1999), pp. 2020-2028. ISSN 0098-7484.

Kroboth, P.D., Salek, F.S., Pittenger, A.L., Fabian, T.J., & Frye R.F. (1999). DHEA and DHEA-S: a Review. *Journal of Clinical Pharmacology*, Vol.39, No.4, (April 1999), pp. 327-348, ISSN 0091-2700.

Kuipers, H., Wijnen, J.A, Hartgens, F. & Willems, S.M. (1991). Influence of Anabolic Steroids on Body Composition, Blood Pressure, Lipid Profile and Liver Function in Bodybuilders. *International Journal of Sports Medicine*, Vol.12, No.4, (August), pp. 413-418, ISSN 0172-4622.

Leder, B.Z., Longcope, C., Catlin, D.H., Ahrens, B., Schonefeld, D.A. & Finkelstein, J.S. (2000). Oral Androstenedione Administration and Serum Testosterone Concentration in Young Men. *JAMA*, Vol.284, No.6, (February 2000), pp. 779-782. ISSN 0098-7484.

Lindstrom, M., Nilsson, A.L., Katzman, P.L., Janzon, L., & Dymling, J.F. (1990). Use of Anabolic-Androgenic Steroids Among Body Builders - Frequency and Attitudes. *Journal of Internal Medicine*, Vol.227, No.6, (June 1990), pp. 407-411, ISSN 0954-6820.

Mohan, P.F. & Cleary, M.P. (1988). Effects of Short-Term DHEA Administration on Liver Metabolism of Lean and Obese Rats. *American Journal of Physiology*, Vol.255, No1. (July 1988), pp. E1-E8, ISSN 0002-9513.

Morales, A.J., Haubrich, R.H., Hwang, J.Y., Asakura, H., & Yen, S.S. (1998). The Effect of Six Months Treatment with a 100 mg Daily Dose of Dehydroepiandrosterone (DHEA) on Circulating Sex Steroids, Body Composition and Muscle Strength in Age-Advanced Men and Women. *Clinical Endocrinology*, Vol.49, No.4, (October 1998), pp. 421-432, ISSN 0300-0664.

Mulcahey, M.K., Schiller, J.R. & Hulstyn, M.J. (2010). Anabolic Steroid Use in Adolescents: Identification of those at Risk and Strategies for Prevention. *The Physician and Sportsmedicinei,* Vol.38, No.3, (October 2010), pp. 105-113, ISSN 0091-3847.

Nestler, J.E., Barlascini, C.O., Clore, J.N., & Blackard, W.G. (1988). Dehydroepiandrosterone Reduces Serum Low Density Lipoprotein Levels and Body Fat but Does Not Alter Insulin Sensitivity in Normal Men. *Journal of Clinical Endocrinology and Metabolism,* Vol.66, No.1, (January 1988), pp. 57-61, ISSN 0021-972X.

Nestler, J.E., Clore, J.N., & Blackard, W.G. (1991). Metabolism and Actions of Dehydroepiandrosterone in Humans. *Journal of Steroid Biochemistry and Molecular Biology,* Vol.40, No.4-6, (June 1991), pp. 599-605, ISSN 0960-0760.

Ostojic, S.M., Calleja-Gonzalez, J. (2009). Ergogenic supplements for endurance performance: science vs. hype. *Proceedings of the Exercise Training Physiology Symposium,* Cordoba, Argentina, June 2009, Available from http://www.sobreentrenamiento.com/CurCE/Simposios/Informacion.asp?sim=PS2

Ostojic, S.M, Calleja-Gonzalez, J. & Jourkesh, M. (2010). Effects of short-term dehydroepiandrosterone supplementation on body composition in young athletes. *Chinese Journal of Physiology,* Vol.53, No.1, (February 2010), pp. 19-25, ISSN 0304-4920.

Saartok, T., Dahlberg, E. & Gustafsson, J.A. (1984). Relative Binding Affinity of Anabolic-Androgenic Steroids: Comparison of the Binding to the Androgen Receptors in Skeletal Muscle and in Prostate, as well as to Sex Hormone-Binding Globuline. *Endocrinology,* Vol. 114, No.6, (June 1984), pp. 2100-2106, ISSN 0013-7227.

Schwingel, P.A., Cotrim, H.P., Salles, B.R., Almeida, C.E., dos Santos, C.R. Jr, Nachef, B., Andrade, A.R., & Zoppi, C.C. (2011). Anabolic–androgenic steroids: a possible new risk factor of toxicantassociated fatty liver disease. *Liver International,* Vol.31, No.3, (March 2011), pp. 348–353, ISSN 1478-3223.

Smurawa, T.M. & Congeni, J.A. (2007). Testosterone Precursors: Use and Abuse in Pediatric Athletes. *Pediatric Clinics of North America,* Vol.54, No.4, (August 2007), pp. 787-796, ISSN 0031-3955.

Sturmi, J.E. & Diorio, D.J. (1998). Anabolic Agents. *Clinics in Sports Medicine,* Vol.17, No.2, (April 1998), pp. 261-282, ISSN 0278-5919

Svec, F., & Porter, J.R. (1998). The Actions of Exogenous Dehydroepiandrosterone in Experimenatl Animals and Humans. *Proceedings of the Society for Experimental Biology and Medicine,* Vol.218, No.3, (July), pp. 174-191, ISSN 0037-9727.

Tagliaferro, A.R., Davies, J.R., Truchon, S. & Van Hamont, N. (1986). Effects of Dehydroepiandrosterone Acetate on Metabolism, Body Weight, and Composition of male and Female Rats. *Journal of Nutrition,* Vo.116, No.10, (October 1986), pp. 1977-1983, ISSN 0022-3166.

Tricker, R., O'Neill, M.R. & Cook, D. (1989). The Incidence of Anabolic Steroid Use Among Competitive Bodybuilders. *Journal of Drug Education,* Vol.19, No.4, (April 1989), pp. 313-325, ISSN 0047-2379

Usiskin, K.S., Butterworth, S., Clore, J.N., Arad, Y., Ginsberg, H.N., Blackard, W.G., & Nestler, J.E. (1990). Lack of Effect of Dehydroepiandrosterone in Obese Men. *International Journal of Obesity,* Vol.14, No.5, (May 1990), pp. 457-463, ISSN 0307-0565.

Vogiatzi, M.G., Boeck, M.A., Vlachopapadopoulou, E., el-Rashid, R., & New, M.I. (1996). Dehydroepiandrosterone in Morbidly Obese Adolescents: Effects on Weight, Body Composition, Lipids, and Insulin Resistance. *Metabolism*, Vol.45, No.8, (August 1996), pp. 1011-1015, ISSN 0026-0495.

Von Muhlen, D., Laughlin, G.A., Kritz-Silverstain, D., Bergstrom, J., and Bettencourt, R. (2008). Effect of Dehydroepiandrosterone Supplementation on Bone Mineral Density, Bone Markers, and Body Composition in Older Adults: The DAWN Trial. *Osteoporosis International*, Vol.19, No.5, (May 2008), pp. 699-707, ISSN 0937-941X

Wallace, M.B., Lim, J., Cutler, A. & Bucci, L. (1999). Effects of Dehydroepiandrosterone vs. Androstenedione Supplementation in Men. *Medicine and Science in Sports and Exercise*, Vol.31, No.12, (Decemebr 1999), pp. 1788-1792, ISSN 0195-9131.

Welle, S., Jozefowicz, R., & Statt, M. (1990). Failure of Dehydroepiandrosterone to Influence Energy and Protein Metabolism in Humans. *Journal of Clinical Endocrinology and Metabolism*, Vol.71, No.5, (November 1990), pp. 1259-1264, ISSN 0021-972X.

Wilson, J.D. (1988). Androgen Abuse by Athletes. *Endocrinology Review*, Vol.9, No.2, (May 1988), pp. 181-199, ISSN 0163-769X.

Windsor, R. & Dumitru, D. (1989). Prevalence of anabolic steroid use by male and female adolescents. *Medicine and Science in Sports and Exercise*, Vol.21, No.5, (October 1989), pp. 494-497, ISSN 0195-9131.

Wolf, O.T., Neumann, O., Hellhammer, D.H., Geiben, A.C., Strasburger, C.J., Dressendörfer, R.A., Pirke, K.M., & Kirschbaum, C. (1997). Effects of a Two-Week Physiological Dehydroepiandrosterone Substitution on Cognitive Performance and Well-Being in Healthy Elderly Women and Men. *Journal of Clinical Endocrinology and Metabolism*, Vol.82, No.7, (July 1997), pp. 2363-2367, ISSN 0021-972X.

Wroble, R.R, Gray, M. & Rodrigo, J. (2002). Anabolic Steroids and Pre-adolescent Athletes: Prevalence, Knowledge, and Attitudes. *Sport Journal*, Vol.5, No.3, (March 2002), pp. 1-8, ISSN 1543-9518.

Yamada, Y., Sekihara, H., Omura, M., Yanase, T., Takayanagi, R., Mune, T., Yasuda, K., Ishizuka, T., Ueshiba, H., Miyachi, Y., Iwasaki, T., Nakajima, A., & Nawata, H. (2007). Changes in Serum Sex Hormone Profiles after Short-Term Low-Dose Administration of Dehydroepiandrosterone (DHEA) to Young And Elderly Persons. *Endocrine Journal*, Vol.54, No.1, (February 2007), pp. 153-162, ISSN 0918-8959.

Yen, S.S., Morales, A.J., & Khorram, O. (1995). Replacement of DHEA in aging men and women. Potential remedial effects. *Annals of the New York Academy of Sciences*, Vol.774, (December 1995), pp. 128-142, ISSN 0077-8923.

Yesalis, C.E., Streit, A.L., Vicary, J.R., Friedl, K.E., Brannon, D. & Buckley, W. (1989). Anabolic Steroid Use: Indications of Habituation Among Adolescents. *Journal of Drug Education*, Vol.19, No.2, (April 1989), pp. 103-116, ISSN 0047-2379.

Yesalis, C.E., Bahrke M,S. (1995). Anabolic-Androgenic Steroids: Current Issues. *Sports Medicine*, Vol.19, No. 5, (May 1995), pp. 326-340, ISSN 0112-1642

Yesalis, C.E. (1999). Medical, Legal and Societal Implications of Androstenedione Use. *JAMA*, Vol.281, No.21 (June 1999), pp. 2043-2044, ISSN 0098-7484.

Yesalis, C.E. & Bahrke, M.S. (2000). Doping among adolescent athletes. *Baillière's best practice & research. Clinical endocrinology & metabolism*, Vol.14, No.1, (March 2000), pp. 25-35, ISSN 0950-351X.

Ziegenfuss, T.N., Berardi, J.M., Lowery, L.M & Antonio, J. (2002). Effects of Prohormone Supplementation in Humans: A Review. *Canadian Journal of Applied Physiology*, Vol.27, No.6, (December 2002), pp. 628-645, ISSN 1066-7814.

3

11β-Hydroxysteroid Dehydrogenase Type 1 and the Metabolic Syndrome

Cidália D. Pereira, Maria J. Martins, Isabel Azevedo and Rosário Monteiro
Dept. of Biochemistry (U38/FCT), Faculty of Medicine, University of Porto, Portugal

1. Introduction

In the past few years, efforts are being made to unravel the mechanisms endowed with the metabolic disturbances associated with obesity that predispose to the metabolic syndrome (MetSyn). The special pathogenic role of liver and visceral adipose tissue (VAT) functions has been particularly intriguing, and many hypotheses have been advanced to explain this association. Tissue-specific actions of glucocorticoids (GCs) go far beyond the circulating levels of the hormones and can be controlled by local intracellular enzymes. In the past few years, evidence is being gathered not only on the relevance of such enzymes to GC physiological actions but also on their involvement in the pathophysiology of certain chronic disease states, in which circulating GC levels are not necessarily altered. These enzymes are 11β-hydroxysteroid dehydrogenases (11β-HSDs, EC 1.1.1.146) which interconvert inactive GCs, such as cortisone and dehydrocorticosterone, and the active hormones, cortisol and corticosterone.

2. Brief overview of the hypothalamus-pituitary-adrenal (HPA) axis

The regulation of tissue GC levels is critical for the maintenance of homeostasis, playing a central role in essential physiological processes, such as stress responses, energy metabolism, electrolyte levels, blood pressure, immunity, cell proliferation and differentiation and cognitive functions (Atanasov & Odermatt, 2007). Cortisol release by the adrenal gland is under the control of the HPA axis. Briefly, corticotrophin releasing hormone (CRH) is produced by parvicellular hypothalamic neurons and acts on anterior pituitary cells increasing the production and release of adenocorticotrophic hormone (ACTH) into the blood stream in a pulsatile fashion and with circadian rhythm: peak in the morning and valley later in the afternoon (Gathercole & Stewart, 2010; White B., 2008b). Cortisol is synthesized in the cells of the zona fasciculata of the adrenal cortex. Under the influence of ACTH, cholesterol esters, stored in the foamy cytoplasm of these cells, are unsterified by cholesterol ester hydrolase and converted to cortisol (Tomlinson et al., 2004; White B., 2008a). GCs are able to bind and activate GC receptors (GR) and mineralocorticoid receptors (MR), which are ligand-regulated nuclear receptors and members of the steroid hormone receptor family (Gathercole & Stewart, 2010). Cortisol and the principal GC in rodents, corticosterone, are active steroids whereas cortisone and 11-dehydrocorticosterone, the latter in rodents, are inactive (Tomlinson et al., 2004). Cortisol is metabolized in the liver through conjugation with glucuronide and sulfate for posterior renal excretion (Tomlinson et al., 2004; White B., 2008a). Moreover, in the liver, 5α- and 5β-reductases inactivate cortisol and cortisone, in conjunction with 3α-HSD, to tetrahydrometabolites: 5α-tetrahydrocortisol (5α-THF), 5β-tetrahydrocortisol (5β-THF) and tetrahydrocortisone (THE) (Campino et al., 2010).

3. 11β-HSDs – enzymology, tissue expression and physiological role

3.1 11β-HSD type 2 (11β-HSD2)

Because cortisol and aldosterone have the same *in vitro* affinity for the MR (Gathercole & Stewart, 2010), 11β-HSD2, that catalyzes the inactivation of cortisol to inert cortisone, in humans, or of corticosterone to 11-dehydrocorticosterone, in rodents, avoids MR actions of GCs. 11β-HSD2 was the first isoform to be identified and is a NAD^+ dependent dehydrogenase. 11β-HSD2 is present in high amounts in the distal convoluted tubule of the kidney, colon, salivary and sweat glands as well as in other locations such as the human placenta and vascular wall to avoid deleterious actions of active GC overstimulation (Anagnostis et al., 2009; Andrews et al., 2003; Edwards et al., 1988; Ferrari, 2010; Funder et al., 1988; Gathercole & Stewart, 2010; Palermo et al., 2004). The importance of 11β-HSD2 activity is illustrated in the case of congenital deficiency of 11β-HSD2 in humans (Gathercole & Stewart, 2010; Stewart et al. 1996), transgenic deletion in mice (Kotelevtsev et al., 1999) or by its pharmacological inhibition which produces the apparent mineralocorticoid excess (AME) syndrome in which the lack of cortisol inactivation in the kidney allows its mineralocorticoid action, producing sodium retention, hypertension and hypokalemia, despite normal circulating levels of cortisol and an intact HPA axis (Anagnostis et al., 2009; Andrews et al., 2003; Edwards et al., 1988; Gathercole & Stewart, 2010; Monder et al., 1986; Mune et al., 1995; Palermo et al., 2004; Quinkler & Stewart, 2003; Stewart et al., 1996; Walker & Andrew, 2006). Thus AME has been considered 'Cushing's disease of the kidney' where there are normal circulating levels of cortisol but a tissue-specific excess at the site of MR action (Stewart, 2005).

3.2 11β-HSD type 1 (11β-HSD1)

Pre-receptor metabolism of GCs by 11β-HSD1 amplifies intracellular levels of GCs, through the reduction of inactive cortisone in humans (11-dehydrocorticosterone in rodents) back into active cortisol (corticosterone in rodents) (Anagnostis et al., 2009; Espindola-Antunes & Kater, 2007). 11β-HSD1 is mostly expressed in the liver, adipose tissue (AT), bone, lung and central nervous system. However, its expression can be present in other tissues including pancreas, kidney cortex, adrenal cortex, cardiac myocytes, bone, placenta, uterus, testis, oocytes and luteinized glanulosa cells of the ovary, eye, pituitary, fibroblasts and immune, skeletal and smooth muscle cells (Anagnostis et al., 2009; Bujalska et al., 1997; Cooper & Stewart, 2009; Espindola-Antunes & Kater, 2007; Stewart & Krozowski, 1999; Tomlinson et al., 2004; Whorwood et al. 2001). This enzyme is located in the endoplasmic reticulum, facing the lumen (Gathercole & Stewart, 2010), where there is a high concentration of NADPH owing to the activity of hexose-6-phosphate dehydrogenase (H6PDH), that regenerates NADPH from $NADP^+$ (Atanasov et al., 2008; Bujalska et al., 2005; Draper et al., 2003).

11β-HSD1 is bidirectional, able to act as both a reductase (activating GCs) and a dehydrogenase (inactivating GCs) (Cooper & Stewart, 2009; Tomlinson et al., 2004). However, its main function is as a reductase on intact cells such as hepatocytes (Jamieson et al., 1995), myocytes (Whorwood et al., 2001) and adipocytes (Bujalska et al., 2002a; Bujalska et al., 2002b), supported by a higher affinity for cortisone than cortisol (Stewart et al., 1994). *In vitro*, when deprived of NADPH regeneration (Seckl & Walker, 2001; Walker & Andrew, 2006) or in certain physiological or developmental states, it may work as a dehydrogenase. For example, in human omental adipose stromal cells, 11β-HSD1 switches from a dehydrogenase to a reductase upon differentiation (Bujalska et al., 2002a; Bujalska et al., 2002b). In the H6PDH null mouse, hepatic or AT, 11β-HSD1 acts mainly as a dehydrogenase (Bujalska et al., 2008b; Lavery et al., 2006). Most studies on the regulation of 11β-HSD1 have been performed on rodent tissues showing that GCs, CCAAT/enhancer binding proteins, peroxisome proliferator-activated receptor (PPAR) agonists and some pro-inflammatory cytokines [tumor necrosis factor-α (TNF-α) and interleukin-1β] increase 11β-HSD1 expression. On the other hand, growth hormone (via insulin-like growth factor-1) and liver X receptor (LXR) agonists inhibit its expression. Some other factors that may influence 11β-HSD1 expression include sex steroids, insulin and thyroid hormone, but effects vary in different tissues and between species (Tomlinson et al., 2004).

Human 11β-HSD1 congenital deficiency has been described as the apparent cortisone reductase deficiency syndrome (Phillipov et al., 1996). The phenotype is related to the lack of regeneration of cortisol in peripheral tissues with compensatory activation of the HPA axis. This results in increased secretion of androgens by the adrenals, and affected females present hirsutism and oligomenorrhea. 11β-HSD1 congenital deficiency does not appear to protect against obesity. The syndrome does not seem to arise only from mutations of HSD11B1, but rather from the co-inheritance of deleterious mutations in both HSD11B1 and H6PDH (Draper et al., 2003), decreasing NADPH supply and switching 11β-HSD1 to the dehydrogenase activity (Lavery et al., 2006).

4. Chronic GC deficiency or excess

The involvement of GCs in human obesity, particularly visceral obesity, and its related metabolic complications, is becoming increasingly evident. As we will discuss further, this is evident not only in subjects with disturbances in the HPA axis, but also in conditions where tissue GCs are locally modified. To illustrate the first case, two conditions reflect the involvement of circulating cortisol on body weight regulation in opposite extremes: Addison's disease (hypocortisolism) and Cushing's syndrome (hypercortisolism) (Rutters et al., 2010). As to the second case, the clinical entity that aggregates visceral obesity along with several metabolic abnormalities in glucose and lipid metabolism as well as in blood pressure, and known as the MetSyn (Reaven, 2011), may constitute the best example. Chronically elevated GC levels cause obesity, type 2 diabetes mellitus (T2DM), heart disease, mood disorders and memory impairments (Wamil & Seckl, 2007). This is demonstrated in Cushing's syndrome, in which elevated GC levels are a result of increased pathological secretion from the adrenal cortex (endogenous) or from prolonged anti-inflammatory GC treatment (iatrogenic) (Newell-Price et al., 2006). A particular case of Cushing's syndrome is Cushing´s disease that consists of hypercortisolism driven by increased ACTH secretion from pituitary adenoma (Cushing, 1932; Stewart, 2005). Patients with Cushing's syndrome are hypertensive, have visceral obesity, insulin resistance (IR; 50% develop T2DM or impaired glucose tolerance) and may present hepatic steatosis (Stewart, 2005), muscle weakness, dyslipidemia, mood disturbances and infertility as well as features more specific to Cushing's syndrome (e.g. easy bruising, facial plethora and violaceous striae) (Carroll & Findling, 2010; Newell-Price et al., 2006).

The increase of AT in states of GC excess, such as Cushing's syndrome, may not seem straightforward. Indeed, one might predict from cortisol metabolic actions that it would increase the availability of energetic substrates, as is seen with its lipolysis-stimulating effects. However, in these settings, particularly if there is positive energy balance, the chronic increase in GCs is concomitant with the increase in insulin (Dallman et al., 2004). This favors fatty acid re-esterification over lipolysis, which, along with pro-adipogenic effects of insulin and GCs (Rosen & MacDougald, 2006), increases AT depots. This is seen particularly on VAT depots, rather than other AT locations, probably for two reasons: higher expression of GR (Bronnegard et al., 1990) and increased reactivation of circulating cortisone due to high 11β-HSD1 expression and/or activity (Alberti et al., 2007; Simonyte et al., 2009).
Diagnostic features of GC excess in Cushing's syndrome overlap many of the MetSyn components suggesting that GCs may contribute to the pathogenesis of both states (Anagnostis et al., 2009; M. Wang, 2011). It has been demonstrated that circulating cortisol concentrations are higher in patients with MetSyn compared with healthy subjects, both in basal conditions and during dynamic stimulation (Duclos et al., 2005; Misra et al., 2008; Phillips et al., 1998; Sen et al., 2008; Weigensberg et al., 2008). Furthermore, increased 11β-HSD1 activity in VAT may generate increased cortisol levels within AT and liver and thereby promote features of the MetSyn (Walker & Andrew, 2006). This effect has been termed 'Cushing's disease of the omentum' (Bujalska et al., 1997; Stewart, 2005).

5. MetSyn definition

In the past few decades, there has been a worldwide increase in the prevalence of obesity and associated metabolic disorders including glucose intolerance, IR, dyslipidemia and hypertension. In the clinical practice, the presence of these conditions defines the MetSyn, which comprises an increased risk of atherosclerotic cardiovascular events and T2DM (or is associated with T2DM) and, additionally, is characterized by a pro-inflammatory and a pro-thrombotic state and occurrence of non-alcoholic fatty liver disease (NAFLD) (Feldeisen & Tucker, 2007; Gathercole & Stewart, 2010; Johnson & Weinstock, 2006; Reaven, 2011).
Distinct organizations have established their own definitions of the MetSyn: the World Health Organization (WHO), in 1998, the Adult Treatment Panel III (ATP III) of the National Cholesterol Education Program (NCEP), in 2001 (updated in 2005), and the International Diabetes Federation (IDF), in 2005 (Johnson & Weinstock, 2006; Reaven, 2011). In the attempt to harmonize MetSyn definitions, ATP III and IDF, joined by several other prestigious organizations, reviewed the criteria. Meeting any three of the following criteria is sufficient for the diagnosis: elevated waist circumference (abdominal obesity), triglycerides, blood pressure and fasting glucose (glucose intolerance) and low HDL-cholesterol levels. The cut points for an elevated waist circumference are not the same for all population groups (with population-specific reference values) and drug treatment is sufficient to meet the criteria for the other four components. The latest WHO report states that the 'MetSyn should not be a clinical diagnosis', but rather viewed as 'a pre-morbid condition, and should thus exclude individuals with established T2DM or cardiovascular disease' (Reaven, 2011).

6. 11β-HSD1 and MetSyn components: evidence from human and animal studies

Evidence has been accumulated that strongly argues for an etiological role of 11β-HSD1 in obesity, T2DM and MetSyn (Cooper & Stewart, 2009; Gathercole & Stewart, 2010; London &

Castonguay, 2009; Masuzaki & Flier, 2003; Morton, 2010; Staab & Maser, 2010; Tomlinson & Stewart, 2007; van Raalte et al., 2009; Wamil & Seckl, 2007).

Initial studies in obese humans, that measured the ratio of cortisol to cortisone metabolites in urine as an indirect index of total body 11β-HSD activity, produced inconsistent results (such ratios, however, are inadequate as they may be influenced by other enzymes involved in cortisol metabolism). Recently, more trustworthy results from various more tissue-specific measures were obtained (Andrews et al., 2002; Andrews et al., 2003; Desbriere et al., 2006; Gathercole & Stewart, 2010; Karlsson et al., 2010; Morton, 2010; Paulmyer-Lacroix et al., 2002; Rask et al., 2001; Rask et al., 2002; Sandeep et al., 2005; Stewart & Tomlinson, 2009; R. Stimson et al., 2011; Tomlinson et al., 2008; Valsamakis et al., 2004; Wamil & Seckl, 2007). After studies in men and women, representing a wide range of body compositions and insulin sensitivities (but without T2DM), 11β-HSD1 activity is found selectively increased in the abdominal subcutaneous AT (SAT) in obese humans (Rask et al., 2001; Rask et al., 2002; Sandeep et al., 2005), to a similar degree as the increase in transgenic overexpressing mice (Andrews et al., 2003), but impaired in the liver (Rask et al., 2001; Rask et al., 2002; Stewart et al., 1999). This decrease in hepatic tissue may represent a compensatory mechanism to preserve insulin sensitivity and to decrease hepatic glucose output (Gathercole & Stewart, 2010; Morton, 2010; Valsamakis et al., 2004; Wamil & Seckl, 2007). Increased adipose 11β-HSD1 activity results from increased 11β-HSD1 mRNA expression (Desbriere et al., 2006; Paulmyer-Lacroix et al., 2002) in the abdominal SAT in adipocytes, and also in the VAT in both adipocytes and stroma (Paulmyer-Lacroix et al., 2002). Valsamakis et al. report a lack of inhibition of 11β-HSD1 activity with increasing body mass index (BMI) in diabetic patients *versus* non-diabetic BMI- and age-matched controls (where the inhibition is closely associated with VAT mass), and suggest that a reduction in 11β-HSD1 activity might act as an autocrine protective mechanism to prevent increasing adiposity and increased hepatic glucose output with advancing obesity. This adaptive mechanism of reduced cortisol regeneration does not occur in obesity-associated T2DM and might contribute to the underlying pathogenesis of the disease (Gathercole & Stewart, 2010; Morton, 2010; Valsamakis et al., 2004; Wamil & Seckl, 2007). In contrast, in lean patients with T2DM (controlled by diet alone) a relatively small decrease in hepatic 11β-HSD1 activity, and no change in gluteal SAT enzyme activity, has been reported, but only by one group (Andrews et al., 2002; Andrews et al., 2003). Abdominal SAT 11β-HSD1 expression is higher in obese women with impaired glucose tolerance than in obese women with normal glucose tolerance, despite AT (total and regional) being similar between the two groups, and positively correlated with glucose area under curve levels across an oral glucose tolerance testing (Tomlinson et al., 2008). Whole-body 11β-HSD1 activity is increased in obese men with T2DM, compared to healthy normal-weight control subjects, whereas liver 11β-HSD1 activity is sustained, unlike in euglycemic obesity (R. Stimson et al., 2011). The evidences presented raise the hypothesis that hepatic 11β-HSD1 inhibition in obese people who develop impaired glucose tolerance may protect from progression to T2DM (Gathercole & Stewart, 2010; Morton, 2010; Wamil & Seckl, 2007). Additionally, in line with this, myotubes established from obese T2DM subjects show an increased expression of 11β-HSD1 mRNA compared to healthy obese subjects (Abdallah et al., 2005). SAT 11β-HSD1 mRNA levels decrease during very low calorie diet (16 weeks) and anthropometric measurements and metabolic parameters are associated with 11β-HSD1 mRNA levels in obese subjects without the MetSyn (following the WHO definition). However, in obese subjects with the MetSyn these associations were lost or in the opposite direction. In another cohort, this difference is also observed in skeletal muscle (vastus lateralis) between subjects with T2DM or with normal glucose tolerance (Karlsson et al., 2010).

6.1. Findings of 11β-HSD1 biology from rodent models

6.1.1 The aP2-HSD11B1 transgenic rodent model

Transgenic mice with 2–3-fold overexpression of 11β-HSD1, comparable to that seen in obese humans, in white AT have been generated, exploiting the murine adipocyte fatty acid binding protein (aP2) promoter. These aP2-HSD11B1 transgenic mice have elevated corticosterone levels in the AT, but unaltered systemic plasma concentrations, and many features of the MetSyn: glucose intolerance and IR [exacerbated further by high-fat (HF) feeding], dyslipidemia, apparent leptin resistance, truncal obesity and hypertension associated with activation of the circulating renin-angiotensin system. 11β-HSD1 expression correlates strongly and positively with adipocyte size (London & Castonguay, 2009; Masuzaki & Flier, 2003; Masuzaki et al., 2001; Masuzaki et al., 2003; Morton, 2010; Staab & Maser, 2010; van Raalte et al., 2009; Wamil & Seckl, 2007). TNF-α and leptin are elevated whereas resistin and insulin-sensitizing adiponectin are reduced. aP2-HSD11B1 transgenic mice are hyperphagic and obese, predominantly in the VAT. Expression of the GR-α is higher in VAT compared to SAT, while the expression of the transgene HSD11B1 is similar in all AT depots. The greater effects in VAT may reflect the higher GR and/or higher lipoprotein lipase in mesenteric AT. aP2-HSD11B1 transgenic mice have elevated corticosterone and free fatty acids (FFA) levels in the hepatic portal vein that drains blood from VAT to the liver (Masuzaki et al., 2001; Masuzaki et al., 2003; Morton, 2010; Wamil & Seckl, 2007). The aP2-HSD11B1 model shows that altered AT metabolism of GCs (similar to human MetSyn levels) could be the primary driver of many features of this disease (Masuzaki & Flier, 2003; Masuzaki et al., 2001; Masuzaki et al., 2003; Morton, 2010).

6.1.2 The apolipoprotein E (apoE)-HSD11B1 transgenic rodent model

To examine the impact of elevated liver GCs, mice overexpressing 11β-HSD1 selectively in that tissue under the control of the human apoE promoter have been generated. Transgenic lines with 2- and 5-fold-elevated 11β-HSD1 activity exhibit unaltered systemic corticosterone, modest IR (but lacking glucose intolerance), unaltered AT mass (lacking obesity or central adiposity), hepatic fat accumulation (mainly as triglycerides) and dyslipidemia (elevated circulating FFA and HF diet-induced dyslipidemic cholesterol lipoprotein profile), with increased hepatic lipid synthesis/flux associated with elevated hepatic LXR-α and PPAR-α expression as well as impaired hepatic lipid clearance. Increased expression of GC-inducible cholesterol 7α-hydroxylase present in apoE-HSD11B1 transgenic livers may drive increased bile acid synthesis, contributing to stimulation of LXR-α-regulated pathways (and further potentiation of cholesterol 7α-hydroxylase expression) as well as PPAR-α. ApoE-HSD11B1 transgenic mice also have a marked, transgene-dose-associated hypertension, paralleled by incrementally increased liver angiotensinogen expression. Elevated 11β-HSD1 hepatic expression may relate to the pathogenesis of specific fatty liver, insulin-resistant and hypertensive syndromes without obesity in humans as may occur in, possibly, the metabolically obese normal-weight individual (Paterson et al., 2004).

6.1.3 The HSD11B1 knockout (KO) rodent model

HSD11B1 KO mice have been generated, which are viable and healthy but unable to convert inert 11-dehydrocorticosterone to corticosterone. Despite compensatory adrenal hyperplasia and increased adrenal secretion of corticosterone, on fasting, HSD11B1 KO mice have attenuated activation of the hepatic gluconeogenic enzymes, presumably, because of relative intra-hepatic GC deficiency. The HSD11B1 KO mice resist hyperglycemia provoked by obesity or stress (Kotelevtsev et al., 1997). HSD11B1 KO mice, fed *ad lib*, have markedly lower plasma triglyceride levels, driven by increased hepatic expression of enzymes of fat catabolism and PPAR-α. HSD11B1 KO mice also have increased plasma HDL-cholesterol, with elevated liver mRNA and serum levels of apoAI. Conversely, hepatic Aα-fibrinogen expression is decreased. Upon fasting, the normal elevation of hepatic PPAR-α mRNA is lost in HSD11B1 KO mice, consistent with attenuated GC induction. Despite this, crucial oxidative responses to fasting are maintained. Refeeding (4 h and/or 24 h) shows more rapid and/or marked induction of genes encoding lipogenic enzymes/transcription factors and a more rapid and/or marked suppression of genes for fat catabolism in HSD11B1 KO mice, implying increased liver insulin sensitivity. PPAR-α is suppressed by 4 h of refeeding (similarly in wild type and HSD11B1 KO mice), but PPAR-α levels are higher after 24 h of refeeding in HSD11B1 KO mice when compared to wild type mice, reestablishing the *ad lib*-fed pattern. Concordant with this, 24 h refed HSD11B1 KO mice have higher plasma triglycerides than 24 h refed wild type mice and *ad lib*-fed HSD11B1 KO mice. 24 h Refed HSD11B1 KO mice have lower plasma glucose levels than 24 h refed wild type mice and *ad lib*-fed HSD11B1 KO mice. HSD11B1 KO mice also have improved glucose tolerance. 11β-HSD1 deficiency may produce an improved lipid profile, hepatic insulin sensitization and a potentially atheroprotective phenotype (Morton et al., 2001). HSD11B1 KO mice on the control diet express, compared to wild-type mice, lower leptin, resistin and TNF-α but higher PPAR-γ, adiponectin and uncoupling protein-2 (UCP-2) mRNA levels in epididymal AT, indicating insulin sensitization. On the control diet, in mesenteric VAT, PPAR-γ mRNA is elevated in HSD11B1 KO mice, though leptin, resistin, TNF-α, adiponectin and UCP-2 mRNA levels are unaltered, compared to wild-type mice. With HF feeding, the elevated PPAR-γ mRNA level in control-fed HSD11B1 KO mice is further increased selectively in VAT, what does not happen in the epididymal AT depot of HSD11B1 KO or wild-type mice. HSD11B1 KO mice also show a HF–mediated induction of UCP-2 selectively in VAT, which is greater than that observed in wild-type mice. Isolated adipocytes from HSD11B1 KO mice exhibit higher basal and insulin-stimulated glucose uptake. HSD11B1 KO mice also display reduced VAT accumulation upon HF feeding. HF-fed HSD11B1 KO mice rederived onto the C57BL/6J strain (obesity/T2DM/metabolic disease-susceptible) resist T2DM and weight gain despite consuming more calories. These data provided the first *in vivo* evidence that AT 11β-HSD1 deficiency beneficially alters AT distribution and function (Morton et al., 2004), complementing the just above-described effects of hepatic 11β-HSD1 deficiency or data presented further bellow regarding 11β-HSD1 pharmacological inhibition. Since PPAR-γ ligands cause insulin sensitization and AT redistribution to the periphery, a mechanism for the beneficial AT redistribution is suggested, on the assumption that increased circulating FFA during HF feeding act as endogenous ligands for PPAR-γ receptors. Further, UCP-2 levels are higher in HSD11B1 KO mice AT, consistent with GC and PPAR-γ regulation. This higher PPAR-γ-responsive UCP-2 expression in HSD11B1 KO mice AT may drive increased energy dissipation within the adipocytes (Morton, 2010). Interestingly, when mice are fed a HF diet they preferentially gain weight in peripheral AT rather than in VAT what can be explained by an increased expression of PPAR-γ and UCP-2 in VAT (Morton, 2010; van Raalte et al., 2009; Wamil & Seckl, 2007).

Mice overexpressing the cortisol inactivating enzyme specifically on the AT (aP2-HSD11B2 mice) are phenotypically similar to HSD11B1 KO mice, exception only for food intake, what emphasizes the importance of AT as a target for enzyme inhibition (Wamil & Seckl, 2007). 11β-HSD1 gene deficiency is associated with a number of improvements of adipose and hepatic functions, what highlights the importance of adipose and hepatic 11β-HSD1 in the development of metabolic disease.

6.2 11β-HSD1 and T2DM/IR

A role for 11β-HSD1 in exacerbating IR and T2DM has been proposed. Animals with targeted deletion of HSD11B1 manifest increased hepatic and adipose insulin sensitivity (Kotelevtsev et al., 1997; Morton et al., 2001; Morton et al., 2004), and when backcrossed onto the C57BL/6J strain appear to resist the development of IR in response to HF feeding (Morton et al., 2004). Additionally, specific 11β-HSD1 inhibitors improve insulin sensitivity (glycemic control and/or glucose and/or insulin levels) in animal models (associated or not with HF feeding) of hyperglycemia, obesity (by damage of feeding center or diet-induced), T2DM (also ob/ob) and combined T2DM, dyslipidemia and atherosclerosis (Alberts et al., 2002; Alberts et al., 2003; Barf et al., 2002; Gathercole & Stewart, 2010; Hermanowski-Vosatka et al., 2005; Morgan et al., 2009; Park et al., 2011; X. Zhang et al., 2009b).

It is well known that excess GCs increase IR and can, in susceptible individuals, precipitate T2DM. In line with this, it has been suggested that the increased production of cortisol from VAT seen in obesity could drain through the portal circulation to the liver and pancreas contributing to IR (Cooper & Stewart, 2009; Masuzaki et al., 2001; Morton, 2010; R. Stimson et al., 2009; Walker & Andrew, 2006; Wamil & Seckl, 2007). This hypothesis was investigated *in vivo* in humans by Stimson et al. by quantifying, for the first time, selectively, the contributions of SAT, visceral tissues and liver to whole-body cortisol production by 11β-HSD1. Stimson et al. confirmed that splanchnic cortisol production is substantial, originating entirely from the 11β-HSD1 activity in the liver. However, although release of cortisol by 11β-HSD1 into the portal vein, which drains a number of visceral organs, is not detected, a significant cortisol release into veins draining exclusively SAT has been found. So, cortisol release from SAT into the systemic circulation is unlikely to have effects in other organs because the feedback control by the HPA axis will adjust adrenal cortisol secretion to maintain circulating cortisol concentrations. Therefore, the most likely impact of this source of cortisol will be intracrine or paracrine in the local AT environment (R. Stimson et al., 2009).

Skeletal muscle represents a key target tissue for insulin-stimulated glucose uptake, metabolism and utilization (Abdul-Ghani & DeFronzo, 2010; Benito, 2011; Van Cromphaut, 2009). There are just a few studies regarding 11β-HSD1 in skeletal muscle from T2DM, although with non-consensual results (Cooper & Stewart, 2009). Whorwood et al. found, with kinetic analysis, that 11β-HSD1, in intact cultured human skeletal myoblasts (from both lean-moderately overweight and obese adult men, few with T2DM but without therapy), acts exclusively as a reductase and is down-regulated by insulin, which may maintain insulin sensitivity in skeletal muscle tissue by diminishing GC antagonism of insulin action (Whorwood et al., 2001). Cortisone reduces glucose uptake in myotubes established from obese T2DM men (treated either by diet alone or in combination with sulfonylurea or metformin, withdrawn one week before performing the biopsy), what could be mediated by an increased mRNA 11β-HSD1 expression (previously mentioned) emphasizing that the local conversion of inactive to active GCs may be important in IR pathogenesis (Abdallah et al., 2005). Accordingly, Zhang et al., in an animal model of T2DM (Wistar rats with HF feeding, combined with multiple low dose streptozotocin injection), report increased 11β-

HSD1 mRNA and protein levels in skeletal muscle extracts of the diabetic animals *versus* the non-diabetic animals, what may be related to disturbances in insulin signaling pathway observed in the skeletal muscle (M. Zhang et al., 2009a). Jang et al. demonstrated that the activities of skeletal muscle 11β-HSD1 and 11β-HSD2 (in vastus lateralis biopsies) are altered in T2DM patients (treated by diet alone or oral hypoglycemic agents) *versus* healthy age- and sex-matched controls (altogether overweight and obese subjects): 11β-HSD1 activity is reduced and 11β-HSD2 activity is higher in T2DM subjects (negative correlation between both enzyme activities; with similar mRNA levels in T2DM and control subjects for both enzymes), and, more importantly, 11β-HSD1 reductase activity is significantly lower in T2DM subjects whereas 11β-HSD1 dehydrogenase activity is significantly higher in the T2DM group (with very low levels of 11β-HSD1 dehydrogenase activity in both groups). Together these results may indicate a reduced intracellular cortisol generation, potentially conferring metabolic protection (Jang et al., 2007). In what regards the AT, Balachandran et al. demonstrated that insulin stimulates adipocyte 11β-HSD1 activity and expression both *in vitro* (in 3T3-L1 adipocytes) and *in vivo* (Wistar rat white AT) (Balachandran et al., 2008).
Morgan et al. established a strong connection between a key player in insulin signaling, the insulin receptor substrate 1 (IRS1), and 11β-HSD1 in skeletal muscle: in KK/Ta Jcl mice (an hyperglycemic model) treated with A2, inducing selective 11β-HSD1 inhibition, skeletal muscle $pSer^{307}IRS1$ decreases, $pThr^{308}Akt/PKB$ increases and lipogenic and lipolytic gene expression decreases (Morgan et al., 2009). 11β-HSD1 has also been proposed to have effects on insulin secretion itself. Davani et al. report 11β-HSD1 mRNA expression in human and ob/ob mice (non-insulin-dependent diabetes model) pancreatic β-cells, and also characterize the 11β-HSD1 activity in intact pancreatic rodent islets (where the reductive reaction prevails). In ob/ob mice islets, in the absence of carbenoxolone, 11-dehydrocorticosterone markedly inhibits insulin release, whereas a reversal of this effect is noted in the presence of carbenoxolone, indicating an important role of 11β-HSD1 in the regulation of insulin release (Davani et al., 2000). A more recent report describes a similar effect of dehydrocorticosterone on insulin release in human and murine pancreatic cells, but it appears that enzyme expression is absent in β-cells, with this effect being mediated indirectly through expression within α-cells. This α-cell expression additionally inhibits insulin-stimulated glucagon secretion (Cooper & Stewart, 2009; Swali et al., 2008).

6.3 11β-HSD1 and hypertension

GC hormones act on the cardiovascular system (Nussinovitch et al., 2010; Raff & Findling, 2003; Walker et al., 2000; Wallerath et al., 1999). Cortisol and 11β-HSDs have been implicated in hypertension (Anagnostis et al., 2009; Andrews et al., 2003; Campino et al., 2010; Cicala & Mantero, 2010; Edwards et al., 1988; Ferrari, 2010; Franks et al., 2004; Funder et al., 1988; Gathercole & Stewart, 2010; Y. Liu et al., 2008; Malavasi et al., 2010; Masuzaki et al., 2003; Millis, 2011; Monder et al., 1989; Morales et al., 2008; Mune et al., 1995; Palermo et al., 2004; Paterson et al., 2004; Quinkler & Stewart, 2003; Raff & Findling, 2003; S. Shah et al., 2011; Stewart et al., 1996; Walker & Andrew, 2006; Walker et al., 1993; Wallerath et al., 1999; White et al., 1997).
The fact that 11β-HSD2 is important in protecting MR in the distal nephron from stimulation by GCs revealed its role in the regulation of arterial blood pressure. Pharmacological inhibition or genetic deficiency of 11β-HSD2 leads to the development of hypertension (Anagnostis et al., 2009; Andrews et al., 2003; Edwards et al., 1988; Ferrari, 2010; Funder et al., 1988; Gathercole & Stewart, 2010; Palermo et al., 2004; Walker et al., 1993; White et al.,

1997). HSD11B2 can be epigenetically regulated, what is also involved in hypertension development (Millis, 2011). In the same line, defects and polymorphisms in HSD11B2 have also been shown to play a role in human hypertension and cardiovascular disease [e.g. essential hypertension (Soro et al., 1995; Walker et al., 1993) and 'salt-sensitive' hypertension (Lovati et al., 1999)] (Bailey et al., 2008; Cooper & Stewart, 2009; Henschkowski et al., 2008). Campino et al. reported a high percentage of alterations in the cortisol metabolism at the pre-receptor level in hypertensive patients, previously misclassified as having essential hypertension, where 18% of the patients present reduced 11β-HSD2 activity or imbalance of 11β-HSD1 activity in comparison to 11β-HSD2 (Campino et al., 2010). As referred above, hypertension is induced in mice genetically modified to overexpress 11β-HSD1 either in the liver or AT (Masuzaki et al., 2003; Paterson et al., 2004). HSD11B1 polymorphisms have been described, affecting enzyme expression and activity *in vitro* and/or *in vivo*, and/or being associated with hypertension (Franks et al., 2004; Malavasi et al., 2010; Morales et al., 2008). Variants of HSD11B1 were associated with the risk of hypertension in Pima Indians (Franks et al., 2004). Liu et al. showed that suppression of 11β-HSD1 expression in the renal medulla attenuates salt-induced hypertension in Dahl salt-sensitive rats (Y. Liu et al., 2008). Taking into consideration that diet is one important factor on MetSyn development, it is interesting to mention that in Dahl salt-sensitive hypertensive rats, fed a high-salt diet for 4 weeks, peri-renal AT corticosterone concentration and 11β-HSD1 activity as well as GR, 11β-HSD1 and TNF-α expression increase when compared with Dahl salt-resistant rats fed the same diet (Usukura et al., 2009).

6.4 11β-HSD1 and NAFLD

NAFLD is being increasingly recognized as a common liver disorder that represents the hepatic manifestation of the MetSyn. NAFLD is more frequent among people with T2DM and obesity, and it is almost universal amongst T2DM patients who are morbidly obese (Bellentani et al., 2000; Fabbrini et al., 2010; Gupte et al., 2004; Konopelska et al., 2009; Ratziu et al., 2010; Wree et al., 2010). Non-alcoholic steatohepatitis (NASH) is the progressive form of liver injury that carries a risk of progressive fibrosis, cirrhosis and end-stage liver disease. There is strong evidence that IR and increased FFA are a major cause of NASH (Brunt, 2004; Konopelska et al., 2009; Ratziu et al., 2010; Scheen & Luyckx, 2002). Inflammation plays an important additional role with increased production of reactive oxygen species and pro-inflammatory cytokines. In addition, several studies support a link between VAT and NASH (Kern et al., 2003; Konopelska et al., 2009; McCullough & Falck-Ytter, 1999). Konopelska et al., for the first time in patients with elevated liver enzymes (that after liver biopsies had histological diagnosis of normality, steatosis, NASH and other forms of hepatitis or cirrhosis), found no association between increased liver fat accumulation or different stages of liver inflammation and hepatic 11β-HSD1 expression, suggesting that, probably, there is no major role of this enzyme in the inflammatory process from fatty liver to NASH in humans (Konopelska et al., 2009). In contrast, as mentioned before, transgenic mice with hepatic overexpression of 11β-HSD1 develop fatty liver and dyslipidemia (Paterson et al., 2004). 11β-HSD1 expression correlated positively with H6PDH expression in the liver and negatively with waist-to-hip ratio in women (this being in accordance to obesity results we have mentioned previously). No evaluation of 11β-HSD1 and H6PDH protein or activity levels was done (Konopelska et al., 2009).

Given all the above evidences, 11β-HSD1 has thus emerged as a major potential drug target for the treatment of obesity and its associated metabolic abnormalities.

7. 11β-HSD1 inhibition studies

Several and distinct selective 11β-HSD1 inhibitors are being produced, developed and tested *in vitro, ex vivo* and *in vivo*, in normal animals, rodent models of metabolic alterations or disease (hyperglycemia, dyslipidemia, atherosclerosis, IR, T2DM, obesity, diet-induced obesity and/or MetSyn) and some of them already in humans, healthy or not (Alberts et al., 2002; Alberts et al., 2003; Barf et al., 2002; Bhat et al., 2008; Bujalska et al., 2008a; Cho et al., 2009; Cooper & Stewart, 2009; Coppola et al., 2005; Courtney et al., 2008; Feig et al., 2011; Gathercole & Stewart, 2010; Ge et al., 2010; Hale et al., 2008; Hale & Wang, 2008; Hermanowski-Vosatka et al., 2005; Hollis & Huber, 2011; Hughes et al., 2008; Hult et al., 2006; Johansson et al., 2008; Julian et al., 2008; J. Liu et al., 2011; Morgan et al., 2009; Morgan & Tomlinson, 2010; Morton, 2010; Park et al., 2011; Rosenstock et al., 2010; S. Shah et al., 2011; U. Shah et al., 2010; Siu et al., 2009; Stewart & Tomlinson, 2009; Tiwari, 2010; Tu et al., 2008; van Raalte et al., 2009; Véniant et al., 2010; S. J. Wang et al., 2006; Webster et al., 2010; Yuan et al., 2007; X. Zhang et al., 2009b). Besides inhibition of 11β-HSD1 reductase activity, increase of 11β-HSD1 dehydrogenase (oxidase) activity, without inhibition of 11β-HSD2, may provide a better therapeutic strategy for T2DM, obesity and MetSyn (Ge et al., 2010). 11β-HSD1 is also inhibited by natural compounds, such as an active ingredient of various Chinese herbs (emodin), derivatives or analogues of the licorice root, coffee extract, flavanone (and the monohydroxylated flavonoid 2'-hydroxyflavanone), endogenous steroids and their metabolites and bile acids (Andrews et al., 2003; Atanasov et al., 2006; Chalbot & Morfin, 2006; Classen-Houben et al., 2009; Diederich et al., 2000; Feng et al., 2010; Gathercole & Stewart, 2010; Hollis & Huber, 2011; Latif et al., 2005; Livingstone & Walker, 2003; Maeda et al., 2010; Monder et al., 1989; Morris et al., 2004; Odermatt & Nashev, 2010; Sandeep et al., 2005; Schweizer et al., 2003; Su et al., 2007; Taylor et al., 2008; Tomlinson et al., 2007; van Raalte et al., 2009; Walker et al., 1995a; Wamil & Seckl, 2007). Glycyrrhetinic acid, the active pharmacological ingredient of the licorice root and some of its derivatives, as well as its steroidal synthetic analogue carbenoxolone (hemisuccinate derivative of glycyrrhetinic acid) are inhibitors of both 11β-HSD1 and 11β-HSD2 (the magnitude of the effect being dependent on *in vitro versus in vivo* environment, dose, administration mode, tissue and specie as well as compound structure) (Abdallah et al., 2005; Andrews et al., 2003; Classen-Houben et al., 2009; Gathercole & Stewart, 2010; Hollis & Huber, 2011; Jellinck et al., 1993; Livingstone & Walker, 2003; Monder et al., 1989; Sandeep et al., 2005; Su et al., 2007; Taylor et al., 2008; Tomlinson et al., 2007; van Raalte et al., 2009; Walker et al., 1995a; Wamil & Seckl, 2007). Both 7-oxygenated steroids and 7-ketocholesterol modulate 11-HSD1 activity (Balázs et al., 2009; Odermatt & Nashev, 2010; Wamil et al., 2008; Wamil & Seckl, 2007). From all the bile salts tested *in vitro* and found to inhibit 11β-HSD1, Diederich et al. reported that chenodesoxycholic acid does not affect *in vivo* the activity of 11β-HSD1 when given in therapeutic doses to healthy men (Diederich et al., 2011).

7.1 Human 11β-HSD1 inhibition studies

In a study with carbenoxolone it is observed, in healthy non-diabetic men, a small (although significant) increase in whole body insulin sensitivity (Hollis & Huber, 2011; Walker et al., 1995a). Walker et al. infered that carbenoxolone, by inhibiting hepatic 11β-HSD1 and reducing intra-hepatic cortisol concentration, increases hepatic insulin sensitivity and decreases hepatic glucose production (Walker et al., 1995b). Further developing their research on carbenoxolone 11β-HSD1 inhibition, Walker et al. report decreased glucagon-stimulated glucose production and glycogenolysis in T2DM men (non-obese normotensive, treated with diet alone), but not in healthy subjects, and decreased total cholesterol in healthy subjects, but not in T2DM patients. Carbenoxolone has no effect on gluconeogenesis, peripheral glucose uptake or insulin-mediated reduction of plasma FFA (Andrews et al., 2003). So, as just described, carbenoxolone enhances hepatic insulin sensitivity in healthy men and in non-obese normotensive T2DM. However, Sandeep et al. describe later, in non-diabetic obese men, a highly effective inhibition of whole-body 11β-HSD turnover by carbenoxolone, but without inhibiting the conversion of cortisone to cortisol in SAT or modifying insulin sensitivity (Sandeep et al., 2005). Nevertheless, 11β-HSD1 inhibition in AT by carbenoxolone has been reported. After both a single dose and posterior 72 h of continuous treatment with carbenoxolone, in healthy male volunteers, Tomlinson et al. observe a decrease not only on serum cortisol generation, after oral administration of cortisone acetate (although only significantly for continuous treatment), but also on cortisol concentrations, after oral cortisone acetate, and glycerol concentrations, after oral prednisone, both within SAT interstitial fluid (in the latter location being indicative of inhibition of GC-mediated lipolysis) (Tomlinson et al., 2007). It is important to mention that 11β-HSD2 inhibition, with licorice or carbenoxolone, can lead to cortisol-dependent mineralocorticoid excess, with hypertension, sodium retention, hypokalemia and fluid retention (Andrews et al., 2003; Edwards et al., 1988; Ferrari, 2010; Gathercole & Stewart, 2010; Palermo et al., 2004; Stewart et al., 1990; Stewart et al., 1987). 11β-HSD2 is expressed principally in the distal nephron, where it inactivates cortisol to cortisone and thereby protects MR from cortisol (Andrews et al., 2003; Edwards et al., 1988; Ferrari, 2010; Funder et al., 1988; Palermo et al., 2004). PF-915275 is a potent and selective 11β-HSD1 inhibitor, without adverse side effects in a wide range of orally tested doses, that is selective for the human and primate enzymes (Bhat et al., 2008; Courtney et al., 2008). A modest pharmacodynamic effect of PF-915275 on 11β-HSD1 activity in the healthy human liver is reported, but experiments to assess its inhibitory effect in the AT have not been performed (Courtney et al., 2008; Hollis & Huber, 2011). So far, to our knowledge, there are no reports of PF-915275 activity in patients with T2DM or MetSyn (or any of the associated components). Bhat et al. showed, in normal cynomolgus monkeys, that PF-915275 dose-dependently inhibits 11β-HSD1-mediated conversion of prednisone to prednisolone and reduces insulin levels (Bhat et al., 2008). Hollis et al. reviewed the clinical results obtained with the selective 11β-HSD1 inhibitor INCB13739. In patients with T2DM inadequately controlled with metformin, INCB13739 treatment achieves significant reductions in hemoglobin A1c, fasting plasma glucose and HOMA-IR (homeostasis model assessment-IR), and improves hyperlipidemia and hypertriglyceridemia (when present). Adverse events (occurring in $\geq 3\%$: nasopharyngitis, headache, diarrhea, cough, nausea, arthralgia and upper respiratory tract infection) were similar across all treatment groups. Interestingly, those positive effects are observed primarily in subjects categorized as obese (BMI > 30 kg/m^2) and not in subjects categorized as overweight (BMI ≤ 30 kg/m^2), underscoring the likely importance of AT 11β-HSD1 activity to the cardiometabolic sequelae of obesity (Hollis & Huber, 2011; Rosenstock et al., 2010). Feig et al. showed that 11β-HSD1 selective inhibition with MK-0916 is generally well tolerated in patients with T2DM and MetSyn (NCEP ATP III-defined) (Feig et al., 2011; S. Shah et al., 2011). Although no significant improvement in fasting plasma glucose is observed with MK-0916 compared to placebo, modest improvements in hemoglobin A1c, body weight and blood pressure are observed (Feig et al., 2011). These patients were only mildly hypertensive, with 55% receiving ongoing anti-hypertensive therapy, and yet treatment with MK-0916 led to reductions from baseline of 7.9 and 5.4 mmHg in systolic and diastolic blood pressure, respectively, relative to placebo (Feig et al., 2011; S. Shah et al., 2011). Further developing the research on 11β-HSD1 selective inhibition, Shah et al. reported that, in overweight-to-obese hypertensive patients, reduction in trough sitting diastolic blood pressure with MK-0736 is not statistically significant. Nonetheless, MK-0736 is well tolerated and appears to modestly improve other blood pressure endpoints as well as LDL-cholesterol and body weight. The 24 h ambulatory blood pressure measurements data (from the subset of patients who participated in ambulatory blood pressure measurements) suggest that MK-0736 has blood pressure-lowering efficacy over a 24 h period not adequately represented by measuring sitting diastolic blood pressure and sitting systolic blood pressure, notably a greater blood pressure-lowering effect during daytime than during night-time (S. Shah et al., 2011). 11β-HSD1 inhibitors may improve a number of metabolic disturbances, unlike current available anti-diabetic compounds, that occur in obesity, T2DM and/or MetSyn patients, as seen from genetically engineered animal studies (Kotelevtsev et al., 1997; Morton et al., 2001; Morton et al., 2004) as well as from animal (Alberts et al., 2002; Alberts et al., 2003; Barf et al., 2002; Cooper & Stewart, 2009; Feng et al., 2010; Gathercole & Stewart, 2010; Hermanowski-Vosatka et al., 2005; Johansson et al., 2008; J. Liu et al., 2011; Livingstone & Walker, 2003; Morgan et al., 2009; Park et al., 2011; Taylor et al., 2008; Véniant et al., 2010; S. J. Wang et al., 2006; X. Zhang et al., 2009b) and human 11β-HSD1 inhibition studies (Andrews et al., 2003; Courtney et al., 2008; Feig et al., 2011; Gathercole & Stewart, 2010; Hollis & Huber, 2011; Morton, 2010; Rosenstock et al., 2010; Sandeep et al., 2005; S. Shah et al., 2011; Tomlinson et al., 2007; van Raalte et al., 2009; Walker et al., 1995a; Wamil & Seckl, 2007). Taking this into account, pharmacological inhibition of 11β-HSD1 to lower intracellular cortisol concentrations in the liver and AT, without altering circulating cortisol concentrations or responses to stress, is an exciting potential therapy in those conditions and likely to be most effective in obese T2DM patients (Andrews et al., 2003; Courtney et al., 2008; Feig et al., 2011; Gathercole & Stewart, 2010; Hollis & Huber, 2011; Morton, 2010; Rosenstock et al., 2010; Sandeep et al., 2005; S. Shah et al., 2011; R. Stimson et al., 2011; Tomlinson et al., 2007; van Raalte et al., 2009; Walker et al., 1995a; Wamil & Seckl, 2007).

8. Conclusion

According to the rising prevalence of the MetSyn and the burden of its associated cardiometabolic complications, the study of the mechanisms of disease as well as of possible prophylactic and therapeutic approaches is becoming increasingly necessary. The recognition of the involvement of GCs and 11β-HSD1, as likely etiological factors, adds new avenues for MetSyn management. Lately, research focusing on 11β-HSD1 inhibition has shown promising results. The role of dietary patterns on MetSyn development and of dietary components on 11β-HSD1 modulation for the prevention and/or treatment of metabolic disorders is now starting to be unraveled and may be a worthwhile investigation.

9. References

Abdallah, B., Beck-Nielsen, H. & Gaster, M. (2005). Increased expression of 11beta-hydroxysteroid dehydrogenase type 1 in type 2 diabetic myotubes. *Eur J Clin Invest*, Vol.35, No.10, (Oct), pp. 627-634, ISSN: 0014-2972

Abdul-Ghani, M. & DeFronzo, R. (2010). Pathogenesis of insulin resistance in skeletal muscle. *J Biomed Biotechnol*, Vol.2010, pp. 476279, ISSN: 1110-7251

Alberti, L., Girola, A., Gilardini, L., et al. (2007). Type 2 diabetes and metabolic syndrome are associated with increased expression of 11beta-hydroxysteroid dehydrogenase 1 in obese subjects. *Int J Obes (Lond)*, Vol.31, No.12, (Dec), pp. 1826-1831, ISSN: 0307-0565

Alberts, P., Engblom, L., Edling, N., et al. (2002). Selective inhibition of 11beta-hydroxysteroid dehydrogenase type 1 decreases blood glucose concentrations in hyperglycaemic mice. *Diabetologia*, Vol.45, No.11, (Nov), pp. 1528-1532, ISSN: 0012-186X

Alberts, P., Nilsson, C., Selen, G., et al. (2003). Selective inhibition of 11 beta-hydroxysteroid dehydrogenase type 1 improves hepatic insulin sensitivity in hyperglycemic mice strains. *Endocrinology*, Vol.144, No.11, (Nov), pp. 4755-4762, ISSN: 0013-7227

Anagnostis, P., Athyros, V., Tziomalos, K., et al. (2009). Clinical review: The pathogenetic role of cortisol in the metabolic syndrome: a hypothesis. *J Clin Endocrinol Metab*, Vol.94, No.8, (Aug), pp. 2692-2701, ISSN: 1945-7197

Andrews, R., Herlihy, O., Livingstone, D., et al. (2002). Abnormal cortisol metabolism and tissue sensitivity to cortisol in patients with glucose intolerance. *J Clin Endocrinol Metab*, Vol.87, No.12, (Dec), pp. 5587-5593, ISSN: 0021-972X

Andrews, R., Rooyackers, O. & Walker, B. (2003). Effects of the 11 beta-hydroxysteroid dehydrogenase inhibitor carbenoxolone on insulin sensitivity in men with type 2 diabetes. *J Clin Endocrinol Metab*, Vol.88, No.1, (Jan), pp. 285-291, ISSN: 0021-972X

Atanasov, A., Dzyakanchuk, A., Schweizer, R., et al. (2006). Coffee inhibits the reactivation of glucocorticoids by 11beta-hydroxysteroid dehydrogenase type 1: a glucocorticoid connection in the anti-diabetic action of coffee? *FEBS Lett*, Vol.580, No.17, (Jul 24), pp. 4081-4085, ISSN: 0014-5793

Atanasov, A., Nashev, L., Gelman, L., et al. (2008). Direct protein-protein interaction of 11beta-hydroxysteroid dehydrogenase type 1 and hexose-6-phosphate dehydrogenase in the endoplasmic reticulum lumen. *Biochim Biophys Acta*, Vol.1783, No.8, (Aug), pp. 1536-1543, ISSN: 0006-3002

Atanasov, A. & Odermatt, A. (2007). Readjusting the glucocorticoid balance: an opportunity for modulators of 11beta-hydroxysteroid dehydrogenase type 1 activity? *Endocr Metab Immune Disord Drug Targets*, Vol.7, No.2, (Jun), pp. 125-140, ISSN: 1871-5303

Bailey, M., Paterson, J., Hadoke, P., et al. (2008). A switch in the mechanism of hypertension in the syndrome of apparent mineralocorticoid excess. *J Am Soc Nephrol*, Vol.19, No.1, (Jan), pp. 47-58, ISSN: 1533-3450

Balachandran, A., Guan, H., Sellan, M., et al. (2008). Insulin and dexamethasone dynamically regulate adipocyte 11beta-hydroxysteroid dehydrogenase type 1. *Endocrinology*, Vol.149, No.8, (Aug), pp. 4069-4079, ISSN: 0013-7227

Balázs, Z., Nashev, L., Chandsawangbhuwana, C., et al. (2009). Hexose-6-phosphate dehydrogenase modulates the effect of inhibitors and alternative substrates of 11beta-hydroxysteroid dehydrogenase 1. *Mol Cell Endocrinol*, Vol.301, No.1-2, (Mar 25), pp. 117-122, ISSN: 0303-7207

Barf, T., Vallgarda, J., Emond, R., et al. (2002). Arylsulfonamidothiazoles as a new class of potential antidiabetic drugs. Discovery of potent and selective inhibitors of the

11beta-hydroxysteroid dehydrogenase type 1. *J Med Chem*, Vol.45, No.18, (Aug 29), pp. 3813-3815, ISSN: 0022-2623

Bellentani, S., Saccoccio, G., Masutti, F., et al. (2000). Prevalence of and risk factors for hepatic steatosis in Northern Italy. *Ann Intern Med*, Vol.132, No.2, (Jan 18), pp. 112-117, ISSN: 0003-4819

Benito, M. (2011). Tissue specificity on insulin action and resistance: past to recent mechanisms. *Acta Physiol (Oxf)*, Vol.201, No.3, (Mar), pp. 297-312, ISSN: 1748-1716

Bhat, B., Hosea, N., Fanjul, A., et al. (2008). Demonstration of proof of mechanism and pharmacokinetics and pharmacodynamic relationship with 4'-cyano-biphenyl-4-sulfonic acid (6-amino-pyridin-2-yl)-amide (PF-915275), an inhibitor of 11 -hydroxysteroid dehydrogenase type 1, in cynomolgus monkeys. *J Pharmacol Exp Ther*, Vol.324, No.1, (Jan), pp. 299-305, ISSN: 1521-0103

Bronnegard, M., Arner, P., Hellstrom, L., et al. (1990). Glucocorticoid receptor messenger ribonucleic acid in different regions of human adipose tissue. *Endocrinology*, Vol.127, No.4, (Oct), pp. 1689-1696, ISSN: 0013-7227

Brunt, E. (2004). Nonalcoholic steatohepatitis. *Semin Liver Dis*, Vol.24, No.1, (Feb), pp. 3-20, ISSN: 0272-8087

Bujalska, I., Draper, N., Michailidou, Z., et al. (2005). Hexose-6-phosphate dehydrogenase confers oxo-reductase activity upon 11 beta-hydroxysteroid dehydrogenase type 1. *J Mol Endocrinol*, Vol.34, No.3, (Jun), pp. 675-684, ISSN: 0952-5041

Bujalska, I., Gathercole, L., Tomlinson, J., et al. (2008a). A novel selective 11beta-hydroxysteroid dehydrogenase type 1 inhibitor prevents human adipogenesis. *J Endocrinol*, Vol.197, No.2, (May), pp. 297-307, ISSN: 1479-6805

Bujalska, I., Hewitt, K., Hauton, D., et al. (2008b). Lack of hexose-6-phosphate dehydrogenase impairs lipid mobilization from mouse adipose tissue. *Endocrinology*, Vol.149, No.5, (May), pp. 2584-2591, ISSN: 0013-7227

Bujalska, I., Kumar, S. & Stewart, P. (1997). Does central obesity reflect "Cushing's disease of the omentum"? *Lancet*, Vol.349, No.9060, (Apr 26), pp. 1210-1213, ISSN: 0140-6736

Bujalska, I., Walker, E., Hewison, M., et al. (2002a). A switch in dehydrogenase to reductase activity of 11 beta-hydroxysteroid dehydrogenase type 1 upon differentiation of human omental adipose stromal cells. *J Clin Endocrinol Metab*, Vol.87, No.3, (Mar), pp. 1205-1210, ISSN: 0021-972X

Bujalska, I., Walker, E., Tomlinson, J., et al. (2002b). 11Beta-hydroxysteroid dehydrogenase type 1 in differentiating omental human preadipocytes: from de-activation to generation of cortisol. *Endocr Res*, Vol.28, No.4, (Nov), pp. 449-461, ISSN: 0743-5800

Campino, C., Carvajal, C., Cornejo, J., et al. (2010). 11beta-Hydroxysteroid dehydrogenase type-2 and type-1 (11beta-HSD2 and 11beta-HSD1) and 5beta-reductase activities in the pathogenia of essential hypertension. *Endocrine*, Vol.37, No.1, (Feb), pp. 106-114, ISSN: 1559-0100

Carroll, T. & Findling, J. (2010). The diagnosis of Cushing's syndrome. *Rev Endocr Metab Disord*, Vol.11, No.2, (Jun), pp. 147-153, ISSN: 1573-2606

Chalbot, S. & Morfin, R. (2006). Dehydroepiandrosterone metabolites and their interactions in humans. *Drug Metabol Drug Interact*, Vol.22, No.1, pp. 1-23, ISSN: 0792-5077

Cho, Y., Kim, C. & Cheon, H. (2009). Cell-based assay for screening 11beta-hydroxysteroid dehydrogenase 1 inhibitors. *Anal Biochem*, Vol.392, No.2, (Sep 15), pp. 110-116, ISSN: 1096-0309

Cicala, M. & Mantero, F. (2010). Hypertension in Cushing's syndrome: from pathogenesis to treatment. *Neuroendocrinology*, Vol.92 Suppl 1, pp. 44-49, ISSN: 1423-0194

Classen-Houben, D., Schuster, D., Da Cunha, T., et al. (2009). Selective inhibition of 11beta-hydroxysteroid dehydrogenase 1 by 18alpha-glycyrrhetinic acid but not 18beta-glycyrrhetinic acid. *J Steroid Biochem Mol Biol*, Vol.113, No.3-5, (Feb), pp. 248-252, ISSN: 1879-1220

Cooper, M. & Stewart, P. (2009). 11Beta-hydroxysteroid dehydrogenase type 1 and its role in the hypothalamus-pituitary-adrenal axis, metabolic syndrome, and inflammation. *J Clin Endocrinol Metab*, Vol.94, No.12, (Dec), pp. 4645-4654, ISSN: 1945-7197

Coppola, G., Kukkola, P., Stanton, J., et al. (2005). Perhydroquinolylbenzamides as novel inhibitors of 11beta-hydroxysteroid dehydrogenase type 1. *J Med Chem*, Vol.48, No.21, (Oct 20), pp. 6696-6712, ISSN: 0022-2623

Courtney, R., Stewart, P., Toh, M., et al. (2008). Modulation of 11beta-hydroxysteroid dehydrogenase (11betaHSD) activity biomarkers and pharmacokinetics of PF-00915275, a selective 11betaHSD1 inhibitor. *J Clin Endocrinol Metab*, Vol.93, No.2, (Feb), pp. 550-556, ISSN: 0021-972X

Cushing, H. (1932). The basophil adenomas of the pituitary body and their clinical manifestations (pituitary basophilism). *Bull Johns Hopkins Hospital*, Vol.50, pp. 137-195, ISSN: 0097-1383

Dallman, M., la Fleur, S., Pecoraro, N., et al. (2004). Minireview: glucocorticoids--food intake, abdominal obesity, and wealthy nations in 2004. *Endocrinology*, Vol.145, No.6, (Jun), pp. 2633-2638, ISSN: 0013-7227

Davani, B., Khan, A., Hult, M., et al. (2000). Type 1 11beta -hydroxysteroid dehydrogenase mediates glucocorticoid activation and insulin release in pancreatic islets. *J Biol Chem*, Vol.275, No.45, (Nov 10), pp. 34841-34844, ISSN: 0021-9258

Desbriere, R., Vuaroqueaux, V., Achard, V., et al. (2006). 11beta-hydroxysteroid dehydrogenase type 1 mRNA is increased in both visceral and subcutaneous adipose tissue of obese patients. *Obesity (Silver Spring)*, Vol.14, No.5, (May), pp. 794-798, ISSN: 1930-7381

Diederich, S., Grossmann, C., Hanke, B., et al. (2000). In the search for specific inhibitors of human 11beta-hydroxysteroid-dehydrogenases (11beta-HSDs): chenodeoxycholic acid selectively inhibits 11beta-HSD-I. *Eur J Endocrinol*, Vol.142, No.2, (Feb), pp. 200-207, ISSN: 0804-4643

Diederich, S., Quinkler, M., Mai, K., et al. (2011). In vivo activity of 11beta-hydroxysteroid dehydrogenase type 1 in man: effects of prednisolone and chenodesoxycholic acid. *Horm Metab Res*, Vol.43, No.1, (Jan), pp. 66-71, ISSN: 1439-4286

Draper, N., Walker, E., Bujalska, I., et al. (2003). Mutations in the genes encoding 11beta-hydroxysteroid dehydrogenase type 1 and hexose-6-phosphate dehydrogenase interact to cause cortisone reductase deficiency. *Nat Genet*, Vol.34, No.4, (Aug), pp. 434-439, ISSN: 1061-4036

Duclos, M., Marquez Pereira, P., Barat, P., et al. (2005). Increased cortisol bioavailability, abdominal obesity, and the metabolic syndrome in obese women. *Obes Res*, Vol.13, No.7, (Jul), pp. 1157-1166, ISSN: 1071-7323

Edwards, C., Stewart, P., Burt, D., et al. (1988). Localisation of 11 beta-hydroxysteroid dehydrogenase--tissue specific protector of the mineralocorticoid receptor. *Lancet*, Vol.2, No.8618, (Oct 29), pp. 986-989, ISSN: 0140-6736

Espindola-Antunes, D. & Kater, C. (2007). Adipose tissue expression of 11beta-hydroxysteroid dehydrogenase type 1 in Cushing's syndrome and in obesity. *Arq Bras Endocrinol Metabol*, Vol.51, No.8, (Nov), pp. 1397-1403, ISSN: 0004-2730

Fabbrini, E., Sullivan, S. & Klein, S. (2010). Obesity and nonalcoholic fatty liver disease: biochemical, metabolic, and clinical implications. *Hepatology*, Vol.51, No.2, (Feb), pp. 679-689, ISSN: 1527-3350

Feig, P., Shah, S., Hermanowski-Vosatka, A., et al. (2011). Effects of an 11beta-hydroxysteroid dehydrogenase type 1 inhibitor, MK-0916, in patients with type 2 diabetes mellitus and metabolic syndrome. *Diabetes Obes Metab*, Vol.13, No.6, (Jun), pp. 498-504, ISSN: 1463-1326

Feldeisen, S. & Tucker, K. (2007). Nutritional strategies in the prevention and treatment of metabolic syndrome. *Appl Physiol Nutr Metab*, Vol.32, No.1, (Feb), pp. 46-60, ISSN: 1715-5312

Feng, Y., Huang, S., Dou, W., et al. (2010). Emodin, a natural product, selectively inhibits 11beta-hydroxysteroid dehydrogenase type 1 and ameliorates metabolic disorder in diet-induced obese mice. *Br J Pharmacol*, Vol.161, No.1, (Sep), pp. 113-126, ISSN: 1476-5381

Ferrari, P. (2010). The role of 11beta-hydroxysteroid dehydrogenase type 2 in human hypertension. *Biochim Biophys Acta*, Vol.1802, No.12, (Dec), pp. 1178-1187, ISSN: 0006-3002

Franks, P., Knowler, W., Nair, S., et al. (2004). Interaction between an 11betaHSD1 gene variant and birth era modifies the risk of hypertension in Pima Indians. *Hypertension*, Vol.44, No.5, (Nov), pp. 681-688, ISSN: 1524-4563

Funder, J., Pearce, P., Smith, R., et al. (1988). Mineralocorticoid action: target tissue specificity is enzyme, not receptor, mediated. *Science*, Vol.242, No.4878, (Oct 28), pp. 583-585, ISSN: 0036-8075

Gathercole, L. & Stewart, P. (2010). Targeting the pre-receptor metabolism of cortisol as a novel therapy in obesity and diabetes. *J Steroid Biochem Mol Biol*, Vol.122, No.1-3, (Oct), pp. 21-27, ISSN: 1879-1220

Ge, R., Huang, Y., Liang, G., et al. (2010). 11beta-hydroxysteroid dehydrogenase type 1 inhibitors as promising therapeutic drugs for diabetes: status and development. *Curr Med Chem*, Vol.17, No.5, pp. 412-422, ISSN: 1875-533X

Gupte, P., Amarapurkar, D., Agal, S., et al. (2004). Non-alcoholic steatohepatitis in type 2 diabetes mellitus. *J Gastroenterol Hepatol*, Vol.19, No.8, (Aug), pp. 854-858, ISSN: 0815-9319

Hale, C., Veniant, M., Wang, Z., et al. (2008). Structural characterization and pharmacodynamic effects of an orally active 11beta-hydroxysteroid dehydrogenase type 1 inhibitor. *Chem Biol Drug Des*, Vol.71, No.1, (Jan), pp. 36-44, ISSN: 1747-0285

Hale, C. & Wang, M. (2008). Development of 11beta-HSD1 inhibitors for the treatment of type 2 diabetes. *Mini Rev Med Chem*, Vol.8, No.7, (Jun), pp. 702-710, ISSN: 1389-5575

Henschkowski, J., Stuck, A., Frey, B., et al. (2008). Age-dependent decrease in 11beta-hydroxysteroid dehydrogenase type 2 (11beta-HSD2) activity in hypertensive patients. *Am J Hypertens*, Vol.21, No.6, (Jun), pp. 644-649, ISSN: 0895-7061

Hermanowski-Vosatka, A., Balkovec, J., Cheng, K., et al. (2005). 11beta-HSD1 inhibition ameliorates metabolic syndrome and prevents progression of atherosclerosis in mice. *J Exp Med*, Vol.202, No.4, (Aug 15), pp. 517-527, ISSN: 0022-1007

Hollis, G. & Huber, R. (2011). 11beta-Hydroxysteroid dehydrogenase type 1 inhibition in type 2 diabetes mellitus. *Diabetes Obes Metab*, Vol.13, No.1, (Jan), pp. 1-6, ISSN: 1463-1326

Hughes, K., Webster, S. & Walker, B. (2008). 11-Beta-hydroxysteroid dehydrogenase type 1 (11beta-HSD1) inhibitors in type 2 diabetes mellitus and obesity. *Expert Opin Investig Drugs*, Vol.17, No.4, (Apr), pp. 481-496, ISSN: 1744-7658

Hult, M., Shafqat, N., Elleby, B., et al. (2006). Active site variability of type 1 11beta-hydroxysteroid dehydrogenase revealed by selective inhibitors and cross-species comparisons. *Mol Cell Endocrinol*, Vol.248, No.1-2, (Mar 27), pp. 26-33, ISSN: 0303-7207

Jamieson, P., Chapman, K., Edwards, C., et al. (1995). 11 beta-hydroxysteroid dehydrogenase is an exclusive 11 beta- reductase in primary cultures of rat hepatocytes: effect of physicochemical and hormonal manipulations. *Endocrinology*, Vol.136, No.11, (Nov), pp. 4754-4761, ISSN: 0013-7227

Jang, C., Obeyesekere, V., Dilley, R., et al. (2007). Altered activity of 11beta-hydroxysteroid dehydrogenase types 1 and 2 in skeletal muscle confers metabolic protection in subjects with type 2 diabetes. *J Clin Endocrinol Metab*, Vol.92, No.8, (Aug), pp. 3314-3320, ISSN: 0021-972X

Jellinck, P., Monder, C., McEwen, B., et al. (1993). Differential inhibition of 11 beta-hydroxysteroid dehydrogenase by carbenoxolone in rat brain regions and peripheral tissues. *J Steroid Biochem Mol Biol*, Vol.46, No.2, (Aug), pp. 209-213, ISSN: 0960-0760

Johansson, L., Fotsch, C., Bartberger, M., et al. (2008). 2-amino-1,3-thiazol-4(5H)-ones as potent and selective 11beta-hydroxysteroid dehydrogenase type 1 inhibitors: enzyme-ligand co-crystal structure and demonstration of pharmacodynamic effects in C57Bl/6 mice. *J Med Chem*, Vol.51, No.10, (May 22), pp. 2933-2943, ISSN: 0022-2623

Johnson, L. & Weinstock, R. (2006). The metabolic syndrome: concepts and controversy. *Mayo Clin Proc*, Vol.81, No.12, (Dec), pp. 1615-1620, ISSN: 0025-6196

Julian, L., Wang, Z., Bostick, T., et al. (2008). Discovery of novel, potent benzamide inhibitors of 11beta-hydroxysteroid dehydrogenase type 1 (11beta-HSD1) exhibiting oral activity in an enzyme inhibition ex vivo model. *J Med Chem*, Vol.51, No.13, (Jul 10), pp. 3953-3960, ISSN: 1520-4804

Karlsson, C., Jernas, M., Olsson, B., et al. (2010). Differences in associations between HSD11B1 gene expression and metabolic parameters in subjects with and without impaired glucose homeostasis. *Diabetes Res Clin Pract*, Vol.88, No.3, (Jun), pp. 252-258, ISSN: 1872-8227

Kern, P., Di Gregorio, G., Lu, T., et al. (2003). Adiponectin expression from human adipose tissue: relation to obesity, insulin resistance, and tumor necrosis factor-alpha expression. *Diabetes*, Vol.52, No.7, (Jul), pp. 1779-1785, ISSN: 0012-1797

Konopelska, S., Kienitz, T., Hughes, B., et al. (2009). Hepatic 11beta-HSD1 mRNA expression in fatty liver and nonalcoholic steatohepatitis. *Clin Endocrinol (Oxf)*, Vol.70, No.4, (Apr), pp. 554-560, ISSN: 1365-2265

Kotelevtsev, Y., Brown, R., Fleming, S., et al. (1999). Hypertension in mice lacking 11beta-hydroxysteroid dehydrogenase type 2. *J Clin Invest*, Vol.103, No.5, (Mar), pp. 683-689, ISSN: 0021-9738

Kotelevtsev, Y., Holmes, M., Burchell, A., et al. (1997). 11beta-hydroxysteroid dehydrogenase type 1 knockout mice show attenuated glucocorticoid-inducible responses and resist hyperglycemia on obesity or stress. *Proc Natl Acad Sci U S A*, Vol.94, No.26, (Dec 23), pp. 14924-14929, ISSN: 0027-8424

Latif, S. A., Pardo, H., Hardy, M., et al. (2005). Endogenous selective inhibitors of 11beta-hydroxysteroid dehydrogenase isoforms 1 and 2 of adrenal origin. *Mol Cell Endocrinol*, Vol.243, No.1-2, (Nov 24), pp. 43-50, ISSN: 0303-7207

Lavery, G., Walker, E., Draper, N., et al. (2006). Hexose-6-phosphate dehydrogenase knock-out mice lack 11 beta-hydroxysteroid dehydrogenase type 1-mediated glucocorticoid generation. *J Biol Chem*, Vol.281, No.10, (Mar 10), pp. 6546-6551, ISSN: 0021-9258

Liu, J., Wang, L., Zhang, A., et al. (2011). Adipose tissue-targeted 11beta-hydroxysteroid dehydrogenase type 1 inhibitor protects against diet-induced obesity. *Endocr J*, Vol.58, No.3, (Mar 31), pp. 199-209, ISSN: 1348-4540

Liu, Y., Singh, R., Usa, K., et al. (2008). Renal medullary 11 beta-hydroxysteroid dehydrogenase type 1 in Dahl salt-sensitive hypertension. *Physiol Genomics*, Vol.36, No.1, (Dec 12), pp. 52-58, ISSN: 1531-2267

Livingstone, D. & Walker, B. (2003). Is 11beta-hydroxysteroid dehydrogenase type 1 a therapeutic target? Effects of carbenoxolone in lean and obese Zucker rats. *J Pharmacol Exp Ther*, Vol.305, No.1, (Apr), pp. 167-172, ISSN: 0022-3565

London, E. & Castonguay, T. (2009). Diet and the role of 11beta-hydroxysteroid dehydrogenase-1 on obesity. *J Nutr Biochem*, Vol.20, No.7, (Jul), pp. 485-493, ISSN: 1873-4847

Lovati, E., Ferrari, P., Dick, B., et al. (1999). Molecular basis of human salt sensitivity: the role of the 11beta-hydroxysteroid dehydrogenase type 2. *J Clin Endocrinol Metab*, Vol.84, No.10, (Oct), pp. 3745-3749, ISSN: 0021-972X

Maeda, Y., Naganuma, S., Niina, I., et al. (2010). Effects of bile acids on rat hepatic microsomal type I 11beta-hydroxysteroid dehydrogenase. *Steroids*, Vol.75, No.2, (Feb), pp. 164-168, ISSN: 1878-5867

Malavasi, E., Kelly, V., Nath, N., et al. (2010). Functional effects of polymorphisms in the human gene encoding 11 beta-hydroxysteroid dehydrogenase type 1 (11 beta-HSD1): a sequence variant at the translation start of 11 beta-HSD1 alters enzyme levels. *Endocrinology*, Vol.151, No.1, (Jan), pp. 195-202, ISSN: 1945-7170

Masuzaki, H. & Flier, J. (2003). Tissue-specific glucocorticoid reactivating enzyme, 11 beta-hydroxysteroid dehydrogenase type 1 (11 beta-HSD1)--a promising drug target for the treatment of metabolic syndrome. *Curr Drug Targets Immune Endocr Metabol Disord*, Vol.3, No.4, (Dec), pp. 255-262, ISSN: 1568-0088

Masuzaki, H., Paterson, J., Shinyama, H., et al. (2001). A transgenic model of visceral obesity and the metabolic syndrome. *Science*, Vol.294, No.5549, (Dec 7), pp. 2166-2170, ISSN: 0036-8075

Masuzaki, H., Yamamoto, H., Kenyon, C., et al. (2003). Transgenic amplification of glucocorticoid action in adipose tissue causes high blood pressure in mice. *J Clin Invest*, Vol.112, No.1, (Jul), pp. 83-90, ISSN: 0021-9738

McCullough, A. & Falck-Ytter, Y. (1999). Body composition and hepatic steatosis as precursors for fibrotic liver disease. *Hepatology*, Vol.29, No.4, (Apr), pp. 1328-1330, ISSN: 0270-9139

Millis, R. (2011). Epigenetics and hypertension. *Curr Hypertens Rep*, Vol.13, No.1, (Feb), pp. 21-28, ISSN: 1534-3111

Misra, M., Bredella, M., Tsai, P., et al. (2008). Lower growth hormone and higher cortisol are associated with greater visceral adiposity, intramyocellular lipids, and insulin resistance in overweight girls. *Am J Physiol Endocrinol Metab*, Vol.295, No.2, (Aug), pp. E385-392, ISSN: 0193-1849

Monder, C., Shackleton, C., Bradlow, H., et al. (1986). The syndrome of apparent mineralocorticoid excess: its association with 11 beta-dehydrogenase and 5 beta-reductase deficiency and some consequences for corticosteroid metabolism. *J Clin Endocrinol Metab*, Vol.63, No.3, (Sep), pp. 550-557, ISSN: 0021-972X

Monder, C., Stewart, P., Lakshmi, V., et al. (1989). Licorice inhibits corticosteroid 11 beta-dehydrogenase of rat kidney and liver: in vivo and in vitro studies. *Endocrinology*, Vol.125, No.2, (Aug), pp. 1046-1053, ISSN: 0013-7227

Morales, M., Carvajal, C., Ortiz, E., et al. (2008). [Possible pathogenetic role of 11 beta-hydroxysteroid dehydrogenase type 1 (11betaHSD1) gene polymorphisms in arterial hypertension]. *Rev Med Chil*, Vol.136, No.6, (Jun), pp. 701-710, ISSN: 0034-9887

Morgan, S., Sherlock, M., Gathercole, L., et al. (2009). 11beta-hydroxysteroid dehydrogenase type 1 regulates glucocorticoid-induced insulin resistance in skeletal muscle. *Diabetes*, Vol.58, No.11, (Nov), pp. 2506-2515, ISSN: 1939-327X

Morgan, S. & Tomlinson, J. (2010). 11beta-hydroxysteroid dehydrogenase type 1 inhibitors for the treatment of type 2 diabetes. *Expert Opin Investig Drugs*, Vol.19, No.9, (Sep), pp. 1067-1076, ISSN: 1744-7658

Morris, D., Souness, G., Latif, S., et al. (2004). Effect of chenodeoxycholic acid on 11beta-hydroxysteroid dehydrogenase in various target tissues. *Metabolism*, Vol.53, No.6, (Jun), pp. 811-816, ISSN: 0026-0495

Morton, N. (2010). Obesity and corticosteroids: 11beta-hydroxysteroid type 1 as a cause and therapeutic target in metabolic disease. *Mol Cell Endocrinol*, Vol.316, No.2, (Mar 25), pp. 154-164, ISSN: 1872-8057

Morton, N., Holmes, M., Fievet, C., et al. (2001). Improved lipid and lipoprotein profile, hepatic insulin sensitivity, and glucose tolerance in 11beta-hydroxysteroid dehydrogenase type 1 null mice. *J Biol Chem*, Vol.276, No.44, (Nov 2), pp. 41293-41300, ISSN: 0021-9258

Morton, N., Paterson, J., Masuzaki, H., et al. (2004). Novel adipose tissue-mediated resistance to diet-induced visceral obesity in 11 beta-hydroxysteroid dehydrogenase type 1-deficient mice. *Diabetes*, Vol.53, No.4, (Apr), pp. 931-938, ISSN: 0012-1797

Mune, T., Rogerson, F., Nikkila, H., et al. (1995). Human hypertension caused by mutations in the kidney isozyme of 11 beta-hydroxysteroid dehydrogenase. *Nat Genet*, Vol.10, No.4, (Aug), pp. 394-399, ISSN: 1061-4036

Newell-Price, J., Bertagna, X., Grossman, A., et al. (2006). Cushing's syndrome. *Lancet*, Vol.367, No.9522, (May 13), pp. 1605-1617, ISSN: 1474-547X

Nussinovitch, U., de Carvalho, J., Pereira, R., et al. (2010). Glucocorticoids and the cardiovascular system: state of the art. *Curr Pharm Des*, Vol.16, No.32, pp. 3574-3585, ISSN: 1873-4286

Odermatt, A. & Nashev, L. (2010). The glucocorticoid-activating enzyme 11beta-hydroxysteroid dehydrogenase type 1 has broad substrate specificity: Physiological and toxicological considerations. *J Steroid Biochem Mol Biol*, Vol.119, No.1-2, (Mar), pp. 1-13, ISSN: 1879-1220

Palermo, M., Quinkler, M. & Stewart, P. (2004). Apparent mineralocorticoid excess syndrome: an overview. *Arq Bras Endocrinol Metabol*, Vol.48, No.5, (Oct), pp. 687-696, ISSN: 0004-2730

Park, J., Rhee, S., Kang, N., et al. (2011). Anti-diabetic and anti-adipogenic effects of a novel selective 11beta-hydroxysteroid dehydrogenase type 1 inhibitor, 2-(3-benzoyl)-4-hydroxy-1,1-dioxo-2H-1,2-benzothiazine-2-yl-1-phenylethanone (KR-66344). *Biochem Pharmacol*, Vol.81, No.8, (Apr 15), pp. 1028-1035, ISSN: 1873-2968

Paterson, J., Morton, N., Fievet, C., et al. (2004). Metabolic syndrome without obesity: Hepatic overexpression of 11beta-hydroxysteroid dehydrogenase type 1 in transgenic mice. *Proc Natl Acad Sci U S A*, Vol.101, No.18, (May 4), pp. 7088-7093, ISSN: 0027-8424

Paulmyer-Lacroix, O., Boullu, S., Oliver, C., et al. (2002). Expression of the mRNA coding for 11beta-hydroxysteroid dehydrogenase type 1 in adipose tissue from obese patients: an in situ hybridization study. *J Clin Endocrinol Metab*, Vol.87, No.6, (Jun), pp. 2701-2705, ISSN: 0021-972X

Phillipov, G., Palermo, M. & Shackleton, C. (1996). Apparent cortisone reductase deficiency: a unique form of hypercortisolism. *J Clin Endocrinol Metab*, Vol.81, No.11, (Nov), pp. 3855-3860, ISSN: 0021-972X

Phillips, D., Barker, D., Fall, C., et al. (1998). Elevated plasma cortisol concentrations: a link between low birth weight and the insulin resistance syndrome? *J Clin Endocrinol Metab*, Vol.83, No.3, (Mar), pp. 757-760, ISSN: 0021-972X

Quinkler, M. & Stewart, P. (2003). Hypertension and the cortisol-cortisone shuttle. *J Clin Endocrinol Metab*, Vol.88, No.6, (Jun), pp. 2384-2392, ISSN: 0021-972X

Raff, H. & Findling, J. (2003). A physiologic approach to diagnosis of the Cushing syndrome. *Ann Intern Med*, Vol.138, No.12, (Jun 17), pp. 980-991, ISSN: 1539-3704

Rask, E., Olsson, T., Soderberg, S., et al. (2001). Tissue-specific dysregulation of cortisol metabolism in human obesity. *J Clin Endocrinol Metab*, Vol.86, No.3, (Mar), pp. 1418-1421, ISSN: 0021-972X

Rask, E., Walker, B., Soderberg, S., et al. (2002). Tissue-specific changes in peripheral cortisol metabolism in obese women: increased adipose 11beta-hydroxysteroid dehydrogenase type 1 activity. *J Clin Endocrinol Metab*, Vol.87, No.7, (Jul), pp. 3330-3336, ISSN: 0021-972X

Ratziu, V., Bellentani, S., Cortez-Pinto, H., et al. (2010). A position statement on NAFLD/NASH based on the EASL 2009 special conference. *J Hepatol*, Vol.53, No.2, (Aug), pp. 372-384, ISSN: 0168-8278

Reaven, G. (2011). The metabolic syndrome: time to get off the merry-go-round? *J Intern Med*, Vol.269, No.2, (Feb), pp. 127-136, ISSN: 1365-2796

Rosen, E. & MacDougald, O. (2006). Adipocyte differentiation from the inside out. *Nat Rev Mol Cell Biol*, Vol.7, No.12, (Dec), pp. 885-896, ISSN: 1471-0072

Rosenstock, J., Banarer, S., Fonseca, V., et al. (2010). The 11-beta-hydroxysteroid dehydrogenase type 1 inhibitor INCB13739 improves hyperglycemia in patients with type 2 diabetes inadequately controlled by metformin monotherapy. *Diabetes Care*, Vol.33, No.7, (Jul), pp. 1516-1522, ISSN: 1935-5548

Rutters, F., Nieuwenhuizen, A., Lemmens, S., et al. (2010). Hypothalamic-pituitary-adrenal (HPA) axis functioning in relation to body fat distribution. *Clin Endocrinol (Oxf)*, Vol.72, No.6, (Jun), pp. 738-743, ISSN: 1365-2265

Sandeep, T., Andrew, R., Homer, N., et al. (2005). Increased in vivo regeneration of cortisol in adipose tissue in human obesity and effects of the 11beta-hydroxysteroid dehydrogenase type 1 inhibitor carbenoxolone. *Diabetes*, Vol.54, No.3, (Mar), pp. 872-879, ISSN: 0012-1797

Scheen, A. & Luyckx, F. (2002). Obesity and liver disease. *Best Pract Res Clin Endocrinol Metab*, Vol.16, No.4, (Dec), pp. 703-716, ISSN: 1521-690X

Schweizer, R. A., Atanasov, A. G., Frey, B. M., et al. (2003). A rapid screening assay for inhibitors of 11beta-hydroxysteroid dehydrogenases (11beta-HSD): flavanone selectively inhibits 11beta-HSD1 reductase activity. *Mol Cell Endocrinol*, Vol.212, No.1-2, (Dec 30), pp. 41-49, ISSN: 0303-7207

Seckl, J. & Walker, B. (2001). Minireview: 11beta-hydroxysteroid dehydrogenase type 1- a tissue-specific amplifier of glucocorticoid action. *Endocrinology*, Vol.142, No.4, (Apr), pp. 1371-1376, ISSN: 0013-7227

Sen, Y., Aygun, D., Yilmaz, E., et al. (2008). Children and adolescents with obesity and the metabolic syndrome have high circulating cortisol levels. *Neuro Endocrinol Lett*, Vol.29, No.1, (Feb), pp. 141-145, ISSN: 0172-780X

Shah, S., Hermanowski-Vosatka, A., Gibson, K., et al. (2011). Efficacy and safety of the selective 11beta-HSD-1 inhibitors MK-0736 and MK-0916 in overweight and obese patients with hypertension. *J Am Soc Hypertens*, Vol.5, No.3, (May-Jun), pp. 166-176, ISSN: 1933-1711

Shah, U., Boyle, C., Chackalamannil, S., et al. (2010). Azabicyclic sulfonamides as potent 11beta-HSD1 inhibitors. *Bioorg Med Chem Lett*, Vol.20, No.5, (Mar 1), pp. 1551-1554, ISSN: 1464-3405

Simonyte, K., Rask, E., Naslund, I., et al. (2009). Obesity is accompanied by disturbances in peripheral glucocorticoid metabolism and changes in FA recycling. *Obesity (Silver Spring)*, Vol.17, No.11, (Nov), pp. 1982-1987, ISSN: 1930-7381

Siu, M., Johnson, T. O., Wang, Y., et al. (2009). N-(Pyridin-2-yl) arylsulfonamide inhibitors of 11beta-hydroxysteroid dehydrogenase type 1: Discovery of PF-915275. *Bioorg Med Chem Lett*, Vol.19, No.13, (Jul 1), pp. 3493-3497, ISSN: 1464-3405

Soro, A., Ingram, M., Tonolo, G., et al. (1995). Evidence of coexisting changes in 11 beta-hydroxysteroid dehydrogenase and 5 beta-reductase activity in subjects with untreated essential hypertension. *Hypertension*, Vol.25, No.1, (Jan), pp. 67-70, ISSN: 0194-911X

Staab, C. & Maser, E. (2010). 11beta-Hydroxysteroid dehydrogenase type 1 is an important regulator at the interface of obesity and inflammation. *J Steroid Biochem Mol Biol*, Vol.119, No.1-2, (Mar), pp. 56-72, ISSN: 1879-1220

Stewart, P. (2005). Tissue-specific Cushing's syndrome uncovers a new target in treating the metabolic syndrome--11beta-hydroxysteroid dehydrogenase type 1. *Clin Med*, Vol.5, No.2, (Mar-Apr), pp. 142-146, ISSN: 1470-2118

Stewart, P. & Krozowski, Z. (1999). 11 beta-Hydroxysteroid dehydrogenase. *Vitam Horm*, Vol.57, pp. 249-324, ISSN: 0083-6729

Stewart, P., Krozowski, Z., Gupta, A., et al. (1996). Hypertension in the syndrome of apparent mineralocorticoid excess due to mutation of the 11 beta-hydroxysteroid dehydrogenase type 2 gene. *Lancet*, Vol.347, No.8994, (Jan 13), pp. 88-91, ISSN: 0140-6736

Stewart, P., Murry, B. & Mason, J. (1994). Human kidney 11 beta-hydroxysteroid dehydrogenase is a high affinity nicotinamide adenine dinucleotide-dependent enzyme and differs from the cloned type I isoform. *J Clin Endocrinol Metab*, Vol.79, No.2, (Aug), pp. 480-484, ISSN: 0021-972X

Stewart, P. & Tomlinson, J. (2009). Selective inhibitors of 11beta-hydroxysteroid dehydrogenase type 1 for patients with metabolic syndrome: is the target liver, fat, or both? *Diabetes*, Vol.58, No.1, (Jan), pp. 14-15, ISSN: 1939-327X

Stewart, P. M., Boulton, A., Kumar, S., et al. (1999). Cortisol metabolism in human obesity: impaired cortisone-->cortisol conversion in subjects with central adiposity. *J Clin Endocrinol Metab*, Vol.84, No.3, (Mar), pp. 1022-1027, ISSN: 0021-972X

Stewart, P. M., Wallace, A. M., Atherden, S. M., et al. (1990). Mineralocorticoid activity of carbenoxolone: contrasting effects of carbenoxolone and liquorice on 11 beta-hydroxysteroid dehydrogenase activity in man. *Clin Sci (Lond)*, Vol.78, No.1, (Jan), pp. 49-54, ISSN: 0143-5221

Stewart, P. M., Wallace, A. M., Valentino, R., et al. (1987). Mineralocorticoid activity of liquorice: 11-beta-hydroxysteroid dehydrogenase deficiency comes of age. *Lancet*, Vol.2, No.8563, (Oct 10), pp. 821-824, ISSN: 0140-6736

Stimson, R., Andersson, J., Andrew, R., et al. (2009). Cortisol release from adipose tissue by 11beta-hydroxysteroid dehydrogenase type 1 in humans. *Diabetes*, Vol.58, No.1, (Jan), pp. 46-53, ISSN: 1939-327X

Stimson, R., Andrew, R., McAvoy, N., et al. (2011). Increased whole-body and sustained liver cortisol regeneration by 11beta-hydroxysteroid dehydrogenase type 1 in obese men with type 2 diabetes provides a target for enzyme inhibition. *Diabetes*, Vol.60, No.3, (Mar), pp. 720-725, ISSN: 1939-327X

Su, X., Vicker, N., Lawrence, H., et al. (2007). Inhibition of human and rat 11beta-hydroxysteroid dehydrogenase type 1 by 18beta-glycyrrhetinic acid derivatives. *J Steroid Biochem Mol Biol*, Vol.104, No.3-5, (May), pp. 312-320, ISSN: 0960-0760

Swali, A., Walker, E., Lavery, G., et al. (2008). 11beta-Hydroxysteroid dehydrogenase type 1 regulates insulin and glucagon secretion in pancreatic islets. *Diabetologia*, Vol.51, No.11, (Nov), pp. 2003-2011, ISSN: 0012-186X

Taylor, A., Irwin, N., McKillop, A. M., et al. (2008). Sub-chronic administration of the 11beta-HSD1 inhibitor, carbenoxolone, improves glucose tolerance and insulin sensitivity in mice with diet-induced obesity. *Biol Chem*, Vol.389, No.4, (Apr), pp. 441-445, ISSN: 1431-6730

Tiwari, A. (2010). INCB-13739, an 11beta-hydroxysteroid dehydrogenase type 1 inhibitor for the treatment of type 2 diabetes. *IDrugs*, Vol.13, No.4, (Apr), pp. 266-275, ISSN: 2040-3410

Tomlinson, J., Finney, J., Gay, C., et al. (2008). Impaired glucose tolerance and insulin resistance are associated with increased adipose 11beta-hydroxysteroid dehydrogenase type 1 expression and elevated hepatic 5alpha-reductase activity. *Diabetes*, Vol.57, No.10, (Oct), pp. 2652-2660, ISSN: 1939-327X

Tomlinson, J., Sherlock, M., Hughes, B., et al. (2007). Inhibition of 11beta-hydroxysteroid dehydrogenase type 1 activity in vivo limits glucocorticoid exposure to human adipose tissue and decreases lipolysis. *J Clin Endocrinol Metab*, Vol.92, No.3, (Mar), pp. 857-864, ISSN: 0021-972X

Tomlinson, J. & Stewart, P. (2007). Modulation of glucocorticoid action and the treatment of type-2 diabetes. *Best Pract Res Clin Endocrinol Metab*, Vol.21, No.4, (Dec), pp. 607-619, ISSN: 1521-690X

Tomlinson, J., Walker, E., Bujalska, I., et al. (2004). 11beta-hydroxysteroid dehydrogenase type 1: a tissue-specific regulator of glucocorticoid response. *Endocr Rev*, Vol.25, No.5, (Oct), pp. 831-866, ISSN: 0163-769X

Tu, H., Powers, J. P., Liu, J., et al. (2008). Distinctive molecular inhibition mechanisms for selective inhibitors of human 11beta-hydroxysteroid dehydrogenase type 1. *Bioorg Med Chem*, Vol.16, No.19, (Oct 1), pp. 8922-8931, ISSN: 1464-3391

Usukura, M., Zhu, A., Yoneda, T., et al. (2009). Effects of a high-salt diet on adipocyte glucocorticoid receptor and 11-beta hydroxysteroid dehydrogenase 1 in salt-sensitive hypertensive rats. *Steroids*, Vol.74, No.12, (Nov), pp. 978-982, ISSN: 1878-5867

Valsamakis, G., Anwar, A., Tomlinson, J., et al. (2004). 11beta-hydroxysteroid dehydrogenase type 1 activity in lean and obese males with type 2 diabetes mellitus. *J Clin Endocrinol Metab*, Vol.89, No.9, (Sep), pp. 4755-4761, ISSN: 0021-972X

Van Cromphaut, S. (2009). Hyperglycaemia as part of the stress response: the underlying mechanisms. *Best Pract Res Clin Anaesthesiol*, Vol.23, No.4, (Dec), pp. 375-386, ISSN: 1521-6896

van Raalte, D., Ouwens, D. & Diamant, M. (2009). Novel insights into glucocorticoid-mediated diabetogenic effects: towards expansion of therapeutic options? *Eur J Clin Invest*, Vol.39, No.2, (Feb), pp. 81-93, ISSN: 1365-2362

Véniant, M. M., Hale, C., Hungate, R. W., et al. (2010). Discovery of a potent, orally active 11beta-hydroxysteroid dehydrogenase type 1 inhibitor for clinical study: identification of (S)-2-((1S,2S,4R)-bicyclo[2.2.1]heptan-2-ylamino)-5-isopropyl-5-methylthiazol-4(5 H)-one (AMG 221). *J Med Chem*, Vol.53, No.11, (Jun 10), pp. 4481-4487, ISSN: 1520-4804

Walker, B. & Andrew, R. (2006). Tissue production of cortisol by 11beta-hydroxysteroid dehydrogenase type 1 and metabolic disease. *Ann N Y Acad Sci*, Vol.1083, (Nov), pp. 165-184, ISSN: 0077-8923

Walker, B., Connacher, A., Lindsay, R., et al. (1995a). Carbenoxolone increases hepatic insulin sensitivity in man: a novel role for 11-oxosteroid reductase in enhancing glucocorticoid receptor activation. *J Clin Endocrinol Metab*, Vol.80, No.11, (Nov), pp. 3155-3159, ISSN: 0021-972X

Walker, B., Connacher, A. A., Lindsay, R. M., et al. (1995b). Carbenoxolone increases hepatic insulin sensitivity in man: a novel role for 11-oxosteroid reductase in enhancing glucocorticoid receptor activation. *J Clin Endocrinol Metab*, Vol.80, No.11, (Nov), pp. 3155-3159, ISSN: 0021-972X

Walker, B., Soderberg, S., Lindahl, B., et al. (2000). Independent effects of obesity and cortisol in predicting cardiovascular risk factors in men and women. *J Intern Med*, Vol.247, No.2, (Feb), pp. 198-204, ISSN: 0954-6820

Walker, B., Stewart, P., Shackleton, C., et al. (1993). Deficient inactivation of cortisol by 11 beta-hydroxysteroid dehydrogenase in essential hypertension. *Clin Endocrinol (Oxf)*, Vol.39, No.2, (Aug), pp. 221-227, ISSN: 0300-0664

Wallerath, T., Witte, K., Schafer, S., et al. (1999). Down-regulation of the expression of endothelial NO synthase is likely to contribute to glucocorticoid-mediated hypertension. *Proc Natl Acad Sci U S A*, Vol.96, No.23, (Nov 9), pp. 13357-13362, ISSN: 0027-8424

Wamil, M., Andrew, R., Chapman, K., et al. (2008). 7-oxysterols modulate glucocorticoid activity in adipocytes through competition for 11beta-hydroxysteroid dehydrogenase type. *Endocrinology*, Vol.149, No.12, (Dec), pp. 5909-5918, ISSN: 0013-7227

Wamil, M. & Seckl, J. (2007). Inhibition of 11beta-hydroxysteroid dehydrogenase type 1 as a promising therapeutic target. *Drug Discov Today*, Vol.12, No.13-14, (Jul), pp. 504-520, ISSN: 1359-6446

Wang, M. (2011). Inhibitors of 11beta-hydroxysteroid dehydrogenase type 1 in antidiabetic therapy. *Handb Exp Pharmacol*, No.203, pp. 127-146, ISSN: 0171-2004

Wang, S. J., Birtles, S., de Schoolmeester, J., et al. (2006). Inhibition of 11beta-hydroxysteroid dehydrogenase type 1 reduces food intake and weight gain but maintains energy expenditure in diet-induced obese mice. *Diabetologia*, Vol.49, No.6, (Jun), pp. 1333-1337, ISSN: 0012-186X

Webster, S. P., Binnie, M., McConnell, K. M., et al. (2010). Modulation of 11beta-hydroxysteroid dehydrogenase type 1 activity by 1,5-substituted 1H-tetrazoles. *Bioorg Med Chem Lett*, Vol.20, No.11, (Jun 1), pp. 3265-3271, ISSN: 1464-3405

Weigensberg, M., Toledo-Corral, C. & Goran, M. (2008). Association between the metabolic syndrome and serum cortisol in overweight Latino youth. *J Clin Endocrinol Metab*, Vol.93, No.4, (Apr), pp. 1372-1378, ISSN: 0021-972X

White B. (2008a). *The endocrine and reproductive systems – The adrenal gland* (6th ed.), Mosby Elsevier, ISBN: 978-0-323-04582-7, Philadelphia

White B. (2008b). *The endocrine and reproductive systems – The hypothalamus and the pituitary gland* (6th ed.), Mosby Elsevier, ISBN: 978-0-323-04582-7, Philadelphia

White, P., Mune, T., Rogerson, F., et al. (1997). 11 beta-Hydroxysteroid dehydrogenase and its role in the syndrome of apparent mineralocorticoid excess. *Pediatr Res*, Vol.41, No.1, (Jan), pp. 25-29, ISSN: 0031-3998

Whorwood, C., Donovan, S., Wood, P., et al. (2001). Regulation of glucocorticoid receptor alpha and beta isoforms and type I 11beta-hydroxysteroid dehydrogenase expression in human skeletal muscle cells: a key role in the pathogenesis of insulin resistance? *J Clin Endocrinol Metab*, Vol.86, No.5, (May), pp. 2296-2308, ISSN: 0021-972X

Wree, A., Kahraman, A., Gerken, G., et al. (2010). Obesity affects the liver - the link between adipocytes and hepatocytes. *Digestion*, Vol.83, No.1-2, pp. 124-133, ISSN: 1421-9867

Yuan, C., St Jean, D. J., Jr., Liu, Q., et al. (2007). The discovery of 2-anilinothiazolones as 11beta-HSD1 inhibitors. *Bioorg Med Chem Lett*, Vol.17, No.22, (Nov 15), pp. 6056-6061, ISSN: 0960-894X

Zhang, M., Lv, X., Li, J., et al. (2009a). Alteration of 11beta-hydroxysteroid dehydrogenase type 1 in skeletal muscle in a rat model of type 2 diabetes. *Mol Cell Biochem*, Vol.324, No.1-2, (Apr), pp. 147-155, ISSN: 1573-4919

Zhang, X., Zhou, Z., Yang, H., et al. (2009b). 4-(Phenylsulfonamidomethyl)benzamides as potent and selective inhibitors of the 11beta-hydroxysteroid dehydrogenase type 1 with efficacy in diabetic ob/ob mice. *Bioorg Med Chem Lett*, Vol.19, No.15, (Aug 1), pp. 4455-4458, ISSN: 1464-3405

Antiandrogenic and Estrogenic Compounds: Effect on Development and Function of Male Reproductive System

Anna Hejmej, Małgorzata Kotula-Balak and Barbara Bilińska
Department of Endocrinology, Institute of Zoology, Jagiellonian University
Poland

1. Introduction

In the last 50 years the increase in the frequency of male reproductive abnormalities has been observed in human (Auger et al., 1995; Bergström et al., 1996; Carlsen et al., 1992; Skakkebaek et al., 2001; Thonneau et al., 2003). Epidemiological studies have shown increasing trends in the incidence of cryptorchidism (undescended testis) and hypospadias (abnormal location of the urethral opening) in several regions of Australia, Europe, and the United States (Acerini et al., 2009; Boisen et al., 2004; Källén et al., 1986; Nassar et al., 2007; Paulozzi, 1999; Toppari et al., 2001). Moreover, several reports indicated that semen quality have declined during last century (Auger et al., 1995; Carlsen et al., 1992; Swan et al., 2000; Sharpe & Irvine, 2004). Decreasing sperm concentration and percentage of motile spermatozoa, and increasing number of spermatozoa with morphological alterations were observed in European population between 1940 and 1990. For instance, it has been found that the prevalence of an abnormally low sperm count in young men reaches even 15-20% (Andersson et al., 2008; Jørgensen et al., 2006, 2011). In earlier study by Jørgensen et al. (2001) significant geographical variations in semen quality have been also described. Although, the reason for these regional differences is not fully elucidated, some data indicate that a correlation exists between impaired semen quality and exposure to pesticides used in agricultural areas (Swan et al., 2003). Interestingly, it has been noticed that in the industrial areas, where peoples are exposed to high levels of industrial chemicals, the birth sex ratio can be altered; in some region of Canada male birth sex ratio (i.e. number of male births per total number of births) have reached only 0.3 during the period 1990 - 2003 (Mackenzie et al., 2005).

In 2001 Skakkebaeck and co-workers have suggested that cryptorchidism, hypospadias, testicular cancer and oligozoospermia are interrelated disorders comprising a single syndrome, called the testicular dysgenesis syndrome (TDS) (Skakkebaeck et al., 2001; Skakkebaeck & Jørgensen, 2005). This idea arose from the observation that cryptorchidism and hypospadias are closely linked to testicular cancer, because in men with a history of one of these anomalies significantly increased risk of testicular cancer was described (Davenport et al., 1997; Dieckmann & Pichlmeier, 2004; Sharpe & Irvine, 2004). Moreover, oligozoospermia is frequently found in men, who develop testicular cancer (Møller & Skakkebaek, 1999). The disorders included in TDS are believed to result from disruption of hormone synthesis or action during fetal development of reproductive system. Indeed, numerous experimental studies have demonstrated that prenatal exposure to some environmental chemicals may disrupt the endocrine system in males and thus interfere with hormone-dependent development (Delbès et al., 2006; Fisher, 2004a; Gray et al., 2006).

Male reproductive system anomalies have been also reported in wild living animals (Vos et al., 2000). In fish, sexual reversal, decreased sperm count and motility, and spermatogenesis impairment were noticed (Barnhoorn et al., 2004; Jobling et al., 2002; Vajda et al., 2008). Feminization and abnormal gonadal development were observed in reptiles and birds (De Solla et al., 1998, 2006; Fry, 1995; Guillette et al., 1994), whereas in mammals, such as panthers or polar bears cryptorchidism and reduced size of reproductive organs were found (Mansfield & Land, 2002; Sonne et al., 2006). An interesting example of the species in which environmental pollutants may be the cause of reproductive system abnormalities is Sitka Black-Tailed Deer. It was reported that in the population living in the Aliulik Peninsula of Kodiak Island extraordinary high percentage (75%) of the males exhibited cryptorchidism when compared with males living elsewhere on the Kodiak Archipelago, among which only 12% were cryptorchid (Bubenik et al., 2001; Veeramachaneni et al., 2006a). Additionally, abnormal antlers and testicular neoplasia were frequently observed in cryptorchid deer from Aliulik Peninsula. The authors hypothesized that it was likely that testis and antler dysgenesis resulted from exposure of pregnant female (or alternatively, historic exposure of founders) to some estrogenic endocrine disrupting agent(s) present in the environment (Veeramachaneni et al., 2006a).

Although the substances affecting endocrine system were studied from 1950', the term "endocrine disruptor" was introduced in 1991 at Wingspread Conference, organized to evaluate the adverse effects observed in wildlife in the Great Lakes region in North America (Colborn & Clement, 1992; Colborn et al., 1993). According the World Health Organization (2006) endocrine disruptor (ED) is "an exogenous chemical substance or mixture that alters the function(s) of the endocrine system and thereby causes adverse effects to an organism, its progeny, or a (sub)population". In 2009, The Endocrine Society presented the Scientific Statement in which endocrine disruptor was defined as "a compound, either natural or synthetic, which through environmental or inappropriate developmental exposure alters the hormonal and homeostatic systems that enable the organism to communicate with and respond to its environment" (Diamanti-Kandarakis et al., 2009).

2. Role of androgens and estrogens in male reproductive tract development and function

Androgens are steroid hormones that play a central role in the development and function of male reproductive system (Dohle et al., 2003). The principal androgens are testosterone and dihydrotestosterone (DHT). High amounts of testosterone are produced in the testes from early stages of fetal development until birth. During prenatal period testosterone is necessary for the differentiation of Wolffian duct into the epididymis, vas deferens and seminal vesicles. It is also involved in the process of testis descent. DHT, synthesized from testosterone by the action of 5α-reductase, mediates the masculinization of external genitalia and prostate. Studies by Welsh et al. (2008) revealed the existence of a fetal "masculinization programming window", a period within which androgens action is necessary to ensure correct later development of the male reproductive system. Blockade of androgen action only during this critical period by using androgen receptor antagonists (e.g., flutamide) suppresses development of the male accessory glands and disrupts testis descent leading to cryptorchidism (Macleod et al., 2010; Welsh et al., 2008). In rat masculinization programming window occurs at 15.5–18.5 gestational days, whereas in human it spans from approximately 8 to 14 weeks of gestation (Welsh et al., 2008). In neonates testosterone level is high for a short time, then its production decreases and is maintained at low level until puberty, when rising androgen level mediate growth and function of accessory sex glands, initiation of spermatogenesis and development of secondary male sex characteristics. In mature males androgen action is essential for the maintenance of male phenotype and fertility (Dohle et al., 2003).

The discovery that aromatase (the enzyme converting androgens to estrogens) and estrogen receptors α and β (ERα and ER β) are expressed in male reproductive tract and studies on transgenic mouse models with inactivated estrogen receptor α (α ERKO) or aromatase genes (ArKO) led to the conclusion that not only androgens, but also estrogens are important for development and physiology of male reproductive system (Bilinska et al., 1997; Carreau et al., 2003; Levallet et al., 1998; Lubahn et al., 1993; Kuiper et al., 1996; Robertson et al., 1999). It was demonstrated that during fetal and neonatal life estrogens are involved in control of gametogenesis, promoting germ cell and seminiferous tubule development, and in the regulation of fetal Leydig cell steroidogenesis (Albrecht et al., 2009; Delbés et al., 2005; Vigueras-Villaseñor et al, 2006). Aromatase and ERs are transiently expressed in the hippocampus of newborn males, suggesting that estrogens are involved in brain masculinization (McEwen & Alves, 1999). In the reproductive system of adult males the role of ERs is associated with the maintenance of fluid reabsorption in the excurrent ducts of the testis (Hess, 2000; Hess et al., 1997). Data from studies on male mice with knockout of ERα suggested that long-term atrophy of the testes, observed in these animals, was caused by backpressure of the accumulating luminal fluids. Moreover, estrogens appear to have direct effects on the Leydig cell, controlling testosterone synthesis, and possibly on the seminiferous epithelium (Akingbemi et al., 2003; Hess, 2003). In male, estrogens play also a physiological role in non-reproductive tissues and organs such as bone and cardiovascular system (Oettel, 2002).

Although endogenous estrogens are necessary for normal male fertility, excessive production of these hormones or exposure to exogenous estrogens during fetal or neonatal life could produce adverse outcomes, affecting reproductive system development and adult reproductive functions. Destructive effects of estrogen overexposure on the development of post-meiotic germ cells and testicular atrophy was observed in rodents and humans (Gancarczyk et al., 2004; Toyama et al., 2001; Williams et al., 2001). Moreover, cryptorchidism, spermatogenic arrest, Leydig cell hyperplasia, and decreased serum follicle-stimulating hormone (FSH) and testosterone levels have been reported in the transgenic mouse model with aromatase overexpression (Fowler et al., 2000; Li et. al., 2001).

3. Antiandrogens

Antiandrogens are defined as chemicals that interfere with androgen action or production. The compounds shown to have antiandrogenic properties include pharmaceuticals (e.g., flutamide, ketoconazole) as well as environmental contaminants: pesticides (e.g., vinclozolin, linuron) and industrial chemicals (e.g., di(n-butyl) phthalate).

3.1 Flutamide as a model antiandrogen

Flutamide, a pharmaceutical used in therapy of androgen-dependent prostate cancer, and its active metabolite hydroxyflutamide, are non-steroidal synthetic androgen receptor (AR) antagonists, which display pure antiandrogenic activity, without exerting agonistic or any other hormonal activity (Neri, 1989; Singh et al., 2000). Flutamide is regarded as a model antiandrogen and in experimental studies it is often used as a positive control in screening assays used for the identification of endocrine disruptors (O'Connor et al., 1998).

In utero exposure to flutamide was shown to alter reproductive development and function in male rat offspring (Mikkila et al., 2006). Recently, it was reported that flutamide interferes with desert hedgehog (Dhh) signaling in the fetal testis, resulting in impaired fetal Leydig cell differentiation. Leydig cell dysfunction was reflected by suppressed levels of insulin-like factor 3 (Insl-3) and testosterone and reduced expression of steroidogenic enzymes, cytochrome P450scc and 3β-hydroxysteroid dehydrogenase (3β-HSD) (Brokken et al., 2009). Insufficient levels of testosterone and Insl-3 in the fetal testis could, in turn, prevent full masculinization. Decrease in gonad and accessory sex glands weight, cryptorchidism, testicular histological lesions and increased germ cell apoptosis have been reported in adult male rats exposed to flutamide during fetal period, indicating that flutamide exerts long-term antiandrogenic effects (Omezzine et al., 2003).

In our recent studies flutamide (50 mg/kg bw) was injected into pregnant gilts during gestational days 20–28 and 80–88, and into male piglets on postnatal days 2–10. We found no changes in testicular morphology of neonatal pigs *in utero* exposed to flutamide, whereas in prepubertal males some of the seminiferous tubules were altered, exhibiting reduced number of Sertoli cells and dilated lumina (Durlej et al., 2011; Kopera et al., 2010). Testes of adult pigs exposed to flutamide *in utero* exhibited moderate alterations of the spermatogenic process: seminiferous tubules showed degeneration of germ cells and their extensive sloughing into the lumen of the seminiferous tubules, however all generations of germ cells could be recognized in the seminiferous epithelium. Testes of neonatally exposed boars contained severely altered seminiferous tubules, exhibiting drastic increase in the number of apoptotic germ cells, hypospermatogenesis or spermatogenic arrest at the spermatocyte level. Alterations of normal histological structure were accompanied by decreased expression and/or disturbed localization of intercellular junction proteins, connexin 43, N-cadherin, β-catenin and ZO-1 in the seminiferous epithelium (Hejmej et al., 2011a; Kopera et al., 2011). Also interstitial tissue was adversely affected; Leydig cells displayed hyperplasia or hypertrophy, increased expression of aromatase and reduced expression of LH receptor. Dysfunction of Leydig cells led to disruption of androgen-estrogen balance (Kotula-Balak et al., submitted for publication). These data suggest that in pigs flutamide acting during fetal, and especially, neonatal period can reprogram the development of testicular cells, leading to morphological and functional alterations of the testis at adulthood.

Interestingly, flutamide exposure has also long-term effects on sperm morphology. Our data showed that in sperm derived from neonatally-treated boars either flattened head or abnormal sperm with altered shape of the acrosome and abnormal packaging of sperm chromatin were frequently observed. Prepuberal treatment with flutamide resulted in an increased number of sperm displaying abnormal midpiece or tail defects (Lydka et al., submitted for publication)

Several studies demonstrated the effects of short-term androgen blockage induced by the administration of flutamide to immature or mature males. In immature rats structure of interstitial tissue and seminiferous epithelium, and the expressions of steroidogenesis-related genes, *Cyp11a1* and *StAR*, were significantly affected by flutamide treatment (Vo et al., 2009). When administered to pubertal animals, flutamide accelerated testes maturation, causing degeneration and detachment of primary spermatocytes and round spermatids (Maschio et al., 2010). In adult males, germ-cell degeneration, alterations in ectoplasmic specialization between the Sertoli cell and spermatids, and premature detachment of spermatids, as well as increase in the relative volume of Leydig cells were observed (Anahara et al., 2008; Maschio et al., 2008). Moreover, our *in vitro* results showed that pig sperm incubated with hydroxyflutamide (50 and 100 μg/mL) displayed disorders in sperm phospholipid membrane, decreased oxidative capability of sperm mitochondria and decreased sperm membrane integrity (Lydka et al., submitted for publication)

3.2 Environmental antiandrogens

3.2.1 Pesticides: procymidone, vinclozolin, prochloraz, linuron and p,p'DDE

Procymidone is used as a fungicide for the control of plant diseases. High quantities of this compound were found in rice, tomatoes and grapes (Gebara et al., 2011; US Environmental Protection Agency annual report, 1994). When administered to pregnant rats, the male pups displayed a reduced anogenital distance, nipple retention, hypospadias, cleft phallus, and reduced sex accessory gland size (Gray et al., 1999; Ostby et al., 1999). Moreover, in prostate and seminal vesicles fibrosis, cellular infiltration and epithelial hyperplasia were observed (Ostby et al., 1999). Chronic treatment of male rats with procymidone inhibited the negative feedback exerted by androgens on the hypothalamus and/or the pituitary, causing enhanced luteinizing hormone (LH) secretion and Leydig cell steroidogenesis, and in consequence, increased serum testosterone level (Hosokawa et al., 1993; Svechnikov et al., 2005). Such a long-term hyperstimulation of Leydig cells induces Leydig cell tumors (Murakami et al., 1995).

Vinclozolin is a dicarboximide fungicide used in the control of *Botrytis cinerea*, *Sclerotinia sclerotiorum*, and *Moniliniam spp* on vegetables, fruits and ornamental plants. Vinclozolin and its two active metabolites, M1 and M2, compete for androgen binding to AR and inhibit AR transactivation and androgen-dependent gene expression (Wong et al., 1995). Administration of vinclozolin to pregnant rats resulted in abnormalities of androgen-regulated sexual differentiation in male offspring, including reduced anogenital distance, nipple retention, hypospadias, cryptorchidism, decreased sex accessory gland growth as well as in induction of prostate inflammation and reduced sperm production at adulthood (Cowin et al., 2010; Gray et al. 1994; 1999). Vinclozolin has also been implicated in epigenetic modifications of male reproductive tract via changes in DNA methyltransferase expression (Anway et al., 2008; Anway & Skinner, 2008). The most sensitive period of rat fetal development to the effects of vinclozolin was found to be gestational days 16-17, whereas less severe malformations were seen in males exposed during gestational days 14–15 and 18–19 (Wolf et al. 2000). Peripubertal exposure resulted in delayed pubertal maturation, decreased sex accessory gland and epididymal growth concomitantly with increased serum levels of LH and testosterone (Monosson et al., 1999).

Prochloraz is an imidazole fungicide widely used in gardening and agriculture which acts as both AR antagonist and inhibitor of fetal testosterone production. In addition to antiandrogenic action, prochloraz antagonizes the estrogen receptor, agonizes the aryl hydrocarbon (Ah) receptor and suppresses aromatase activity (Andersen et al., 2002; Vinggaard et al., 2006). Gestational exposure significantly reduces testosterone production by inhibiting activity of cytochrome P450c17, decreases reproductive organ weights, increases nipple retention and induces malformations (e.g., hypospadias) in androgen-dependent tissues of male offspring (Blystone et al. 2007; Laier et al., 2006; Noriega et al., 2005; Vinggaard et al., 2005).

Linuron is a herbicide employed to control of weeds in crops and potatoes (Gray et al., 2006). It binds AR and inhibits dihydrotestosterone induced gene expression *in vitro* (Lambright et al., 2000). Fetal exposure to linuron resulted in epididymal and testicular abnormalities, reduced anogenital distance and nipple retention; however, in contrast to other AR antagonists, it does not induce hypospadias and cryptorchidism. Moreover, linuron was shown to decrease testosterone production by fetal Leydig cells (McIntyre et al., 2000, 2002a, 2002b; Wilson et al., 2009). Thus its mechanism of action resembles those of phthalates (Gray et al., 2006). Interestingly, when administered to sexually immature and mature rats, linuron decreased weights of accessory sex organs, increased serum estradiol and LH levels, and produced Leydig cell tumors (Cook et al., 1993).

p,p'-DDE (dichlorodiphenyldichloroethylene) is a metabolite of the persistent pesticide, DDT (dichlorodiphenyltrichloroethane). DTT is now banned in most countries, since in 1960' it was discovered that it has endocrine disrupting properties and causes birth defects in human and animals. However, it is still used in some regions to prevent malaria and other tropical diseases spread by insects (van den Berg et al., 2009). p,p'-DDE acts as AR antagonist both *in vivo* and *in vitro* (Kelce et al., 1995). Fetal treatment with this compound was shown to affect male development, leading to reduced anogenital distance, nipple retention and hypospadias (You et al., 1998). Recently, it was reported that p,p'-DDE induces testicular apoptosis in pubertal rats through the involvement of Fas/FasL, mitochondria and endoplasmic reticulum-mediated pathways (Shi et al., 2011).

3.2.2 Phthalates

The diesters of 1,2-benzenedicarboxylic acid, called phthalates, are widely used as plasticizers in the production of toys, medical devices, rainwear, food packaging, and certain cosmetics (Schettler, 2006). Di-n-butyl phthalate (DBP) and di(2-ethylhexyl) phthalate (DEHP) and their metabolites have been shown to cause antiandrogenic effects, however, without binding to AR (Frederiksen et al., 2007). Although, the exact mechanism of action is not yet fully elucidated, it was demonstrated that phthalates interfere with Leydig cell function, reducing the expression of most of genes involved in testosterone biosynthesis (Barlow et al., 2003). Fetal exposure to phthalates results in reduced anogenital distance, hypospadias, cryptorchidism, malformed epididymis, and nipple retention (Mylchreest et al., 1999, 2002; Mylchreest & Foster, 2000). At the histological level, multinucleated gonocytes, detachment of gonocytes from the seminiferous epithelium, Sertoli cell-only tubules and Leydig cell hyperplasia were found in the testes of males exposed to DEHP and DBP (Fisher et al., 2003; Mylchreest et al., 2002; Parks et al., 2000). Some of these alterations were permanent and affected testicular function in adulthood, resulting in low testosterone level and reduced sperm count. It is worth noting that histological changes induced in rat by *in utero* exposure to phthalates resemble those observed in patients with TDS (Fisher, 2004a).

4. Xenoestrogens

Compounds with estrogenic activity, called xenoestrogens, comprise a broad range of synthetic chemicals (e.g., diethylstilbestrol, bisphenol-A, octylphenol, nonylphenol), naturally occurring phytoestrogens (e.g., genistein, resveratrol) and heavy metals (e.g., cadmium, lead, and boron).

4.1 Diethylstilbestrol (DES)

DES is synthetic potent non-steroidal estrogen used as a supplement in cattle and poultry feed and as a pharmaceutical (Rubin, 2007). DES was given to pregnant women to prevent miscarriages or premature deliveries from about 1940 to 1970. It was restricted in 1971 because of increased risk of a rare reproductive tract cancer, vaginal clear cell adenocarcinoma, in daughters of women who had taken DES (Gill et al., 1979; Melnick et al., 1987). Further studies have reported multiple adverse effects in males and females as a result of prenatal DES exposure. In males decreased fertility and anatomical malformations of reproductive organs such as cryptorchidism, epididymal cysts and prostatic squamous metaplasia were observed (Driscoll & Taylor, 1980; Marselos & Tomatis, 1992; Mittendorf, 1995).

Nowadays, experimental animals exposed to DES during fetal and neonatal development are useful models for studying mechanisms of endocrine disruption caused by exogenous estrogenic compounds (Diamanti-Kandarakis et al., 2009). In male mice exposed to DES during gestation, cryptorchidism, hypospadias, as well as underdeveloped epididymis, vas deferens and seminal vesicles were observed (McLachlan et al., 2001). Similarly, neonatal treatment of male rats with DES induced a wide range of reproductive abnormalities, including delay of testicular descent, retardation of pubertal spermatogenesis, reduction in testis weight, infertility, and gross morphological alterations in the rete testis, efferent ducts, epididymis and accessory sex glands (Atanassova et al., 1999, 2000; Fisher et al., 1999; McKinnell et al, 2001; Williams et al., 2001). Testes of adult rats neonatally exposed to DES displayed suppression of Leydig cell development and steroidogenesis, reduced Sertoli cell proliferation and spermatogenic impairment. It was shown that DES has both direct and pituitary-mediated effects on the developing testis, leading to decreased expression of AR and reduced FSH level (Sharpe et al., 1998, 2003). Studies on transgenic mouse models with inactivated ERs suggest that DES elicits its toxic effects in the male reproductive tract through an ERα-mediated mechanism (Prins et al., 2001).

4.2 Environmental xenoestrogens

4.2.1 Industrial xenoestrogens: bisphenol A and alkylphenols

Bisphenol A (BPA) is one of the most important industrial chemicals, which worldwide production is over 500 000 tons per year. It is found mainly in plastic food containers, baby bottles, the resins lining food cans, dental sealants, cardboards, and as an additive in other plastics (Richter et al., 2007). BPA is structurally similar to DES and can act by binding to ERα and ERβ, and through other mechanisms, since some effects differ from those observed in response to activation of estrogen receptors. *In vivo* and *in vitro* experiments revealed that BPA mimics estrogen action, however it is also able to antagonize the activity of estradiol, acting as a selective estrogen receptor modulator (SERM) (Welshons et al., 2006). In high concentrations BPA can bind to AR and inhibit the androgen action (Lee et al., 2003). Although BPA is approximately 1000- to 2000-fold less potent than estradiol, exposure to environmentally relevant doses impacts the reproductive system development and function in male rodents (Richter et al., 2007). It was demonstrated that rodents exposed to BPA during fetal and/or neonatal life had decreased weights of the epididymis and seminal vesicles, but increased weights of the prostate and preputial glands, decreased epithelial height in the efferent ducts and decreased levels of testicular testosterone (Akingbemi et al., 2004; Fisher et al., 1999; vom Saal et al., 1998). Alterations in ectoplasmic specialization between the Sertoli cell and spermatids, abnormalities in the acrosomal granule and nucleus of spermatids, reduced percentage of motile sperm, and increased incidence of sperm malformations were also observed (Aikawa et al., 2004; Toyama et al., 2004). Similar changes in the seminiferous epithelium and reduced fertility were found in adult males treated with BPA (Toyama et al., 2004). BPA was found to act directly on Leydig cell steroidogenesis, affecting the expression of cytochrome cytochrome P450 17α-hydroxylase/C_{17-20} lyase (P450c17) and aromatase enzymes and interfering with LH receptor-ligand binding (Akingbemi et al., 2004; Svechnikov et al., 2010).

Alkylphenols, such as 4-nonylphenol and 4-*tert*-octylphenol, are used to manufacture the alkylphenol polyethoxylates, non-ionic surfactants used as detergents, plasticizers, emulsifiers and modifiers in paints, pesticides, textiles, and personal care products. Alkylphenols present in the environment, mainly in wastewater and rivers, derive from the release of unreacted alkylphenols during manufacturing as well as from degradation of the alkylphenol polyethoxylates in the environment (Blake et al., 2004; Staples et al., 2001). Currently, alkylphenols have been found in human urine and breast milk (Ademollo et al., 2008; Calafat et al., 2008,). Octylphenol and nonylphenol has been reported to exhibit weak estrogenic activity as demonstrated by its ability to bind and activate the estrogen receptors (Kuiper et al., 1998; Lee, 1998; Safe et al., 2000). Although these chemicals are between 100 and 10000-fold less estrogenic than 17β-estradiol, the widespread use of these compounds causes that they largely contribute to the environmental estrogen pool (Blake & Bookfor, 1997).

Maternal exposure to octylphenol was shown to affect the expression of genes essential for reproductive system development, such as steroidogenic factor-1 (SF-1) and steroidogenic enzymes in rat testes (Majdic et al., 1996, 1997). In the lamb, it was demonstrated to inhibit the secretion of FSH in the fetus with a concomitant decrease in testis size and Sertoli cell number at birth (Sweeney et al., 2000). In adult males exposed *in utero* or neonatally to alkylphenols abnormalities in reproductive organs histology, reduced weight of the testis, epididymis and prostate, reduced testosterone level as well as increased number of abnormal sperm and decreased sperm production were observed (Aydoğan & Barlas, 2006; Jie et al., 2010; Lee, 1998; Yoshida et al., 2001). These alterations may result from both modulation of the hypothalamus-pituitary axis and direct estrogenic action in reproductive tissues (Yoshida et al., 2001). Importantly, all these effects were observed only when relatively high doses (400 mg/kg bw) of alkylphenols were used (Atanassova et al., 2000; Sharpe et al., 2003).

Administration of high doses of alkylphenols to adult males resulted in reduced size and function of the testis, epididymis and male accessory glands, decreased serum LH, FSH and testosterone concentrations, increased apoptosis of germ cells and reduced sperm count (Blake & Boockfor, 1997; Boockfor & Blake, 1997; Han et al., 2004; Gong & Han, 2006; Kim et al., 2007). However, reports on the effects of lower doses (<200 mg/kg bw) of octylphenol on male reproductive system are contradictory (Bian et al., 2006; Kim et al., 2007).

Recently, bank vole, a seasonally breeding rodent, was used to investigate the effects of 4-tert-octylphenol on testes and seminal vesicles, depending on the length of exposure and reproductive status of animals. Adult bank vole males kept under long or short photoperiod were orally administered octylphenol (200 mg/kg bw) for 30 or 60 days. We found that treatment for 30 days had no effect on the reproductive organs, whereas treatment for 60 days adversely influenced sperm morphology as well as weights and histological structure of the testes and seminal vesicles. In these tissues, expression of 3β-HSD and AR, and testosterone levels were decreased, concomitantly with increased expression of aromatase and ERα, and elevated estradiol levels, resulting in androgen-estrogen imbalance. These data indicate that long-term exposure to octylphenol is necessary to affect male reproductive organs histology and hormonal milieu. Furthermore, a subtle difference in the sensitivity to octylphenol between voles kept in different light conditions was noted (Hejmej et al., 2011b). In a further study negative effects of this compound on MA-10 Leydig cells *in vitro* have been reported. In cell cultures treated with different octylphenol concentrations, dose-related changes in the cytoarchitecture of MA-10 cells, including cytoplasm vacuolization and altered size and distribution of lipid droplets, were visible. Moreover, it was shown that high doses attenuate 3β-HSD and AR expression, concomitantly with the reduction of progesterone synthesis. Based on this results it was hypothesized that octylphenol besides binding to ERs may use other potential routes of action such as effects on the AR (Kotula-Balak et al., 2011).

4.2.2 Phytoestrogens

Phytoestrogens are plant compounds, structurally similar to 17β-estradiol and thus exhibiting estrogenic or antiestrogenic activity. There are four main classes of phytoestrogens: isoflavones (genistein, daidzein, biochanin A, naringenin), coumestans (coumestrol), lignans (matairesinol) and stilbene (resveratrol). Phytoestrogens are present in fruits, vegetables and leguminous plants, but the main source of these compounds in human diet are soy-based products, i. a. soy-based infant formula, that contain high concentration of genistein and daidzein (Reinli & Block, 1996; Setchell et al., 1997). It is believed that isoflavones exert beneficial effects in prevention of cancer, cardiovascular diseases and osteoporosis, however it was reported that they can adversely affect development and function of male and female reproductive function (Lee et al., 2004; Suthar et al., 2001). This may be of special concern in case of infants fed with soy formula milk. Although, phytoestrogens binding affinity to the estrogen receptors is 1000-10000-fold lower compared with the 17β-estradiol, in infants, which consume even 9 mg/kg/day of isoflavones, mainly genistein, blood concentrations of the isoflavones exceed 1000 times those of endogenous estradiol and are higher than the amount reported to produce hormonal effects in adult women (Henley & Korach et al., 2010; Schmitt et al., 2001; Setchell et al., 1997). Therefore in recent years multiple studies on animal models were undertaken to elucidate the mechanism of action and the consequences of exposure to genistein. In rodents dietary administration of genistein induced Leydig cell hyperplasia and decrease of testosterone level by down-regulation of the expression of steroidogenic enzymes (e.g., cytochrome P450scc) (Svechnikov et al., 2005). *In vivo* and *in vitro* data indicate that genistein is able to signal through both ERα and ERβ, depending on the specific tissue (Mueller et al., 2004).

In recent years resveratrol, a stilbene found in grapes and wine, has been widely used to prevent cardiovascular diseases, since it was shown to inhibit oxidation of LDL cholesterol,

platelets aggregation and synthesis of eikozanoids (Kris-Etherton et al., 2002). However, resveratrol appeared to have adverse effect on Leydig cell steroidogenesis through suppression of the expression of StAR and cytochrome P450c17 (Svechnikov et al., 2009).
Estrogenic activity is also attributed to several other compounds derived from plants, for example lavender oil and tea tree oil, frequently used in cosmetics, such as lotions, gels, and creams. It is supposed that exposure to these chemicals may induce prepubertal gynecomastia in humans. *In vitro* experiments revealed that apart from estrogenic activity both lavender and tea tree oil possess antiandrogenic properties (Henley et al., 2007; Henley & Korach et al., 2010).
Interestingly, based on the analysis of published data concerning correlations between exposure to different endocrine disruptors and decrease in sperm counts and increase in testicular cancer rate, Safe (2004) suggested that dietary phytoestrogens, rather than synthetic environmental endocrine disruptors may by involved in induction of reproductive tract disorders in human.

4.2.3 Methoxychlor

Methoxychlor was introduced in 1944 to substitute more persistent and more toxic insecticide, DDT. It is used on agricultural crops, livestock, animal feed, grain storage, home gardens, and on pets. Methoxychlor exhibits mixed estrogenic and antiandrogenic activity: the most active estrogenic metabolite is HPTE [2,2-bis-(*p*-hydroxyphenyl)-1, 1, 1-trichloroethane], whereas other metabolites have antiandrogenic activity (Cummings, 1997; Dehal & Kupfer, 1994; Kelce & Wilson, 1997). HPTE has differential effects on ERs, being an ERα agonist and ERβ antagonist (Gaido et al., 1999, 2000). In cultured Leydig cells from immature and adult rats, HPTE was shown to inhibit both basal and hCG-stimulated testosterone production, and these effects were reported to be mediated through the ER (Murono & Derk, 2005). Recently, a direct inhibitory activity of methoxychlor and HPTE on 3β-HSD and 17β-hydroxysteroid dehydrogenase (17β-HSD) was reported (Hu et al., 2011). Exposure to methoxychlor during gestation or neonatal period affected embryonic testis cellular composition, Sertoli and germ cell numbers, germ cell survival and epididymal sperm count, reducing spermatogenic potential of males (Chapin et al., 1997; Johnson et al., 2002; Suzuki et al., 2004). In adult rat testis methoxychlor induced apoptosis via mitochondria- and FasL-mediated pathways (Vaithinathan et al., 2010).

4.2.4 Heavy metals

Numerous heavy metals (e.g., cadmium, lead, arsenic, boron, mercury, antimony, aluminum, cobalt, chromium, lithium) have been demonstrated to adversely affect the reproductive function of human and experimental animals. For example, cadmium, used in battery electrode production, galvanizing, plastics, alloys and paint pigments, has potent estrogen- and androgen-like activities *in vivo* and *in vitro* (Sikka et al., 2008; Takiguchi & Yoshihara, 2006). In mice exposed to cadmium during late gestation and puberty markedly reduced weights of testes, epididymides, prostate and seminal vesicles, and decreased testosterone levels were observed. Moreover, testicular expression of StAR and steroidogenic enzymes, such as cytochrome P450scc, 17*α*-HSD and 17*β*-HSD, was down-regulated (Ji et al., 2010, 2011). In the seminiferous tubules, cadmium caused disruption of the blood-testis barrier and oxidative stress, leading to germ cell degeneration, seminiferous tubules vacuolization, and aberrant morphology and apoptosis of Sertoli cells (de Souza

Predes et al., 2010; Zhang et al., 2010). Epidemiological and animal studies have additionally demonstrated a carcinogenic effect of cadmium on the prostate (Nakamura et al., 2002).
Lead, another metal widespread in the environment, has adverse reproductive effect on the testes and the hypothalamic-pituitary axis. In animal studies, lead has been shown to reduce serum testosterone and FSH levels, disrupt spermatogenesis and induce oxidative cellular damage in epididymis (Foster at al., 1998; Marchlewicz et al., 2004; Sokol et al., 1985). Clinical studies have associated exposure to lead with reduced libido, reduced sperm motility and sperm count, chromosomal damage, infertility, and changes in serum testosterone (Braunstein et al., 1978; Winder, 1989).

5. Mechanisms of action

Endocrine disruptors affect cellular processes by different modes of action. They can act by mimicking the action of naturally produced hormones, blocking their receptors in target cells or altering the synthesis or metabolism of hormones and hormone receptors. It is important to note, that many endocrine disruptors have more than one mechanism of action (e.g., methoxychlor) (Gaido et al., 2000). Some can be metabolized to hormonally active compounds, exhibiting different properties (e.g., DDT and its metabolite DDE) (Kelce et al., 1995). Moreover, even compounds with the same supposed mechanism of action can induce different effects after exposure. It was also demonstrated that action of some xenoestrogens may be different in various tissues; thus they can act as SERMs (e.g., BPA, resveratrol, naringenin) (Gehm et al., 1997; Gould et al., 1998; Yoon et al., 2001).

5.1 Interaction with hormone receptors

Endocrine disruptors can bind to specific hormone receptors and act via agonistic or antagonistic mechanism. Numerous xenoestrogens (e.g., BPA, alkylphenols, genistein) activate estrogen receptors, interacting with their binding pockets (Lehraiki et al., 2011; Mueller, 2004; Singleton & Khan, 2003). It is possible due to structural similarities of these compounds to estradiol. The affinity of xenoestrogens to the estrogen receptor and/or their ability to initiate nuclear retention and transcriptional effects is usually lower than those of estradiol. It is worth noting, however, that weak activity via receptor-dependent pathway does not necessarily predict the potency of the chemical acting via another signaling pathway. Moreover, many xenoestrogenic compounds bioaccumulate in fat tissues, resulting in prolonged exposure (Watson et al., 2011). Several estrogenic chemicals, among others flavonoids and resveratrol, have been shown to interact not only with ERs, but also with aryl hydrocarbon receptor (AhR) (Revel et al., 2003; Van der Heiden, et al., 2009).
Antiandrogens, such as flutamide, vinclozolin, prochloraz and linuron, repress AR-mediated transcriptional activation, by competitive inhibition of endogenous androgens binding to their receptor (Gray et al., 1999; Lambright et al., 2000; Mohler et al., 2009; Noriega et al., 2005; Vinggaard et al., 2002). Binding of antiandrogen may result in a conformational change of ligand binding domain of AR appropriate for the interaction with co-repressors, instead of coactivators (Berrevoets et al., 2002; Hodgson et al., 2008).
Besides classical intracellular steroid hormone receptors, several membrane steroid receptors, capable to mediating non-genomic steroid actions, have been described (Thomas & Dong, 2006; Watson et al., 2007). BPA has been shown to bind to membrane-bound form of ERα (mER) and a transmembrane G protein-coupled receptor 30 (GPR30) (Watson et al., 2005). This GPCR-mediated non-genomic action included activation of cAMP-dependent

protein kinase and cGMP-dependent protein kinase pathways and a rapid phosphorylation of the transcription factor cAMP response-element-binding protein (CREB) (Bouskine et al., 2009). Recent results revealed the possibility that BPA may have adverse effects on spermatogenesis via activation of extracellular signal-related kinases 1 and 2 (ERK1/2) (Izumi et al., 2011). Also alkylphenols and phytoestrogens appear to activate non-genomic pathways, signaling via calcium influx and activation of mitogen-activated protein kinases (MAP kinases) (Bulayeva & Watson, 2004; Wozniak et al., 2005).

5.2 Alterations in synthesis, metabolism and transport of hormones or their receptors

It was reported that some endocrine disruptors can interfere with steroid synthesis or metabolism, acting via non-receptor mediated mechanisms (Fisher, 2004b). Phthalates induce antiandrogenic effects, however they do not interact with the AR (Lehraiki et al., 2009; Stroheker et al., 2005,). It was demonstrated that DBP and DEHP decrease fetal testosterone synthesis by reducing the expression of steroidogenic genes, such as *Cyp17*, *Cyp11a* and *StAR* (Barlow & Foster, 2003; Borch et al., 2006; Howdeshell et al., 2007; Parks et al., 2000). Phthalates were also shown to decrease the expression of Insl-3, a factor produced by fetal Leydig cells. Insl-3 is an important regulator of testicular descent and phthalate-induced reduction of Insl-3 is consistent with the high incidence of cryptorchidism (Gray et al., 2006; Laguë & Tremblay, 2008; Wilson et al., 2004). In contrast to phthalates, *in utero* exposure to prochloraz decreases testosterone production by direct inhibition of the activity of steroidogenic enzymes without affecting the mRNA expression of these enzymes (Blystone et al., 2007; Wilson et al., 2008).

As mentioned above, biosynthesis of estrogens is catalyzed by the enzyme aromatase. Various endocrine disruptors were reported to alter the expression or activity of aromatase, leading to testosterone-estradiol imbalance. Enhanced expression of aromatase was found in testes of males exposed to octylphenol and BPA (Hejmej et al., 2011b; Kim et al., 2010), whereas prochloraz reduced aromatase expression (Vinggaard et al., 2006). Estradiol level can also be influenced by inhibition of SULT 1A1 and 2E1 enzymes, which catalyze inactivation of estrogens by sulphation. It was shown that alkylphenols and phthalates, suppressing these enzymes, cause a rise in the levels of the free active endogenous estrogens (Waring & Harris, 2005).

Some endocrine disruptors may additionally influence the expression levels of hormone receptors, shifting the balance between concentrations of endogenous ligand and its receptor. For instance, it was reported that exposure to DES (McKinnell et al., 2001; Williams et al., 2001) and octylphenol (Hejmej et al., 2011b; Kotula-Balak et al., 2011) results in up-regulation of ERα and down-regulation of AR in male reproductive tissues.

In case of steroid hormones, the level of bioavailable hormone is determined not only by the level of synthesis and metabolism, but also by concentration of steroid hormone-binding globulin (SHBG), protein involved in transport of steroids in the blood. Studies revealed that endocrine disruptors may influence SHBG level, altering the level of free, bioavailable hormone (Bagchi et al., 2009; Sikka & Wang, 2008).

It should be mentioned, that xenoestrogens and antiandrogens affect reproductive functions not only acing directly on reproductive organs, but also disturbing hypothalamus-pituitary-testicular axis. For example, in adult male rats exposed to BPA during pre- and early postnatal periods, LH serum levels showed no changes, whereas FSH and testosterone levels decreased significantly (Cardoso et al., 2011). Secretion of FSH was also reduced following prenatal octylphenol and vinclozolin exposure (Sweeney et al., 2000; Veeramachaneni et al., 2006b).

5.3 Epigenetic mechanisms

Epigenetic modifications are regulators in numerous biological processes, including spermatogenesis. Key mechanism in establishing epigenetic change is DNA methylation, which usually suppresses expression of the gene. Several studies revealed that endocrine disrupting chemicals are implicated in epigenetic programming and DNA methylation (McLachlan, 2001; Skinner & Anway, 2005). Indeed, hypermethylation found in several genes in the sperm DNA (i. a. *Mest*, *Snrpn*, *Peg1* and *Peg3*) was accompanied by the reduction of semen quality (Stouder & Paoloni-Giacobino, 2010). These changes may be heritable, if they occur during certain stages of development (Crews & McLachlan, 2006). It was demonstrated that methoxychlor and vinclozolin when administered during prenatal period interfere with testis development and lead to increased spermatogenic cell apoptosis and decreased fertility in the adult males. These spermatogenic defects were also evident in subsequent generations (Chang et al., 2006; Skinner & Anway, 2005). Also maternal exposure to BPA resulted in postnatal changes in DNA methylation status and altered expression of specific genes in offspring (Bernal & Jirtle, 2010; Kundakovic & Champagne, 2011).

Taken together, estrogenic and antiandrogenic compounds act by multiple mechanisms of toxicity disrupting the interactions among the interconnected signaling pathways in reproductive tissues. Importantly, in the environment organisms are usually exposed to mixtures of multiple endocrine disruptors, which can produce cumulative effects, regardless of the mode of action of the individual mixture component (Gray et al., 2006).

6. Conclusion

Experimental studies clearly suggest that estrogenic and antiandrogenic compounds could cause alterations of sexual differentiation and impairment of male reproductive functions. Although the process of spermatogenesis is directly vulnerable to exposure to endocrine disrupting agents only in sexually mature males, above-mentioned data imply that exposure during the period of reproductive system development may have subsequent impact on the reproductive functions in adulthood. Fetal and neonatal exposures might result in the reprogramming of the developmental process of testicular cells, leading to their irreversible dysfunction. In contrast, adverse effects on the process of spermatogenesis in adulthood can be reversible (Sharpe, 2010; West et al., 2005). It is likely, therefore, that fetal and neonatal periods are of critical importance, when considering the role of hormonally active chemicals in male reproductive functions.

7. Acknowledgment

This work was financially supported by the Foundation for Polish Science, an Academic Grant 2008 (Mistrz Programme) and by the Ministry of Science and Higher Education, Grant N N303816640.

8. References

Acerini, C. L.; Miles, H. L.; Dunger, D. B.; Ong, K. K. & Hughes, I. A. (2009) The descriptive epidemiology of congenital and acquired cryptorchidism in a UK infant cohort *Archives of Disease in Childhood*, Vol.94, No.11, (November 2009), pp. 868-872, ISSN 0003-9888

Ademollo, N.; Ferrara, F.; Delise, M,; Fabietti, F. & Funari, E. (2008) Nonylphenol and octylphenol in human breast milk. *Environment International,* Vol.34, No.7, (October 2008), pp. 984-987, ISSN 0160-4120

Aikawa, H.; Koyama, S.; Matsuda, M.; Nakahashi, K.; Akazome, Y. & Mori, T. (2004) Relief effect of vitamin A on the decreased motility of sperm and the increased incidence of malformed sperm in mice exposed neonatally to bisphenol A. *Cell and Tissue Research,* Vol.315, No.1, (January 2004), pp. 119-124, ISSN 0302-766X

Akingbemi, B. T.; Ge, R.; Rosenfeld, C. S.; Newton, L. G.; Hardy, D. O.; Catterall, J. F.; Lubahn, D. B.; Korach, K. S. & Hardy, M. P. (2003) Estrogen receptor-alpha gene deficiency enhances androgen biosynthesis in the mouse Leydig cell. *Endocrinology,* Vol.144, No.1, (January 2003), pp. 84-93, ISSN 0013-7227

Akingbemi, B. T.; Sottas, C. M.; Koulova, A. I.; Klinefelter, G. R. & Hardy, M. P. (2004) Inhibition of testicular steroidogenesis by the xenoestrogen bisphenol A is associated with reduced pituitary luteinizing hormone secretion and decreased steroidogenic enzyme gene expression in rat Leydig cells. *Endocrinology,* Vol.145, No.2, (February 2004), pp. 592-603, ISSN 0013-7227

Albrecht, E. D.;, Lane, M. V.; Marshall, G. R.; Merchenthaler, I.; Simorangkir, D. R.; Pohl, C. R.; Plant, T.M. & Pepe, G. J. (2009) Estrogen promotes germ cell and seminiferous tubule development in the baboon fetal testis. *Biology of Reproduction,* Vol.81, No.2, (August 2009), pp. 406-414, ISSN 0368-2315

Anahara, R.; Toyama, Y. & Mori, C. (2008) Review of the histological effects of the anti-androgen, flutamide, on mouse testis. *Reproductive Toxicology,* Vol.25, No.2, (February 2008), pp. 139-143, ISSN 0890-6238

Andersen, H. R.; Vinggaard, A. M.; Rasmussen, T. H.; Gjermandsen, I.M. & Bonefeld-Jørgensen, E. C. (2002) Effects of currently used pesticides in assays for estrogenicity, androgenicity, and aromatase activity in vitro. *Toxicology and Applied Pharmacology,* Vol.179, No.1, (February 2002), pp. 1-12, ISSN 0041-008X

Andersson, A.M.; Jørgensen, N.; Main, K.M.; Toppari, J.; Rajpert-De Meyts, E.; Leffers, H.; Juul, A.; Jensen, T.K. & Skakkebaek, N.E. (2008) Adverse trends in male reproductive health: we may have reached a crucial 'tipping point'. *International Journal of Andrology,* Vol.31, No.2, (April 2008), pp. 74-80, ISSN 0105-6263

Anway, M. D. & Skinner, M. K. (2008) Epigenetic programming of the germ line: effects of endocrine disruptors on the development of transgenerational disease. *Reproductive Biomedicine Online,* Vol.16, No.1, (January 2008), pp. 23-25, ISSN 1472-6483

Anway, M. D.; Rekow, S. S. & Skinner, M. K. (2008) Comparative anti-androgenic actions of vinclozolin and flutamide on transgenerational adult onset disease and spermatogenesis. *Reproductive Toxicology,* Vol.26, No.2, (October 2008), pp. 100-106, ISSN 0890-6238

Atanassova, N.; McKinnell, C.; Turner, K. J.; Walker, M.; Fisher, J. S.; Morley, M.; Millar, M. R.; Groome, N. P. & Sharpe, R. M. (2000) Comparative effects of neonatal exposure of male rats to potent and weak (environmental) estrogens on spermatogenesis at puberty and the relationship to adult testis size and fertility: evidence for stimulatory effects of low estrogen levels. *Endocrinology,* Vol.141, No.10, (October 2000), pp. 3898-38907, ISSN *0013-7227*

Atanassova, N.; McKinnell, C.; Walker, M.; Turner, K. J.; Fisher, J. S.; Morley, M.; Millar, M. R.; Groome, N. P. & Sharpe, R. M. (1999) Permanent effects of neonatal estrogen exposure in rats on reproductive hormone levels, Sertoli cell number, and the efficiency of spermatogenesis in adulthood. *Endocrinology,* Vol.140, No.11, (November 1999), pp. 5364-5373, ISSN 1477-7827

Auger, J.; Kunstmann, J. M.; Czyglik, F. & Jouannet, P. (1995). Decline in semen quality among fertile men in Paris during the past 20 years. *The New England Journal of Medicine,* Vol.332, No.5, (February 1995), pp. 281-285, ISSN 0028-4793

Aydoğan, M. & Barlas, N. (2006) Effects of maternal 4-tert-octylphenol exposure on the reproductive tract of male rats at adulthood. *Reproductive Toxicology,* Vol.22, No.3, (October 2006),pp. 455-460, ISSN 0890-6238

Bagchi, G.; Hurst, C. H. & Waxman, D. J. (2009) Interactions of methoxyacetic acid with androgen receptor. *Toxicology and Applied Pharmacology,* Vol.238, No.2, (July 2009), pp. 101-110, ISSN 0041-008X

Barlow, N. J.; Phillips, S. L.; Wallace, D. G.; Sar, M.; Gaido, K. W. & Foster, P. M. (2003) Quantitative changes in gene expression in fetal rat testes following exposure to di(n-butyl) phthalate. *Toxicological Sciences,* Vol.73, No.2, (June 2003), pp. 431-441, ISSN 1096-6080

Barlow, N.J. & Foster, P. M. (2003) Pathogenesis of male reproductive tract lesions from gestation through adulthood following in utero exposure to di(n-butyl) phthalate. *Toxicologic Pathology,* Vol.31, No.4, (July-August 2003), pp. 397-410, ISSN 0940-2993

Barnhoorn, I. E.; Bornman, M. S.; Pieterse, G. M. & van Vuren, J. H. (2004) Histological evidence of intersex in feral sharptooth catfish (Clarias gariepinus) from an estrogen-polluted water source in Gauteng, South Africa. *Environmental Toxicology,* Vol.19, No.6, (December 2004), pp. 603-608, ISSN1520-4081

Bergström, R.; Adami, H.O.; Möhner, M.; Zatonski, W.; Storm, H.; Ekbom, A.; Tretli, S.; Teppo, L.; Akre, O. & Hakulinen, T. (1996) Increase in testicular cancer incidence in six European countries: a birth cohort phenomenon. *The Journal of the National Cancer Institute,* Vol.88, No.11, (June 1996), pp. 727-733, ISSN 0027-8874

Bernal, A. J. & Jirtle, R. L. (2010) Epigenomic disruption: the effects of early developmental exposures. *Birth defects research. Part A, Clinical and molecular teratology,* Vol.88, No.10, (October 2010), pp. 938-944, ISSN 1542-0752

Berrevoets, C. A.; Umar, A. & Brinkmann, A. O. (2002) Antiandrogens: selective androgen receptor modulators. *Molecular and Cellular Endocrinology,* Vol.198, No.1-2, (December 2002), pp. 97-103, ISSN 0303-7207

Bian, Q.; Qian, J.; Xu, L.; Chen, J.; Song, L. & Wang, X. (2006) The toxic effects of 4-tert-octylphenol on the reproductive system of male rats. Food *and Chemical Toxicology,* Vol.44, No.8, (August 2006), pp. 1355-1361, ISSN 0278-6915

Bilinska B.; Lesniak M. & Schmalz, B. (1997) Are ovine Leydig cells able to aromatize androgens? *Reproduction, Fertility and Development,* Vol.9, No.2, 193-199, ISSN, 1031-3613

Blake, C. A. & Boockfor, F. R. (1997) Chronic administration of the environmental pollutant 4-tert-octylphenol to adult male rats interferes with the secretion of luteinizing hormone, follicle-stimulating hormone, prolactin, and testosterone. *Biology of Reproduction,* Vol.57, No.2, (August 1997), pp. 255-266, ISSN 0006-3363

Blake, C. A.; Boockfor, F. R.; Nair-Menon, J. U.; Millette, C. F.; Raychoudhury, S. S. & McCoy, G. L. (2004) Effects of 4-tert-octylphenol given in drinking water for 4 months on the male reproductive system of Fischer 344 rats. *Reproductive Toxicology*, Vol.18, No.1, (January-February 2004), pp. 43-51, ISSN 0890-6238

Blystone, C. R.; Lambright, C. S.; Howdeshell, K. L.; Furr, J.; Sternberg, R. M.; Butterworth, B. C.; Durhanm, E. J.; Makynen, E. A.; Ankley, G. T.; Wilson, V. S.; Leblanc, G. A. & Gray, L. E. Jr. (2007) Sensitivity of fetal rat testicular steroidogenesis to maternal prochloraz exposure and the underlying mechanism of inhibition. *Toxicological Sciences,* Vol.97, No.2, (June 2007),pp. 512-519, ISSN 1096-6080

Blystone, C. R.; Lambright, C. S.; Howdeshell, K. L.; Furr, J.; Sternberg, R. M.; Butterworth, B. C.; Durhan, E. J.; Makynen, E. A.; Ankley, G. T.; Wilson, V. S.; Leblanc, G. A. & Gray, L. E. Jr. (2007) Sensitivity of fetal rat testicular steroidogenesis to maternal prochloraz exposure and the underlying mechanism of inhibition. *Toxicological Sciences*, Vol.97, No.2, (June 2007), pp. 512-519, ISSN 1096-6080

Boisen, K. A.; Kaleva, M.; Main, K. M.; Virtanen, H. E.; Haavisto, A. M.; Schmidt, I. M.; Chellakooty, M.; Damgaard, I. N.; Mau, C.; Reunanen, M.; Skakkebaek, N. E. & Toppari, J. (2004) Difference in prevalence of congenital cryptorchidism in infants between two Nordic countries. *Lancet*, Vol.363, No.9417, (April 2004), pp. 1264-1269, ISSN 0140-6736

Boockfor, F.R. & Blake, C.A. (1997) Chronic administration of 4-tert-octylphenol to adult male rats causes shrinkage of the testes and male accessory sex organs, disrupts spermatogenesis, and increases the incidence of sperm deformities. *Biology of Reproduction,* Vol.57, No.2, (August 1997), pp. 267-277, ISSN 0006-3363

Borch, J.; Metzdorff, S. B.; Vinggaard, A. M.; Brokken, L. & Dalgaard, M. (2006) Mechanisms underlying the anti-androgenic effects of diethylhexyl phthalate in fetal rat testis. *Toxicology,* Vol.223, No.1-2, (June 2006), pp. 144-155, ISSN 0300-483X

Bouskine, A.; Nebout, M.; Brücker-Davis, F.; Benahmed, M. & Fenichel, P. (2009) Low doses of bisphenol A promote human seminoma cell proliferation by activating PKA and PKG via a membrane G-protein-coupled estrogen receptor. Environmental Health *Perspectives,* Vol.117, No.7, (July 2009), pp. 1053-1058, ISSN 0091-6765

Braunstein, G. D.; Dahlgren, J. & Loriaux, D. L. (1978) Hypogonadism in chronically lead-poisoned men. *Infertility,* Vol.1, No.1, pp. 33-51, ISSN 1203-3243

Brokken, L. J.; Adamsson, A.; Paranko, J. & Toppari, J. (2009) Antiandrogen exposure in utero disrupts expression of desert hedgehog and insulin-like factor 3 in the developing fetal rat testis. *Endocrinology,* Vol.150, No.1, (January 2009), pp. 445-451, ISSN *0013-7227*

Bubenik, G. A.; Jacobson, J. P.; Schams, K. D. & Bartoš, L. (2001) Cryptorchidism, hypogonadism and antler malformation in black-tailed deer (Odocoileus hemionus sitkensis) of Kodiak Island. *Zeitschrift für Jagdwissenschaft*, Vol.47, No.4, (December 2001), pp. 241–252, ISSN 0044-2887

Bulayeva, N. N. & Watson, C. S. (2004) Xenoestrogen-induced ERK-1 and ERK-2 activation via multiple membrane-initiated signaling pathways. *Environmental Health Perspectives,* (November 2004), Vol.112, No.15, pp.1481-1487, ISSN 0091-6765

Calafat, A.M.; Ye, X.; Wong, L. Y.; Reidy, J. A.; Needham, L. L. (2008) Exposure of the U.S. population to bisphenol A and 4-tertiary-octylphenol: 2003-2004. *Environmental Health Perspectives,* Vol.116, No.1, (January 2008), pp. 39-44, ISSN 0091-6765

Cardoso, N.; Pandolfi, M.; Lavalle, J.; Carbone, S.; Ponzo, O.; Scacchi, P. & Reynoso, R. (2011) Probable gamma-aminobutyric acid involvement in bisphenol A effect at the hypothalamic level in adult male rats. *Journal of Physiology & Biochemistry,* (June 2011), doi: 10.1007/s13105-011-0102-6, ISSN 1138-7548

Carlsen, E.; Giwercman, A.; Keiding, N. & Skakkebaek, N. E. (1992) Evidence for decreasing quality of semen during past 50 years. *British Medical Journal,* Vol.305, No.6854, (September 1992), pp. 609-613, ISSN 09598138

Carreau, S.; Lambard, S.; Delalande, C.; Denis-Galeraud, I.; Bilinska, B. & Bourguiba, S. (2003) Aromatase expression and role of estrogens in male gonad : a review. *Reproductive Biology and Endocrinology,* Vol.1: 35, (April 2003), ISSN 1477-7827

Chang, H. S.; Anway, M. D.; Rekow, S. S. & Skinner, M. K. (2006) Transgenerational epigenetic imprinting of the male germline by endocrine disruptor exposure during gonadal sex determination. *Endocrinology,* Vol.147, No.12, (December 2006), pp. 5524-5541, ISSN 0013-7227

Chapin, R. E.; Harris, M. W.; Davis, B. J.; Ward, S. M.; Wilson, R. E.; Mauney, M. A.; Lockhart, A. C.; Smialowicz, R. J.; Moser, V. C.; Burka, L. T. & Collins, B. J. (1997) The effects of perinatal/juvenile methoxychlor exposure on adult rat nervous, immune, and reproductive system function. *Fundamental and Applied Toxicology,* Vol.40, No.1, (November 1997), pp. 138-157, ISSN 0272-0590

Colborn, T. & Clement, C. (Eds.). (1992) *Chemically-induced alterations in sexual and functional development - the wildlife/human connection,* Princeton Scientific Pub., ISBN 0-911131-35-3, Princeton

Colborn, T.; vom Saal, F. S. & Soto, A. M. (1993) Developmental effects of endocrine-disrupting chemicals in wildlife and humans. *Environmental Health Perspectives,* Vol.101, No.5, (October 1993), pp. 378-384, ISSN 0091-6765

Cook, J. C.; Mullin, L. S.; Frame, S. R. & Biegel, L. B. (1993) Investigation of a mechanism for Leydig cell tumorigenesis by linuron in rats. *Toxicology and Applied Pharmacology,* (April 1993), Vol.119, No.2, pp. 195-204, ISSN 0041-008X

Cowin, P. A.; Gold, E.; Aleksova, J.; O'Bryan, M. K.; Foster, P. M.; Scott, H. S. & Risbridger, G. P. (2010) Vinclozolin exposure in utero induces postpubertal prostatitis and reduces sperm production via a reversible hormone-regulated mechanism. *Endocrinology,* Vol.151, No.2, (February 2010), pp. 783-792, ISSN 0013-7227

Crews, D. & McLachlan, J. A. (2006) Epigenetics, evolution, endocrine disruption, health, and disease. *Endocrinology,* Vol.147, Suppl.6, (June 2006), pp. S4-10, ISSN 0013-7227

Cummings, A. M. (1997) Methoxychlor as a model for environmental estrogens. *Critical Reviews in Toxicology,* Vol.27, No.4, (July 1997), pp. 367-379, ISSN 1040-8444

Davenport, M. (1997) Risk of testicular cancer in boys with cryptorchidism. Study was based on small number of cancers. *British Medical Journal,* Vol.315, No.7120, (November 1997), pp. 1462-1463, ISSN 09598138

Davenport, M. (1997) Risk of testicular cancer in boys with cryptorchidism. Study was based on small number of cancers. *British Medical Journal,* Vol.315, No.7120, (November 1997), pp. 1462-1463, ISSN 0959-8138

de Solla, S. R.; Bishop, C.A.; Van der Kraak, G. & Brooks, R. J. (1998) Impact of organochlorine contamination on levels of sex hormones and external morphology of common snapping turtles (Chelydra serpentina serpentina) in Ontario, Canada. *Environmental Health Perspectives,* Vol.106, No.5, (May 1998), pp. 253-260, ISSN 0091-6765 de Solla, S. R.; Martin, P. A.; Fernie, K. J.; Park, B. J. & Mayne, G. (2006) Effects of environmentally relevant concentrations of atrazine on gonadal development of snapping turtles (Chelydra serpentina). *Environmental Toxicology & Chemistry*, Vol.25, No.2, (February 2006), pp. 520-526, ISSN, 0730-7268

de Souza Predes, F.; Diamante, M. A. & Dolder, H. (2010) Testis response to low doses of cadmium in Wistar rats. *International Journal of Experimental Pathology*, Vol.91, No.2, (April 2010), pp.125-131, ISSN 0959-9673

Dehal, S. S. & Kupfer, D. (1994) Metabolism of the proestrogenic pesticide methoxychlor by hepatic P450 monooxygenases in rats and humans. Dual pathways involving novel ortho ring-hydroxylation by CYP2B. *Drug Metabolism and Disposition*, Vol.22, No.6, (November-December 1994), pp. 937-946, ISSN 0090-9556

Delbès, G.; Levacher, C. & Habert, R. (2006) Estrogen effects on fetal and neonatal testicular development. *Reproduction*, Vol.132, No.4, (October 2006), pp. 527-538, ISSN 1470-1626

Delbès, G.; Levacher, C.; Duquenne, C.; Racine, C.; Pakarinen, P. & Habert, R. (2005) Endogenous estrogens inhibit mouse fetal Leydig cell development via estrogen receptor alpha. *Endocrinology*, (May 2005), Vol.146, No.5, pp. 2454-2461, ISSN 0013-7227

Diamanti-Kandarakis, E.; Bourguignon, J. P.; Giudice, L. C.; Hauser, R.; Prins, G. S.; Soto, A. M.; Zoeller, R. T. & Gore, A. C. (2009) Endocrine-disrupting chemicals: an Endocrine Society scientific statement. *Endocrine Reviews*, Vol.30, No.4, (June 2009), pp. 293-342, ISSN 0163-769X

Dieckmann, K. P. & Pichlmeier, U. (2004) Clinical epidemiology of testicular germ cell tumors. *World Journal of Urology* , Vol.22, No.1, (April 2004), pp. 2-14, ISSN 0724-4983

Dohle, G. R.; Smit, M. & Weber, R. F. (2003) Androgens and male fertility. *World Journal of Urology*, Vol.21, No.5, (November 2003), pp. 341-345, ISSN1433-8726

Driscoll, S. G. & Taylor, S. H. (1980) Effects of prenatal maternal estrogen on the male urogenital system. *Obstetrics and Gynecology*, Vol.56, No.5, (November 1980), pp. 537-542, ISSN 0029-7844

Durlej, M.; Kopera, I.; Knapczyk-Stwora, K.; Hejmej, A.; Duda, M.; Koziorowski, M.; Slomczynska, M. & Bilinska, B. (2011) *Acta Histochemica*, Vol.113, No.1, (January 2011), pp. 6-12, ISSN 0065-1281

Fisher, J. S. (2004a) Environmental anti-androgens and male reproductive health: focus on phthalates and testicular dysgenesis syndrome. *Reproduction*, Vol.127, No.3, (March 2004), pp. 305-315, ISSN 1470-1626

Fisher, J. S. (2004b) Are all EDC effects mediated via steroid hormone receptors? *Toxicology*, Vol.205, No.1-2, (December 2004), pp. 33-41, ISSN 0300-483X

Fisher, J. S.; Macpherson, S.; Marchetti, N. & Sharpe, R. M. (2003) Human 'testicular dysgenesis syndrome': a possible model using in-utero exposure of the rat to dibutyl phthalate. *Human Reproduction*, Vol.18, No.7, (July 2003), pp. 1383-1394, ISSN 0268-1161

Fisher, J. S.; Turner, K. J.; Brown, D. & Sharpe, R. M. (1999) Effect of neonatal exposure to estrogenic compounds on development of the excurrent ducts of the rat testis through puberty to adulthood. *Environmental Health Perspectives*, Vol.107, No.5, (May 1999), pp. 397-405, ISSN 0091-6765

Foster, W. G.; Singh, A.; McMahon, A. & Rice, D. C. (1998) Chronic lead exposure effects in the cynomolgus monkey (Macaca fascicularis) testis. *Ultrastructural Pathology,* Vol.22, No.1, (January-February 1998), pp. 63-71, ISSN 0191-3123

Fowler, K. A.; Gill, K.; Kirma, N.; Dillehay, D. L. & Tekmal, R. R. (2000) Overexpression of aromatase leads to development of testicular Leydig cell tumors : an in vivo model for hormone-mediated testicular cancer. *American Journal of Pathology,* Vol.156, No.1, (January 2000), pp. 347-353, ISSN 0002-9440

Frederiksen, H.; Skakkebaek, N. E. & Andersson, A. M. (2007) Metabolism of phthalates in humans. *Molecular Nutrition & Food Research,* Vol.51, No.7, (July 2007), pp. 899-911, ISSN 1613-4125

Fry, D. M. (1995) Reproductive effects in birds exposed to pesticides and industrial chemicals. *Environmental Health Perspectives,* Vol.103, Suppl. 7, (October 1995), pp. 165-171, ISSN 0091-6765

Gaido, K. W.; Leonard, L. S.; Maness, S. C.; Hall, J. M.; McDonnell, D. P.; Saville, B. & Safe, S. (1999) Differential interaction of the methoxychlor metabolite 2,2-bis-(p-hydroxyphenyl)-1,1,1-trichloroethane with estrogen receptors alpha and beta. *Endocrinology,* Vol.140, No.12, (December 1999), pp. 5746-5753, ISSN 0013-7227

Gaido, K. W.; Maness, S. C.; McDonnell, D. P.; Dehal, S. S.; Kupfer, D. & Safe, S. (2000) Interaction of methoxychlor and related compounds with estrogen receptor alpha and beta, and androgen receptor: structure-activity studies. *Molecular Pharmacology,* Vol.58, No.4, (October 2000), pp. 852-858, ISSN 0026-895X

Gancarczyk, M.; Paziewska-Hejmej, A.; Carreau, S.; Tabarowski, Z. & Bilinska, B. (2004) Dose- and photoperiod-dependent effects of 17beta-estradiol and the anti-estrogen ICI 182,780 on testicular structure, acceleration of spermatogenesis, and aromatase immunoexpression in immature bank voles. *Acta Histochemica,* Vol.106, No.4, pp. 269-278, ISSN 0065-1281

Gebara, A. B.; Ciscato, C. H.; Monteiro, S. H. & Souza, G. S. (2011) Pesticide residues in some commodities: dietary risk for children. *Bulletin of Environmental Contamination and Toxicology,* Vol.86, No.5, (May 2011), pp. 506-510, ISSN 0007-4861

Gehm, B. D.; McAndrews, J. M.; Chien, P. Y. & Jameson, J. L. (1997) Resveratrol, a polyphenolic compound found in grapes and wine, is an agonist for the estrogen receptor. *Proceedings of the National Academy of Sciences USA,* Vol.94, No.25, (December 1997), pp. 14138-14143, ISSN 0027-8424

Gill, W. B.; Schumacher, G. F.; Bibbo, M.; Straus, F. H. 2nd & Schoenberg, H. W. (1979) Association of diethylstilbestrol exposure in utero with cryptorchidism, testicular hypoplasia and semen abnormalities. *Journal of Urology,* Vol.122, No.1, (July 1979), pp. 36-39, ISSN1433-8726

Gong, Y. & Han, X. D. (2006) Effect of nonylphenol on steroidogenesis of rat Leydig cells. *Journal of Environmental Science and Health, Part B,* Vol.41, No.5, pp. 705-715, ISSN 0360-1234

Gould, J. C.; Leonard, L. S.; Maness, S. C.; Wagner, B. L.; Conner, K.; Zacharewski, T.; Safe, S.; McDonnell, D. P. & Gaido, K. W. (1998) Bisphenol A interacts with the estrogen receptor alpha in a distinct manner from estradiol. *Molecular and Cellular Endocrinology,* Vol.142, No.1-2, (July 1998), pp. 203-214, ISSN 0303-7207

Gray, L. E. Jr; Ostby, J. S. & Kelce, W. R. (1994) Developmental effects of an environmental antiandrogen: the fungicide vinclozolin alters sex differentiation of the male rat.

Toxicology and Applied Pharmacology, Vol.129, No.1, (November 1994), pp. 46-52,ISSN 0041-008X

Gray, L. E. Jr; Wilson, V. S.; Stoker, T.; Lambright, C.; Furr, J.; Noriega, N.; Howdeshell, K.; Ankley, G. T. & Guillette, L. (2006) Adverse effects of environmental antiandrogens and androgens on reproductive development in mammals. *International Journal of Andrology,* Vol.29, No.1, (February 2006), pp. 96-104, ISSN 0105-6263

Gray, L. E. Jr; Wolf, C.; Lambright, C.; Mann, P.; Price, M.; Cooper, R. L. & Ostby, J. (1999) Administration of potentially antiandrogenic pesticides (procymidone, linuron, iprodione, chlozolinate, p,p'-DDE, and ketoconazole) and toxic substances (dibutyl- and diethylhexyl phthalate, PCB 169, and ethane dimethane sulphonate) during sexual differentiation produces diverse profiles of reproductive malformations in the male rat. *Toxicology and Industrial Health,* (January-March 1999), Vol.15, No.1-2, pp. 94-118, ISSN: 0748-2337

Guillette, L. J. Jr; Gross, T. S.; Masson, G. R.; Matter, J. M.; Percival, H. F. & Woodward, A. R. (1994) Developmental abnormalities of the gonad and abnormal sex hormone concentrations in juvenile alligators from contaminated and control lakes in Florida. *Environmental Health Perspectives,* Vol.102, No.8, (August 1994), pp. 680-688, ISSN 0091-6765

Han, X. D.; Tu, Z. G.; Gong, Y.; Shen, S. N.; Wang, X. Y.; Kang, L. N.; Hou, Y. Y. & Chen, J. X. (2004) The toxic effects of nonylphenol on the reproductive system of male rats. *Reproductive Toxicology,* Vol.19, No.2, (December 2004), pp. 215-221, ISSN 0890-6238

Hejmej, A.; Kopera, I.; Kotula-Balak, M.; Lydka, M.; Lenartowicz, M. & Bilinska, B. (2011a) Are expression and localization of tight and adherens junction proteins in testes of adult boar affected by foetal and neonatal exposure to flutamide? *Reproductive Toxicology,* doi:10.1111/j.1365-2605.2011.01206.x, ISSN 0890-6238

Hejmej, A.; Kotula-Balak, M.; Galas, J. & Bilinska, B. (2011b) Effects of 4-tert-octylphenol on the testes and seminal vesicles in adult male bank voles. *Reproductive Toxicology,* Vol.31, No.1, (January 2011), pp. 95-105, ISSN 0890-6238.

Henley, D. V. & Korach, K. S. (2010) Physiological effects and mechanisms of action of endocrine disrupting chemicals that alter estrogen signaling. *Hormones (Athens),* Vol.9, No.3, (July-September 2010), pp. 191-205, ISSN 1109-3099

Henley, D. V.; Lipson, N.; Korach, K. S. & Bloch, C. A. (2007) Prepubertal gynecomastia linked to lavender and tea tree oils. *New England Journal of Medicine,* Vol.356, No.5, (February 2007), pp. 479-485, ISSN 0028-4793

Hess, R. A. (2000) Oestrogen in fluid transport in efferent ducts of the male reproductive tract. *Reviews of Reproduction,* Vol.5, No.2, (May 2000), pp. 84-92, ISSN 1359-6004

Hess, R. A. (2003) Estrogen in the adult male reproductive tract: a review. *Reproductive Biology and Endocrinology,* Vol.1: 52, (July 2003), ISSN 0196-9781

Hess, R. A.; Bunick, D.; Lee, K. H.; Bahr, J.; Taylor, J. A.; Korach, K. S. & Lubahn, D. B. (1997) A role for oestrogens in the male reproductive system. *Nature,* (December 1997), Vol.390, No.6659, pp. 509-512, ISSN 0028-0836

Hodgson, M. C.; Shen, H. C.; Hollenberg, A. N. & Balk, S. P. (2008) Structural basis for nuclear receptor corepressor recruitment by antagonist-liganded androgen receptor. *Molecular Cancer Therapeutics,* Vol.7, No.10, (October 2008), pp. 3187-3194, ISSN 1535-7163

Hosokawa, S.; Murakami, M.; Ineyama, M.; Yamada, T.; Koyama, Y.; Okuno, Y.; Yoshitake, A.; Yamada, H. & Miyamoto, J. (1993) Effects of procymidone on reproductive organs and serum gonadotropins in male rats. *Journal of Toxicological Sciences*, Vol.18, No.2, (May 1993), pp. 111-124, ISSN 0388-1350

Howdeshell, K. L.; Furr, J.; Lambright, C. R.; Rider, C. V.; Wilson, V. S. & Gray, L. E. Jr. (2007) Cumulative effects of dibutyl phthalate and diethylhexyl phthalate on male rat reproductive tract development: altered fetal steroid hormones and genes. *Toxicological Sciences*, Vol.99, No.1, (September 2007), pp. 190-202, ISSN 1096-6080

Hu, G. X.; Zhao, B.; Chu, Y.; Li, X. H.; Akingbemi, B. T.; Zheng, Z. Q. & Ge, R. S. (2011) Effects of methoxychlor and 2,2-bis(p-hydroxyphenyl)-1,1,1-trichloroethane on 3β-hydroxysteroid dehydrogenase and 17β-hydroxysteroid dehydrogenase-3 activities in human and rat testes. *International Journal of Andrology*, Vol.34, No.2, (April 2011), pp. 138-144, ISSN 0105-6263

Izumi, Y.; Yamaguchi, K.; Ishikawa, T.; Ando, M.; Chiba, K.; Hashimoto, H.; Shiotani, M. & Fujisawa, M. (2011) Molecular changes induced by bisphenol-A in rat Sertoli cell culture. *Systems Biology in Reproductive Medicine*, (May 2011), doi: 10.3109/19396368.2011.574248, ISSN 1939-6368

Ji, Y. L.; Wang, H.; Liu, P.; Wang, Q.; Zhao, X. F.; Meng, X. H.; Yu, T.; Zhang, H.; Zhang, C.; Zhang, Y. & Xu, D. X. (2010) Pubertal cadmium exposure impairs testicular development and spermatogenesis via disrupting testicular testosterone synthesis in adult mice. *Reproductive Toxicology*,Vol.29, No.2, (April 2010), pp. 176-183, ISSN 0890-6238

Ji, Y. L.; Wang, H.; Liu, P.; Zhao, X. F.; Zhang, Y.; Wang, Q.; Zhang, H.; Zhang, C.; Duan, Z. H.; Meng, C. & Xu, D. X. (2011) Effects of maternal cadmium exposure during late pregnant period on testicular steroidogenesis in male offspring. *Toxicology Letters*, Vol.205, No.1, (August 2011), pp. 69-78, ISSN 0378-4274

Jie, X.; Yang, W.; Jie, Y.; Hashim, J. H.; Liu, X. Y.; Fan, Q. Y. & Yan, L. (2010) Toxic effect of gestational exposure to nonylphenol on F1 male rats. *Birth Defects Research Part B Development Reproductive Toxicology*, Vol.89, No.5, (October 2010), pp. 418-428, ISSN 1542-9733

Jobling, S.; Beresford, N.; Nolan, M.; Rodgers-Gray, T.; Brighty, G.C.; Sumpter, J.P. & Tyler, C.R. (2002) Altered sexual maturation and gamete production in wild roach (Rutilus rutilus) living in rivers that receive treated sewage effluents. *Biology of Reproduction*, Vol.66, No.2, (February 2002), pp. 272-281, ISSN 0006-3363

Johnson, L.; Staub, C.; Silge, R. L.; Harris, M. W. & Chapin, R. E. (2002) The pesticide methoxychlor given orally during the perinatal/juvenile period, reduced the spermatogenic potential of males as adults by reducing their Sertoli cell number. *Reproduction, Nutrition and Development*, Vol.42, No.6, (November-December 2002), pp. 573-580, ISSN 0926-5287

Jørgensen, N.; Andersen, A.G; Eustache, F.; Irvine, D. S.; Suominen, J.; Petersen, J. H.; Andersen, A. N.; Auger, J.; Cawood, E. H.; Horte, A.; Jensen, T. K.; Jouannet, P.; Keiding, N.; Vierula, M.; Toppari, J. & Skakkebaek, N. E. (2001) Regional differences in semen quality in Europe. *Human Reproduction*, Vol.16, No.5, (May 2001), pp. 1012-1019, ISSN 1355-4786

Jørgensen, N.; Asklund, C.; Carlsen, E. & Skakkebaek, N. E. (2006) Coordinated European investigations of semen quality: results from studies of Scandinavian young men is a matter of concern. *International Journal of Andrology*, Vol.29, No.1, (February 2006), pp. 54-61, ISSN 0105-6263

Jørgensen, N.; Vierula, M.; Jacobsen, R.; Pukkala, E.; Perheentupa, A.; Virtanen, H. E.; Skakkebaek, N. E. & Toppari, J. (2011) Recent adverse trends in semen quality and testis cancer incidence among Finnish men. *International Journal of Andrology*, (March 2011), doi: 10.1111/j.1365-2605.2010.01133.x. ISSN 0105-6263

Källén, B.; Bertollini, R.; Castilla, E.; Czeizel, A.; Knudsen, L. B.; Martinez-Frias, M. L.; Mastroiacovo, P. & Mutchinick, O. (1986) A joint international study on the epidemiology of hypospadias. *Acta Pediatrica Scandinavica. Supplement*, Vol.324, pp. 1-52, ISSN 0300-8843

Kelce, W. R. & Wilson, E. M. (1997) Environmental antiandrogens: developmental effects, molecular mechanisms, and clinical implications. Journal of Molecular Medicine, Vol.75, No.3, (March 1997), pp. 198-207, ISSN 0946-2716

Kelce, W. R.; Stone, C. R.; Laws, S. C.; Gray, L. E.; Kemppainen, J. A. & Wilson, E. M. (1995) Persistent DDT metabolite p,p'-DDE is a potent androgen receptor antagonist. *Nature*, Vol.375, No.6532, (June 1995), pp. 581-585, ISSN 0028-0836

Kim, J. Y.; Han, E. H.; Kim, H. G.; Oh, K. N.; Kim, S. K.; Lee, K. Y. & Jeong, H. G. (2010) Bisphenol A-induced aromatase activation is mediated by cyclooxygenase-2 up-regulation in rat testicular Leydig cells. *Toxicology Letters*, Vol.193, No.2, (March 2010), pp. 200-208, ISSN 0378-4274

Kim, S. K.; Kim, J. H.; Lee, H. J. & Yoon, Y. D. (2007) Octylphenol reduces the expressions of steroidogenic enzymes and testosterone production in mouse testis. *Environmental Toxicology*, Vol.22, No.5, (October 2007), pp. 449-458, ISSN 1520-4081

Kopera, I.; Durlej, M.; Hejmej, A.; Knapczyk-Stwora K.; Duda, M.; Slomczynska, M. & Bilinska, B. (2011) Differential Expression of Connexin 43 in Adult Pig Testes During Normal Spermatogenic Cycle and After Flutamide Treatment. *Reproduction in Domestic Animals*, doi: 10.1111/j.1439-0531.2011.01783.x, ISSN 0936-6768

Kopera, I.; Durlej, M.; Hejmej, A.; Knapczyk-Stwora K.; Duda, M.; Slomczynska, M.; Koziorowski, M. & Bilinska, B. (2010) Effects of pre- and postnatal exposure to flutamide on connexin 43 expression in testes and ovaries of prepubertal pigs. *European Journal of Histochemistry*, Vol.54, No.2, (April 2010), pp. e15, ISSN 1121-760X

Kotula-Balak, M.; Pochec, E.; Hejmej, A.; Duda, M. & Bilinska, B. (2011) Octylphenol affects morphology and steroidogenesis in mouse tumor Leydig cells. *Toxicology In Vitro*, Vol.25, No.5, (August 2011), pp. 1018-1026, ISSN 0887-2333

Kris-Etherton, P. M.; Hecker, K. D.; Bonanome, A.; Coval, S. M.; Binkoski, A. E.; Hilpert, K. F.; Griel, A. E. & Etherton, T. D. (2002) Bioactive compounds in foods: their role in the prevention of cardiovascular disease and cancer. *American Journal of Medicine* Vol.113, Suppl.9B, (December 2002), pp. 71S-88S, ISSN 0002-9343

Kuiper, G. G.; Enmark, E.; Pelto-Huikko, M.; Nilsson, S. & Gustafsson J. A. (1996) Cloning of a novel receptor expressed in rat prostate and ovary. *The Proceedings of the National Academy of Science U S A*, Vol.93, No.12, (June 1996),pp. 5925-5930, ISSN 0027-8424

Kuiper, G. G.; Lemmen, J. G.; Carlsson, B.; Corton, J. C.; Safe, S. H.; van der Saag, P. T.; van der Burg, B. & Gustafsson, J. A. (1998) Interaction of estrogenic chemicals and phytoestrogens with estrogen receptor beta. *Endocrinology*, Vol.139, No.10, (October 1998), pp. 4252-4263, ISSN 0013-7227

Kundakovic, M. & Champagne, F. A. (2011) Epigenetic perspective on the developmental effects of bisphenol A. *Brain, Behavior, and Immunity,* (February 2011), doi:10.1016/j.bbi.2011.02.005, ISSN 0889-1591

Laguë, E . & Tremblay, J. J. (2008) Antagonistic effects of testosterone and the endocrine disruptor mono-(2-ethylhexyl) phthalate on INSL3 transcription in Leydig cells. *Endocrinology,* Vol.149, No.9, (September 2008), pp. 4688-4694, ISSN 0013-7227

Laier, P.; Metzdorff, S. B.; Borch, J.; Hagen, M. L.; Hass, U.; Christiansen, S.; Axelstad, M.; Kledal, T.; Dalgaard, M.; McKinnell, C,.; Brokken, L. J. & Vinggaard, A. M. (2006) Mechanisms of action underlying the antiandrogenic effects of the fungicide prochloraz. *Toxicology and Applied Pharmacology,* (June 2006), Vol.213, No.2, pp. 160-171, ISSN 0041-008X

Lambright, C.; Ostby, J.; Bobseine, K.; Wilson, V.; Hotchkiss, A. K.; Mann, P. C. & Gray, L. E. Jr. (2000) Cellular and molecular mechanisms of action of linuron: an antiandrogenic herbicide that produces reproductive malformations in male rats. *Toxicological Sciences,* Vol.56, No.2, (August 2000), pp. 389-399, ISSN 1096-6080

Lee, B. J.; Jung, E. Y.; Yun, Y.W.; Kang, J. K.; Baek, I. J.; Yon, J. M.; Lee, Y. B.; Sohn, H. S.; Lee, J. Y.; Kim, K. S. & Nam, S. Y. (2004) Effects of exposure to genistein during pubertal development on the reproductive system of male mice. *Journal of Reproduction and Development,* Vol.50, No.4, (August 2004), pp. 399-409, ISSN 0916-8818

Lee, H. J.; Chattopadhyay, S.; Gong, E. Y.; Ahn, R. S. & Lee, K. (2003) Antiandrogenic effects of bisphenol A and nonylphenol on the function of androgen receptor. *Toxicological Sciences,* Vol.75, No.1, (September 2003), pp. 40-46, ISSN 1096-6080

Lee, P. C. (1998) Disruption of male reproductive tract development by administration of the xenoestrogen, nonylphenol, to male newborn rats. *Endocrine,* Vol.9, No.1, (August 1998), pp. 105-111, ISSN 1355-008X

Lehraiki, A.; Chamaillard, C.; Krust, A.; Habert, R. & Levacher, C. (2011) Genistein impairs early testosterone production in fetal mouse testis via estrogen receptor alpha. *Toxicology In Vitro,* (May 2011), doi:10.1016/j.tiv.2011.05.017, ISSN 0887-2333

Lehraiki, A.; Racine, C.; Krust, A.; Habert, R. & Levacher, C. (2009) Phthalates impair germ cell number in the mouse fetal testis by an androgen- and estrogen-independent mechanism. *Toxicological Sciences,* Vol.111, No.2, (October 2009), pp. 372-382, ISSN 1096-6080

Levallet, J.; Bilinska, B.; Mittre, H.; Genissel, C.; Fresnel, J. & Carreau, S. (1998) Expression and immunolocalization of functional cytochrome P450 aromatase in mature rat testicular cells. *Biology of Reproduction,* Vol.58, No.4, (April 1998), pp. 919-926, ISSN 0006-3363

Li, X.; Nokkala, E.; Yan, W.; Streng, T.; Saarinen, N.; Wärri, A.; Huhtaniemi. I.; Santti. R.; Mäkelä, S. & Poutanen, M. (2001) Altered structure and function of reproductive organs in transgenic male mice overexpressing human aromatase. *Endocrinology;* Vol.142, No.6, (June 2001), pp. 2435-2442, ISSN 0013-7227

Lubahn, D. B.; Moyer, J. S.; Golding, T. S.; Couse, J. F.; Korach, K. S. & Smithies, O. (1993) Alteration of reproductive function but not prenatal sexual development after insertional disruption of the mouse estrogen receptor gene. *The Proceedings of the National Academy of Science U S A,* Vol.90, No.23, (December 1993), pp. 11162-11166, ISSN 0027-8424

Mackenzie, C. A.; Lockridge, A. & Keith, M. (2005) Declining sex ratio in a first nation community. *Environmental Health Perspectives*, Vol.113, No.10, (October 2005), pp. 1295-1298, ISSN 0091-6765

Macleod, D. J.; Sharpe, R. M.; Welsh, M.; Fisken, M.; Scott, H. M.; Hutchison, G. R.; Drake, A. J. & van den Driesche, S. (2010) Androgen action in the masculinization programming window and development of male reproductive organs. *International Journal of Andrology*, Vol.33, No.2, (April 2010), pp. 279-287, ISSN 0105-6263

Majdic, G.; Sharpe, R. M. & Saunders, P. T. (1997) Maternal oestrogen/xenoestrogen exposure alters expression of steroidogenic factor-1 (SF-1/Ad4BP) in the fetal rat testis. *Molecular and Cellular Endocrinology*, Vol.127, No.1, (March 1997), pp. 91-98, ISSN 0303-7207

Majdic, G.; Sharpe, R. M.; O'Shaughnessy, P. J. & Saunders, P. T. (1996) Expression of cytochrome P450 17alpha-hydroxylase/C17-20 lyase in the fetal rat testis is reduced by maternal exposure to exogenous estrogens. *Endocrinology*, Vol.137, No.3, (March 1996), pp. 1063-1070, ISSN 1477-7827

Mansfield, K. G. & Land, E. D. (2002) Cryptorchidism in Florida panthers: prevalence, features, and influence of genetic restoration. *Journal of Wildlife Diseases*, Vol.38, No.4, (October 2002), pp. 693-698, ISSN 0090-3558

Marchlewicz, M.; Michalska, T. & Wiszniewska, B. (2004) Detection of lead-induced oxidative stress in the rat epididymis by chemiluminescence. *Chemosphere*, (December 2004), Vol.57, No.10, pp. 1553-1562, ISSN 0045-6535

Marselos, M. & Tomatis, L. (1992) Diethylstilboestrol: I, Pharmacology, Toxicology and carcinogenicity in humans. *European Journal of Cancer*, Vol.28A, No.6-7, pp. 1182-1189, ISSN 0014-2964

Maschio, L. R.; Cordeiro, R. S.; Taboga, S. R. & Góes, R. M. (2010) Short-term antiandrogen flutamide treatment causes structural alterations in somatic cells associated with premature detachment of spermatids in the testis of pubertal and adult guinea pigs. *Reproduction in Domestic Animals*, (June 2010), Vol.45, No.3, pp. 516-524, ISSN 0936-6768

McEwen, B.S. & Alves, S. E. (1999) Estrogen actions in the central nervous system. *Endocrine Reviews*, Vol.20, No.3, (June 1999), pp. 279-307, ISSN 0163-769X

McIntyre, B. S.; Barlow, N. J.; Sar, M.; Wallace, D. G. & Foster, P. M. (2002a) Effects of in utero linuron exposure on rat Wolffian duct development. *Reproductive Toxicology*, Vol.16, No.2, (March-April 2002),pp. 131-139, ISSN 0890-6238

McIntyre, B. S.; Barlow, N. J.; Wallace, D. G.; Maness, S. C.; Gaido, K. W. & Foster, P. M. (2000) Effects of in utero exposure to linuron on androgen-dependent reproductive development in the male Crl:CD(SD)BR rat. *Toxicology and Applied Pharmacology*, Vol.167, No.2, (September 2000), pp. 87-99, ISSN 0041-008X

McIntyre, B. S.; Barlow, N.J. & Foster, P. M. (2002b) Male rats exposed to linuron in utero exhibit permanent changes in anogenital distance, nipple retention, and epididymal malformations that result in subsequent testicular atrophy. *Toxicological Sciences*, Vol.65, No.1, (January 2002), pp. 62-70, ISSN 1096-6080

McKinnell, C.; Atanassova, N.; Williams, K.; Fisher, J. S.; Walker, M.; Turner, K. J.; Saunders, P. T. K. & Sharpe, R. M. (2001) Suppression of androgen action and the induction of gross abnormalities of the reproductive tract in male rats treated neonatally with diethylstilbestrol. *Journal of Andrology,* Vol.22, No.2, (March-April 2001), pp. 323-338, ISSN 0105-6263

McLachlan, J. A. (2001) Environmental signaling: what embryos and evolution teach us about endocrine disrupting chemicals. *Endocrine Reviews,* Vol.22, No.3, (June 2001), pp. 319-341, ISSN 1945-7189

McLachlan, J. A.; Newbold, R. R.; Burow, M. E. & Li, S. F. (2001) From malformations to molecular mechanisms in the male: three decades of research on endocrine disrupters. *Acta Pathologica, Microbiologica et Immunologica Scandinavica,* Vol.109, No.4, (April 2001), pp. 263-272, ISSN 0903-4641

Melnick, S.; Cole, P.; Anderson, D. & Herbst, A. (1987) Rates and risks of diethylstilbestrol-related clear-cell adenocarcinoma of the vagina and cervix. An update. *New England Journal of Medicine,* Vol.316, No.9, (February 1987), pp. 514-516, ISSN 0028-4793

Mikkilä, T. F.; Toppari, J. & Paranko, J. (2006) Effects of neonatal exposure to 4-tert-octylphenol, diethylstilbestrol, and flutamide on steroidogenesis in infantile rat testis. *Toxicological Sciences,* Vol.91, No.2, (June 2006), pp. 456-466, ISSN 1096-6080

Mittendorf, R. (1995) Teratogen update: carcinogenesis and teratogenesis associated with exposure to diethylstilbestrol (DES) in utero. *Teratology,* Vol.51, No.6, (June 1995), pp. 435-445, ISSN 0040-3709

Mohler, M. L.; Bohl, C. E.; Jones, A.; Coss, C. C.; Narayanan, R.; He, Y.; Hwang, D. J.; Dalton, J. T. & Miller, D. D. (2009) Nonsteroidal selective androgen receptor modulators (SARMs): dissociating the anabolic and androgenic activities of the androgen receptor for therapeutic benefit. *Journal of Medicinal Chemistry,* Vol.52, No.12, (June 2009), pp. 3597-3617, ISSN 0223-5234

Møller, H. & Skakkebaek N. E. (1999) Risk of testicular cancer in subfertile men: case-control study. *British Medical Journal,,* Vol.318, No.7183, (February 1999), pp. 559-562, ISSN 09598138

Monosson, E.; Kelce, W. R.; Lambright, C.; Ostby, J. & Gray, L. E. Jr. (1999) Peripubertal exposure to the antiandrogenic fungicide, vinclozolin, delays puberty, inhibits the development of androgen-dependent tissues, and alters androgen receptor function in the male rat. *Toxicology and Industrial Health,* Vol.15, No.1-2, (January-March 1999), pp. 65-79, ISSN: 0748-2337

Mueller, S. O. (2004) Xenoestrogens: mechanisms of action and detection methods. *Analytical and Bioanalytical Chemistry,* Vol.378, No.3, (February 2004), pp. 582-587, ISSN 1618-2642

Mueller, S. O.; Simon, S.; Chae, K.; Metzler, M. & Korach, K. S. (2004) Phytoestrogens and their human metabolites show distinct agonistic and antagonistic properties on estrogen receptor alpha (ERalpha) and ERbeta in human cells. *Toxicological Sciences,* Vol.80, No.1, (July 2004), pp. 14-25, ISSN 1096-6080

Murakami, M.; Hosokawa, S.; Yamada, T.; Harakawa, M.; Ito, M.; Koyama, Y.; Kimura, J.; Yoshitake, A. & Yamada, H. (1995) Species-specific mechanism in rat Leydig cell tumorigenesis by procymidone. *Toxicology and Applied Pharmacology,* Vol.131, No.2, (April 1995), pp. 244-252, ISSN 0041-008X

Murono, E. P. & Derk, R. C. (2005) The reported active metabolite of methoxychlor, 2,2-bis(p-hydroxyphenyl)-1,1,1-trichloroethane, inhibits testosterone formation by cultured Leydig cells from neonatal rats. *Reproductive Toxicology,* Vol.20, No.4, (November-December 2005), pp. 503-513, ISSN 0890-6238

Mylchreest, E. & Foster, P. M. (2000) DBP exerts its antiandrogenic activity by indirectly interfering with androgen signaling pathways. *Toxicology and Applied Pharmacology,* Vol.168, No.2, (October 2000), pp. 174-175, ISSN 0041-008X

Mylchreest, E.; Sar, M.; Cattley, R. C. & Foster, P. M. (1999) Disruption of androgen-regulated male reproductive development by di(n-butyl) phthalate during late gestation in rats is different from flutamide. *Toxicology and Applied Pharmacology,* Vol.156, No.2, (April 1999), pp. 81-95, ISSN 0041-008X

Mylchreest, E.; Sar, M.; Wallace, D. G. & Foster, P. M. (2002) Fetal testosterone insufficiency and abnormal proliferation of Leydig cells and gonocytes in rats exposed to di(n-butyl) phthalate. *Reproductive Toxicology,* Vol.16, No.1, (Jan-Feb 2002), pp. 19-28, ISSN 0890-6238

Nakamura, K.; Yasunaga, Y.; Ko, D.; Xu, L. L.; Moul, J. W.; Peehl, D. M.; Srivastava, S. & Rhim, J. S. (2002) Cadmium-induced neoplastic transformation of human prostate epithelial cells. *International Journal of Oncology,* Vol.20, No.3, (March 2002), pp. 543-547, ISSN 1019-6439

Nassar, N.; Bower, C. & Barker, A. (2007) Increasing prevalence of hypospadias in Western Australia, 1980-2000. *Archives of disease in childhood,* Vol.92, No.7, (July 2007), pp. 580-584, ISSN 0003-9888

Neri, R. (1989) Pharmacology and pharmacokinetics of flutamide. *Urology,* Vol.34, Suppl.4, (October 1989), pp. 19-21, ISSN 0090-4295

Noriega, N. C.; Ostby, J.; Lambright, C.; Wilson, V. S. & Gray, L. E. Jr. (2005) Late gestational exposure to the fungicide prochloraz delays the onset of parturition and causes reproductive malformations in male but not female rat offspring. *Biology of Reproduction,* Vol.72, No.6, (June 2005), pp. 1324-1335, ISSN 0006-3363

O'Connor, J. C.; Cook, J. C.; Slone, T. W.; Makovec, G. T.; Frame, S. R. & Davis, L. G. (1998) An ongoing validation of a Tier I screening battery for detecting endocrine-active compounds (EACs). *Toxicological Sciences,* Vol.46, No.1, (November 1998), pp. 45-60, ISSN 1096-6080

Oettel, M. (2002) Is there a role for estrogens in the maintenance of men's health? *Aging Male,* (December 2002), Vol.5, No.4, pp. 248-257, ISSN 1368-5538

Omezzine, A.; Chater, S.; Mauduit, C.; Florin, A.; Tabone, E.; Chuzel, F.; Bars, R. & Benahmed, M. (2003) Long-term apoptotic cell death process with increased expression and activation of caspase-3 and -6 in adult rat germ cells exposed in utero to flutamide. *Endocrinology,* Vol.144, No.2, (February 2003), pp. 648-661, ISSN *0013-7227*

Ostby, J.; Kelce, W. R.; Lambright, C.; Wolf, C. J.; Mann, P. & Gray, L. E. Jr. (1999) The fungicide procymidone alters sexual differentiation in the male rat by acting as an androgen-receptor antagonist in vivo and in vitro. *Toxicology and Industrial Health,* Vol.15, No.1-2, (January-March 1999), pp. 80-93, ISSN: 0748-2337

Parks, L. G.; Ostby, J. S.; Lambright, C. R.; Abbott, B. D.; Klinefelter, G. R.; Barlow, N. J. & Gray, L. E. Jr. (2000) The plasticizer diethylhexyl phthalate induces malformations by decreasing fetal testosterone synthesis during sexual differentiation in the male rat. *Toxicological Sciences,* Vol.58, No.2, (December 2000), pp. 339-349, ISSN 1096-6080

Paulozzi, L. J. International trends in rates of hypospadias and cryptorchidism. (1999) *Environmental Health Perspectives,* Vol.107, No.4, (April 1999), pp. 297-302, ISSN 0091-6765

Prins, G. S.; Birch, L.; Couse, J. F.; Choi, I.; Katzenellenbogen, B. & Korach, K. S. (2001) Estrogen imprinting of the developing prostate gland is mediated through stromal estrogen receptor alpha: studies with alphaERKO and betaERKO mice. *Cancer Research,* Vol.61, No.16, (August 2001), pp. 6089-6097, ISSN 0008-5472

Reinli, K. & Block, G. (1996) Phytoestrogen content of foods - a compendium of literature values. *Nutrition and Cancer,* Vol.26, No.2, pp. 123-48, ISSN 0163-5581

Revel, A.; Raanani, H.; Younglai, E.; Xu, J.; Rogers, I.; Han, R.; Savouret, J. F. & Casper, R. F. (2003) Resveratrol, a natural aryl hydrocarbon receptor antagonist, protects lung from DNA damage and apoptosis caused by benzo[a]pyrene. *Journal of Applied Toxicology,* Vol.23, No.4, (July-August 2003), pp. 255-261, ISSN 0260-437X

Richter, C. A.; Birnbaum, L. S.; Farabollini, F.; Newbold, R. R.; Rubin, B. S.; Talsness, C. E.; Vandenbergh, J. G.; Walser-Kuntz, D. R. & vom Saal, F. S. (2007) In vivo effects of bisphenol A in laboratory rodent studies. *Reproductive Toxicology,* Vol.24, No.2, (August-September 2007), pp. 199-224, ISSN 0890-6238

Robertson, K. M.; O'Donnell, L.; Jones, M. E.; Meachem, S. J.; Boon, W. C.; Fisher, C. R.; Graves, K. H.; McLachlan, R. I. & Simpson, E. R. (1999) Impairment of spermatogenesis in mice lacking a functional aromatase (cyp 19) gene. *The Proceedings of the National Academy of Science U S A,* Vol.96, No.14, (July 1999), pp. 7986-7991, ISSN 0027-8424

Rubin, M. M. (2007) Antenatal exposure to DES: lessons learned...future concerns. *Obstetrical and Gynecological Survey,* Vol.62, No.8, (August 2007),pp. 548-555, ISSN 0029-7828

Safe, S. (2004) Endocrine disruptors and human health: is there a problem. *Toxicology,* Vol.205, No.1-2, (December 2004), pp. 3-10, ISSN 0300-483X

Safe, S. H. (2000) Endocrine disruptors and human health--is there a problem? An update. *Environmental Health Perspectives,* Vol.108, No.6, (June 2000), pp. 487-493, ISSN 0091-6765

Scandinavica. Supplement, Vol.324, pp. 1-52, ISSN 0300-8843

Schettler, T. (2006) Human exposure to phthalates via consumer products. *International Journal of Andrology,* Vol.29, No.1, (February 2006), pp. 134-139, ISSN 0105-6263

Schmitt, E.; Dekant, W. & Stopper, H. (2001) Assaying the estrogenicity of phytoestrogens in cells of different estrogen sensitive tissues. *Toxicology In Vitro,* Vol.15, No.4-5, (August-October 2001), pp. 433-439, ISSN 0887-2333

Setchell, K.D.; Zimmer-Nechemias, L.; Cai, J. & Heubi, J. E. (1997) Exposure of infants to phyto-oestrogens from soy-based infant formula. *Lancet,* Vol.350, No.9070, (July 1997), pp. 23-7, ISSN 0140-6736

Sharpe, R. M. & Irvine, D.S. (2004) How strong is the evidence of a link between environmental chemicals and adverse effects on human reproductive health? *British Medical Journal,* Vol.328, No.7437, (February 2004), pp. 447-451, ISSN 09598138

Sharpe, R. M. (2010) Environmental/lifestyle effects on spermatogenesis. *Philosophical transactions of the Royal Society of London. Series B, Biological sciences,* Vol.365, No.1546, (May 2010), pp. 1697-1712, ISSN 1471-2970

Sharpe, R. M.; Atanassova, N.; McKinnell, C.; Parte, P.; Turner, K. J.; Fisher, J. S.; Kerr, J. B.; Groome, N. P.; Macpherson, S.; Millar, M. R. & Saunders P. T. (1998) Abnormalities in functional development of the Sertoli cells in rats treated neonatally with diethylstilbestrol: a possible role for estrogens in Sertoli cell development. *Biology of Reproduction,* Vol.59, No.5, (November 1998), pp. 1084-1094, ISSN 0006-3363

Sharpe, R. M.; Rivas, A.; Walker, M.; McKinnell, C. & Fisher, J. S. (2003) Effect of neonatal treatment of rats with potent or weak (environmental) oestrogens, or with a GnRH antagonist, on Leydig cell development and function through puberty into adulthood. *International Journal of Andrology,* Vol.26, No.1, (February 2003), pp. 26-36, ISSN 0105-6263

Shi, Y. Q.; Li, H. W.; Wang, Y. P.; Liu, C. J. & Yang, K. D. (2011) p,p'-DDE induces apoptosis and mRNA expression of apoptosis-associated genes in testes of pubertal rats. *Environmental Toxicology,* (March 2011), doi: 10.1002/tox.20694, ISSN1520-4081

Sikka, S. C. & Wang, R. (2008) Endocrine disruptors and estrogenic effects on male reproductive axis. *Asian Journal of Andrology,* Vol.10, No.1, (January 2008), pp. 134-145, ISSN 1008-682X

Singh, S. M.; Gauthier, S. & Labrie, F. (2000) Androgen receptor antagonists (antiandrogens): structure-activity relationships. *Current Medical Chemistry* (February 2000), Vol.7, No.2, pp. 211-247, ISSN 0929-8673

Singleton, D. W. & Khan, S. A. (2003) Xenoestrogen exposure and mechanisms of endocrine disruption. *Frontiers in Bioscience,* Vol.8, (January 2003), pp. s110-118, ISSN 1093-9946

Skakkebaek, N. E. & Jørgensen, N. (2005) Testicular dysgenesis and fertility. *Andrologia,* Vol.37, No.6, (December 2005), pp. 217-218, ISSN 0303- 4569

Skakkebaek, N. E.; Rajpert-De Meyts, E. & Main, K. M. (2001) Testicular dysgenesis syndrome: an increasingly common developmental disorder with environmental aspects. *Human Reproduction,* Vol.16, No.5, (May 2001), pp. 972-978, ISSN 0268-1161

Skinner, M.K. & Anway, M. D. (2005) Seminiferous cord formation and germ-cell programming: epigenetic transgenerational actions of endocrine disruptors. *Annals of the New York Academy of Sciences,* Vol.1061, (December 2005), pp. 18-32, ISSN 0077-8923

Sokol, R. Z.; Madding, C. E. & Swerdloff, R. S. (1985) Lead toxicity and the hypothalamic-pituitary-testicular axis. *Biology of Reproduction,* Vol.33, No.3, (October 1985), pp. 722-728, ISSN 0006-3363

Sonne, C.; Leifsson, P. S.; Dietz, R.; Born, E. W.; Letcher, R. J.; Hyldstrup, L.; Riget, F. F.; Kirkegaard, M. & Muir, D. C. (2006) Xenoendocrine pollutants may reduce size of sexual organs in East Greenland polar bears (Ursus maritimus). *Environmental Science &Technology* (September 2006), Vol.40, No.18, pp. 5668-5674, ISSN 0013-936X

Staples, C. A.; Naylor, C. G.; Williams, J. B. & Gledhill, W. E. (2001) Ultimate biodegradation of alkylphenol ethoxylate surfactants and their biodegradation intermediates. *Environmental Toxicology & Chemistry,* Vol.20, No.11, (November 2001), pp. 2450-2455, ISSN 0730-7268

Stouder, C & Paoloni-Giacobino, A. (2010) Specific transgenerational imprinting effects of the endocrine disruptor methoxychlor on male gametes. *Reproduction,* Vol.141, No.2, (February 2011), pp. 207-216, ISSN 1470-1626

Stroheker, T.; Cabaton, N.; Nourdin, G.; Régnier, J. F.; Lhuguenot, J. C. & Chagnon, M. C. (2005) Evaluation of anti-androgenic activity of di-(2-ethylhexyl)phthalate. *Toxicology*, Vol.208, No.1, (March 2005), pp. 115-121, ISSN 0300-483X

Suthar, A.C.; Banavalikar, M. M. & Biyani, M. K. (2001) Pharmacological activities of Genistein, an isoflavone from soy (Glycine max): part II--anti-cholesterol activity, effects on osteoporosis & menopausal symptoms. *Indian Journal of Experimental Biology*, Vol.39, No.6, (June 2001), pp. 520-525, ISSN 0019-5189

Suzuki, M.; Lee, H. C.; Chiba, S.; Yonezawa, T. & Nishihara, M. (2004) Effects of methoxychlor exposure during perinatal period on reproductive function after maturation in rats. *Journal of Reproduction and Development*, Vol.50, No.4, (August 2004), pp. 455-461, ISSN 0916-8818

Svechnikov, K.; Izzo, G.; Landreh, L.; Weisser, J. & Söder, O. (2010) Endocrine disruptors and Leydig cell function. *Journal of Biomedicine and Biotechnology*, Vol.2010: 684504, (August 2010), ISSN 1110-7243

Svechnikov, K.; Spatafora, C.; Svechnikova, I.; Tringali, C. & Söder, O. (2009) Effects of resveratrol analogs on steroidogenesis and mitochondrial function in rat Leydig cells in vitro. *Journal of Applied Toxicology*, Vo.29, No.8, (November 2009), pp. 673-680, ISSN 0260-437X

Svechnikov, K.; Supornsilchai, V.; Strand, M. L.; Wahlgren, A.; Seidlova-Wuttke, D.; Wuttke, W. & Söder, O. (2005) Influence of long-term dietary administration of procymidone, a fungicide with anti-androgenic effects, or the phytoestrogen genistein to rats on the pituitary-gonadal axis and Leydig cell steroidogenesis. *Journal of Endocrinology*, Vol.187, No.1, (October 2005), pp. 117-124, ISSN 0022-0795

Swan, S. H.; Elkin, E.P. & Fenster, L. (2000) The question of declining sperm density revisited: an analysis of 101 studies published 1934-1996. *Environmental Health Perspectives*, Vol.108, Vo.10, (October 2000), pp. 961-966, ISSN 0091-6765

Swan, S. H.; Kruse, R. L.; Liu, F.; Barr, D. B.; Drobnis, E.Z.; Redmon, J. B.; Wang, C.; Brazil, C.; Overstreet, J. W. & Study for Future Families Research Group. (2003) Semen quality in relation to biomarkers of pesticide exposure. *Environmental Health Perspectives*, Vol.111, No.12, (September 2003), pp. 1478-1484, ISSN 0091-6765

Sweeney, T.; Nicol, L.; Roche, J. F. & Brooks, A. N. (2000) Maternal exposure to octylphenol suppresses ovine fetal follicle-stimulating hormone secretion, testis size, and Sertoli cell number. *Endocrinology*, Vol.141, No.7, (July 2000), pp. 2667-2673, ISSN *0013-7227*

Takiguchi, M. & Yoshihara, S. (2006) New aspects of cadmium as endocrine disruptor. *Environmental Sciences*, Vol.13, No.2, pp. 107-116, ISSN 0915-955X

Thomas, P. & Dong, J. (2006) Binding and activation of the seven-transmembrane estrogen receptor GPR30 by environmental estrogens: a potential novel mechanism of endocrine disruption. *Journal of Steroid Biochemistry and Molecular Biology*, Vol.102, No.1-5, (December 2006), pp. 175-179, ISSN 0960-0760

Thonneau, P.F.; Gandia, P. & Mieusset, R. (2003) Cryptorchidism: incidence, risk factors, and potential role of environment; an update. *International Journal of Andrology*, Vol.24, No.2, (March-April 2003), pp. 155-162, ISSN 0105-6263

Toppari, J.; Kaleva, M. & Virtanen, H. E. (2001) Trends in the incidence of cryptorchidism and hypospadias, and methodological limitations of registry-based data. *Human Reproduction Update*, Vol.7, No.3, (May-June 2001), pp. 282-286, ISSN 1355-4786

Toyama, Y.; Hosoi, I.; Ichikawa, S.; Maruoka, M.; Yashiro, E.; Ito, H. & Yuasa, S. (2001) Beta-estradiol 3-benzoate affects spermatogenesis in the adult mouse. *Molecular and Cellular Endocrinology*, Vol.178, No.1-2, (June 2001), pp. 161-168, ISSN 0303-7207

Toyama, Y.; Suzuki-Toyota, F.; Maekawa, M.; Ito, C. & Toshimori, K. (2004) Adverse effects of bisphenol A to spermiogenesis in mice and rats. *Archives of Histology and Cytology*, Vol.67, No.4, (November 2004), pp. 373-381, ISSN 0914-9465

Vaithinathan, S.; Saradha, B. & Mathur, P. P. (2010) Methoxychlor induces apoptosis via mitochondria- and FasL-mediated pathways in adult rat testis. *Chemico-Biological Interactions*, Vol.185, No.2, (April 2010), pp. 110-118, ISSN 0009-2797

Vajda, A.M.; Barber, L. B.; Gray, J. L.; Lopez, E. M.; Woodling, J. D. & Norris, D. O. (2008) Reproductive disruption in fish downstream from an estrogenic wastewater effluent. *Environmental Science &Technology*, Vol.42, No.9, (May 2008), pp. 3407-3414, ISSN 0013-936X

van den Berg, H. (2009) Global status of DDT and its alternatives for use in vector control to prevent disease. *Environmental Health Perspectives*, Vol.117, No.11, (November 2009), pp. 1656-1663, ISSN 0091-6765

Van der Heiden, E.; Bechoux, N.; Muller, M.; Sergent, T.; Schneider, Y. J.; Larondelle, Y.; Maghuin-Rogister, G. & Scippo, M. L. (2009) Food flavonoid aryl hydrocarbon receptor-mediated agonistic/antagonistic/synergic activities in human and rat reporter gene assays. *Analytica Chimica Acta*, Vol.637, No.1-2, (April 2009), pp. 337-345, ISSN 0003-2670

Veeramachaneni, D. N.; Amann, R. P. & Jacobson, J. P. (2006a) Testis and antler dysgenesis in sitka black-tailed deer on Kodiak Island, Alaska: Sequela of environmental endocrine disruption? *Environmental Health Perspectives*, Vol.114, Suppl. 1, (April 2006), pp. 51-59, ISSN 0091-6765

Veeramachaneni, D. N.; Palmer, J. S.; Amann, R. P.; Kane, C. M.; Higuchi, T. T. & Pau, K. Y. (2006b) Disruption of sexual function, FSH secretion, and spermiogenesis in rabbits following developmental exposure to vinclozolin, a fungicide. *Reproduction*, Vol.131, No.4, (April 2006), pp. 805-816, ISSN 1470-1626

Vigueras-Villaseñor, R. M.; Moreno-Mendoza, N. A.; Reyes-Torres, G.; Molina-Ortiz, D.; León, M.C. & Rojas-Castañeda J. C. (2006) The effect of estrogen on testicular gonocyte maturation. *Reproductive Toxicology*, Vol.22, No.3, (October 2006), pp. 513-520, ISSN 0890-6238

Vinggaard, A. M.; Christiansen, S.; Laier, P.; Poulsen, M. E.; Breinholt, V.; Jarfelt, K.; Jacobsen, H.; Dalgaard, M.; Nellemann, C. & Hass, U. (2005) Perinatal exposure to the fungicide prochloraz feminizes the male rat offspring. *Toxicological Sciences*, Vol.85, No.2, (June 2005), pp. 886-897, ISSN 1096-6080

Vinggaard, A. M.; Hass, U.; Dalgaard, M.; Andersen, H.R.; Bonefeld-Jørgensen, E.; Christiansen, S.; Laier, P. & Poulsen, M. E. (2006) Prochloraz: an imidazole fungicide with multiple mechanisms of action. *International Journal of Andrology*, Vol.29, No.1, (February 2006), pp. 186-192, ISSN 0105-6263

Vinggaard, A. M.; Nellemann, C.; Dalgaard, M.; Jørgensen, E. B. & Andersen, H. R. (2002) Antiandrogenic effects in vitro and in vivo of the fungicide prochloraz. *Toxicological Sciences*, Vol.69, No.2, (October 2002), pp. 344-353, ISSN 1096-6080

Vo, T. T.; Jung, E. M.; Dang, V. H.; Yoo, Y. M.; Choi, K. C.; Yu, F. H. & Jeung, E. B. (2009) Di-(2 ethylhexyl) phthalate and flutamide alter gene expression in the testis of immature male rats. *Reproductive Biology and Endocrinology*, Vol.7: 104, (September 2009), ISSN 0196-9781

vom Saal, F. S.; Cooke, P. S.; Buchanan, D. L.; Palanza, P.; Thayer, K. A.; Nagel, S, C.; Parmigiani, S. & Welshons, W. V. (1998) A physiologically based approach to the study of bisphenol A and other estrogenic chemicals on the size of reproductive organs, daily sperm production, and behavior. *Toxicology and Industrial Health*, Vol.14, No.1-2, (January-April 1998), pp. 239-260, ISSN: 0748-2337

Vos, J. G.; Dybing, E.; Greim, H. A.; Ladefoged, O.; Lambré, C.; Tarazona, J. V.; Brandt, I. & Vethaak, A. D. (2000) Health effects of endocrine-disrupting chemicals on wildlife, with special reference to the European situation. *Critical Reviews in Toxicology*, Vol.30, No.1, (January 2000), pp. 71-133, ISSN 1040-8444

Waring, R. H. & Harris, R. M. (2005) Endocrine disrupters: a human risk? *Molecular and Cellular Endocrinology*, Vol.244, No.1-2, (December 2005), pp. 2-9, ISSN 0303-7207

Watson, C. S.; Alyea, R. A.; Jeng, Y. J. & Kochukov, M. Y. (2007) Nongenomic actions of low concentration estrogens and xenoestrogens on multiple tissues. *Molecular and Cellular Endocrinology*, Vol.274, No.1-2, (August 2007), pp. 1-7, ISSN 0303-7207

Watson, C. S.; Bulayeva, N. N.; Wozniak, A. L. & Finnerty, C. C. (2005) Signaling from the membrane via membrane estrogen receptor-alpha: estrogens, xenoestrogens, and phytoestrogens. *Steroids*, Vol.70, No.5-7, (May-June 2005), pp. 364-371, ISSN 0585-2617

Watson, C. S.; Jeng, Y. J. & Guptarak, J. (2011) Endocrine disruption via estrogen receptors that participate in nongenomic signaling pathways. *Journal of Steroid Biochemistry and Molecular Biology*, (February 2011), doi:10.1016/j.jsbmb.2011.01.015, ISSN 0960-0760

Welsh, M.; Saunders, P. T.; Fisken, M.; Scott, H. M.; Hutchison, G.R.; Smith, L.B. & Sharpe, R. M. (2008) Identification in rats of a programming window for reproductive tract masculinization, disruption of which leads to hypospadias and cryptorchidism. *Journal of Clinical Investigation*, (April 2008), Vol.118, No.4, pp. 1479-1490, ISSN 0021-9738

Welshons, W. V.; Nagel, S. C. & vom Saal, F. S. (2006) Large effects from small exposures. III. Endocrine mechanisms mediating effects of bisphenol A at levels of human exposure. *Endocrinology*, Vol.147, Suppl.6, (June 2006),pp. S56-69, ISSN 0013-7227

West, M. C.; Anderson, L. ; McClure, N. & Lewis, S. E. (2005) Dietary oestrogens and male fertility potential. *Human fertility* (*Cambridge)*,Vol.8, No.3, (September 2005), pp. 197-207, ISSN 1464-7273

Williams, K.; McKinnell, C.; Saunders, P. T.; Walker, M.; Fisher, J. S.; Turner, K. J.; Atanassova, N. & Sharpe, M. (2001) Neonatal exposure to potent and environmental oestrogens and abnormalities of the male reproductive system in the rat: evidence for importance of the androgen-oestrogen balance and assessment of the relevance to man. *Human Reproductive Update*, Vol.7, No.3, (May-June 2001), pp. 236-247, ISSN 1355-4786

Wilson, V. S.; Blystone, C. R.; Hotchkiss, A. K.; Rider, C. V. & Gray, L. E. Jr. (2008) Diverse mechanisms of anti-androgen action: impact on male rat reproductive tract development. *International Journal of Andrology*, Vol.31, No.2, (April 2008), pp. 178-187, ISSN 0105-6263

Wilson, V. S.; Lambright, C. R.; Furr, J. R.; Howdeshell, K. L. & Gray, L. E. Jr. (2009) The herbicide linuron reduces testosterone production from the fetal rat testis during both in utero and in vitro exposures. *Toxicology Letters,* Vol.186, No.2, (April 2009), pp. 73-77,ISSN 0378-4274

Wilson, V. S.; Lambright, C.; Furr, J.; Ostby, J.; Wood, C.; Held, G. & Gray, L. E. Jr. (2004) Phthalate ester-induced gubernacular lesions are associated with reduced insl3 gene expression in the fetal rat testis. *Toxicology Letters,* Vol.146, No.3, (February 2004), pp. 207-215, ISSN 0378-4274

Winder, C. (1989) Reproductive and chromosomal effects of occupational exposure to lead in the male. *Reproductive Toxicology,* Vol.3, No.4, pp. 221-233, ISSN 0890-6238

Wolf, C. J.; LeBlanc, G. A.; Ostby, J. S. & Gray, L. E. Jr. (2000) Characterization of the period of sensitivity of fetal male sexual development to vinclozolin. *Toxicological Sciences* Vol.55, No.1, (May 2000), pp. 152-161, ISSN 1096-6080

Wong, C.; Kelce, W. R.; Sar, M. & Wilson, E. M. (1995) Androgen receptor antagonist versus agonist activities of the fungicide vinclozolin relative to hydroxyflutamide. *Journal of Biological Chemistry,* Vol.270, No.34, (August 1995), pp. 19998-20003, ISSN 0021-9258

Wozniak, A. L.; Bulayeva, N. N. & Watson, C. S. (2005) Xenoestrogens at picomolar to nanomolar concentrations trigger membrane estrogen receptor-alpha-mediated Ca2+ fluxes and prolactin release in GH3/B6 pituitary tumor cells. *Environmental Health Perspectives,* Vol.113, No.4, (April 2005), pp. 431-439, ISSN 0091-6765

Yoon, K.; Pallaroni, L.; Stoner, M.; Gaido, K. & Safe, S. (2001) Differential activation of wild-type and variant forms of estrogen receptor alpha by synthetic and natural estrogenic compounds using a promoter containing three estrogen-responsive elements. *Journal of Steroid Biochemistry and Molecular Biology,* Vol.78, No.1, (July 2001), pp. 25-32, ISSN 0960-0760

Yoshida, M.; Katsuda, S.; Takenaka, A.; Watanabe, G.; Taya, K. & Maekawa, A. (2001) Effects of neonatal exposure to a high-dose p-tert-octylphenol on the male reproductive tract in rats. *Toxicology Letters,* Vol.121, No.1, (April 2001), pp. 21-33, ISSN 0378-4274

You, L.; Casanova, M.; Archibeque-Engle, S.; Sar, M.; Fan, L. Q. & Heck, H. A. (1998) Impaired male sexual development in perinatal Sprague-Dawley and Long-Evans hooded rats exposed in utero and lactationally to p,p'-DDE. *Toxicological Sciences,* Vol.45, No.2, (October 1998), pp. 162-173, ISSN 1096-6080

Zhang, M.; He, Z.; Wen, L.; Wu, J.; Yuan, L.; Lu, Y.; Guo, C.; Zhu, L.; Deng, S. & Yuan, H. (2010) Cadmium suppresses the proliferation of piglet Sertoli cells and causes their DNA damage, cell apoptosis and aberrant ultrastructure. *Reproductive Biology and Endocrinology,*Vol.8: 97, (August 2010), ISSN 0196-9781

Part 2

Steroid Clinical Correlation

5

Relationship Between Steroid Hormones and *Helicobacter pylori*

Hirofumi Shimomura
Jichi Medical University
Japan

1. Introduction

Helicobacter pylori is a Gram-negative microaerobic curved-rod possessing polar flagella as the motility organ. This bacterium colonizes human gastric epithelium and causes chronic gastritis and peptic ulcers (Graham, 1991; Warren & Marshall, 1983; Wyatt & Dixon, 1988). Via longer periods of colonization in the human stomach, it also contributes to the development of gastric cancer and marginal zone B-cell lymphoma (Forman, Eurogast Study Group, 1993; Wotherspoon et al., 1991). Approximately half of population in the world is infected with *Helicobacter pylori*, and the majority of infected persons develop atrophic gastritis with or without symptoms. Among *Helicobacter pylori*-infected individuals, about 10% persons develop gastric and duodenal ulcers, 1% to 3% persons develop gastric adenocarcinoma, and 0.1% or less person develops gastric mucosa-associated lymphoid tissue (MALT) lymphoma (Fukase et al., 2008; Peek & Blaser, 2002; Peek & Crabtree, 2006; Stolte et al., 2002; Uemura et al., 2001).

The bacterial species belonging to the genus *Helicobacter* have a unique feature of free-cholesterol (FC) assimilation into the membrane lipid compositions (Haque et al., 1995, 1996). *Helicobacter pylori* aggressively absorbs free-cholesterol supplemented to a medium, or extracts free-cholesterol from the lipid raft of epithelial cell membrane when the organism adhered onto the epithelial cell surface (Wunder et al., 2006). The free-cholesterol assimilated into the *Helicobacter pylori* membranes is glucosylated via the enzymatic action, and the organism utilizes as the membrane lipid components both free-cholesterol itself and the glucosylated cholesterols. Previous study by our group has identified the following three types of glucosyl cholesterols in the membrane lipid compositions of *Helicobacter pylori* (Hirai et al., 1995): cholesteryl-α-D-glucopyranoside (CGL), cholesteryl-6-*O*-tetradecanoyl-α-D-glucopyranoside (CAG), and cholesteryl-6-*O*-phosphatidyl-α-D-glucopyranoside (CPG). One of the enzymes involved in the biosynthesis of glucosyl cholesterols is HP0421 protein, a cholesterol α-glucosyltransferase encoded by HP0421 gene in *Helicobacter pylori* (Lebrun et al., 2006). The HP0421 protein adopts as the glucose source a uridine diphosphate-glucose (UDP-Glc) and catalyzes the dehydration condensation reaction between a 1α-hydroxyl (OH) group of D-glucose (Glc) molecule and a 3β-OH group of free-cholesterol (FC) molecule, and thereby CGL is synthesized. The other enzymes involved in the biosynthesis of CAG and CPG have still not been identified (Fig. 1).

Though it is almost special cases that bacterial species produce glucosyl sterols, plants and fungi universally produce various glucosyl sterols such as glucosyl sitosterol and glucosyl ergosterol (Kim et al., 2002; Oku et al., 2003; Peng et al., 2002; Warnecke et al., 1994, 1997, 1999). As with *Helicobacter pylori*, the bacterial species that produce glucosyl cholesterol have been only reported in *Borrelia hermsi*, *Acholeplasma axanthum*, *Spiroplasma* spp., and *Mycoplasma gallinarum* (Livermore et al., 1978; Mayberry & Smith, 1983; Patel et al., 1978; Smith, 1971). Recent studies have shown that *Borrelia burgdorferi*, *Borrelia garinii*, and *Borrelia afzelii* possess the galactosyl cholesterol that binds to the cholesterol a D-galactose as the sugar molecule in place of a D-glucose (Ben-Menachem et al., 2003; Schröder et al., 2003; Stübs et al., 2009). Plants and fungi carry out the biosynthesis of sterols by themselves, and thereafter attach a D-glucose molecule to the sterols biosynthesized via the catalytic action of sterol β-glucosyltransferase. In contrast, bacterial species including *Helicobacter pylori* do not have the anabolic pathway for cholesterol. Therefore, *Helicobacter pylori* must absorb free-cholesterol from the outside environments to biosynthesize glucosyl cholesterols. In addition, there is the structural difference between glucosyl cholesterols of *Helicobacter pylori* and the other glucosyl sterols. The D-glucose molecule in glucosyl cholesterols of *Helicobacter pylori* is attached to the cholesterol molecule with α-configuration, whereas the D-glucose molecule of phytogenic and fungal glucosyl sterols is attached to the sterol molecule with β-configuration. This structural difference is resulting from the enzymatic action catalyzing the binding of D-glucose into the sterol. In sum, the HP0421 protein of *Helicobacter pylori* catalyzes the α-glucosidic linkage between the 1α-OH group of D-glucose molecule and the 3β-OH group of free-cholesterol molecule, whereas the sterol β-glucosyltransferase of plants and fungi catalyzes the β-glucosidic linkage between the 1β-OH group of D-glucose molecule and the 3β-OH group of free-sterol molecule.

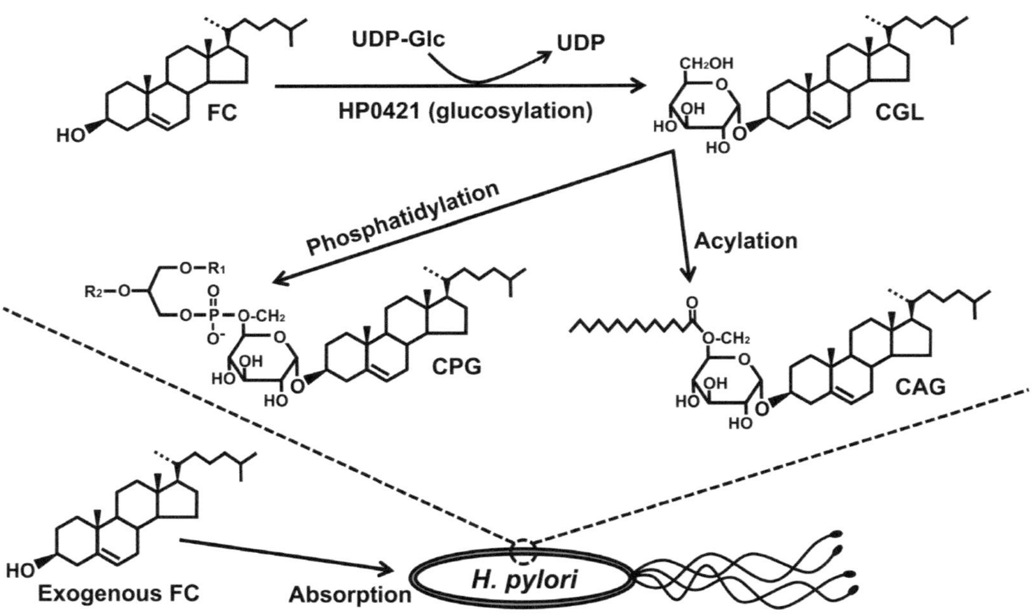

Fig. 1. The free-cholesterol (FC) assimilation of *Helicobacter pylori*

For many years, the biological significance of cholesterol glucosylation in *Helicobacter pylori* remained to be clarified. Recently, it has been, however, elucidated that *Helicobacter pylori* induces the glucosylation of free-cholesterol absorbed into the membranes to evade the host immune systems (Wunder et al., 2006). The HP0421 gene-knockout *Helicobacter pylori* mutant, which lacks the capability to biosynthesize the glucosyl cholesterols and retains free-cholesterol without glucosylation, easily succumbs to the phagocytosis of macrophages, and strongly induces the activation of antigen-specific T cells, compared to the wild type *Helicobacter pylori*. In addition, when the HP0421 gene-knockout mutant is inoculated into the mouse via oral administration, the organism is promptly excluded from the murine gastric epithelium. The abnormal wild type *Helicobacter pylori*, which fails to induce the biosynthesis of enough amount glucosyl cholesterols by artificial insertion of excessive free-cholesterol into the membranes, also succumbs to the phagocytosis of macrophages and induces the activation of antigen-specific T cells, to similar to the cases of HP0421 gene-knockout mutant. In contrast, the normal wild type *Helicobacter pylori* and the HP0421 gene-reconstructed organism resist the phagocytosis of macrophages, control the induction of antigen-specific T cell activation, and colonize longer periods onto the gastric epithelium of mouse. These findings indicate that the glucosylation of free-cholesterol absorbed into the membranes of *Helicobacter pylori* plays an important role in survival and colonization of the organism in host.

However, it remains to be clarified about why *Helicobacter pylori* aggressively absorbs exogenous free-cholesterol into the membranes. If *Helicobacter pylori*, as with the general bacterial species, did not absorb free-cholesterol into the membranes, the organism will not need to glucosylate it. In addition, free-cholesterol is rather harmful for the survival of *Helicobacter pylori*, because the organism possessing free-cholesterol without glucosylation strongly activates the macrophages and the antigen-specific T cells, and is eradicated from the gastric epithelium by inducing the host immune responses. Moreover, whether the free-cholesterol is the only sterol absorbed into the membranes of *Helicobacter pylori* is also unsolved. Our group, thus, assumed that the free-cholesterol (or steroid) absorption in *Helicobacter pylori* has other some physiological role to maintain the viability of the organism.

To elucidate these unsolved points, our group has initiated the investigations as to the capability of *Helicobacter pylori* to use steroid hormones. Steroid hormones, such as sex hormones and corticoids, are typical sterol analogues that are derived from free-cholesterol in mammals. A number of investigations have demonstrated that the enzymes involved in the biosynthesis and the activation of sex hormones are also expressed in human stomach tissue (Javitt et al., 2001; Miki et al., 2002; Takeyama et al., 2000; Turgeon et al., 2001). In addition, the expression of sex hormone receptors has been found in gastric cancer (Kominea et al., 2004; Matsuyama et al., 2002; Takano et al., 2002). These studies indirectly indicate that sex hormones exist in the human stomach environment. We know that *Helicobacter pylori* colonizes the human stomach. In sum, there is possibility that *Helicobacter pylori* has contact with sex hormones in the human stomach. No earlier studies, however, have investigated the assimilation of sex hormones in *Helicobacter pylori*, and/or the influence of sex hormones on the viability of the organism.

Based on the findings from our current basal research, this chapter summarizes the capability of *Helicobacter pylori* to assimilate various sex hormones, and the bactericidal activity of certain sex hormones targeting selectively the *Helicobacter pylori*.

2. The 3β-OH steroids and *Helicobacter pylori*

Of the steroid hormones including steroid pre-hormone, pregnenolone (PN), dehydroepiandrosterone (DEA), and epiandrosterone (EA) possess a hydroxyl group (3β-

OH) with β-configuration at the carbon-3 position of steroid framework, as with free-cholesterol (FC). First of all, our group has, therefore, examined the capability of *Helicobacter pylori* to assimilate the 3β-OH steroid hormones. After *Helicobacter pylori* (10^5 CFU, colony-forming unit/ml) was cultured for 24 hours with pregnenolone (50 μM concentration), dehydroepiandrosterone (50 μM concentration), or epiandrosterone (50 μM concentration) in a serum-free medium (10 ml) with continuous shaking under microaerobic conditions (an atmosphere of 5% O_2, 10% CO_2, and 85% N_2 at 37°C), the membrane lipids of the organisms were purified via the Folch method (Folch et al., 1957) and analyzed by thin-layer chromatography (TLC). This paragraph summarizes the assimilation of 3β-OH steroid hormones in *Helicobacter pylori*.

2.1 Pregnenolone and *Helicobacter pylori*

Though the structure at the carbon-17 position of pregnenolone framework differs from that at the same carbon position of free-cholesterol framework, the membranes of *Helicobacter pylori* aggressively absorbed the exogenous pregnenolone, and the organism induced the glucosylation of this 3β-OH steroid pre-hormone: the TLC analysis detected the three spots of glucosyl pregnenolones equivalent to the three spots of glucosyl cholesterols (CGL, CAG and CPG) in the membrane lipid compositions of *Helicobacter pylori* (Hosoda et al., 2009).

The recombinant HP0421 protein expressed in *Escherichia coli* has been shown to catalyze α-glucosylation of various phytogenic and fungal sterols (Lebrun et al., 2006). Moreover, *Helicobacter pylori* lacks the gene that encodes sterol β-glucosyltransferase in plants and fungi. Therefore, the glucosyl pregnenolones detected in the membrane lipid compositions of *Helicobacter pylori* are easily guessed to be all α-glucosyl pregnenolones. As with free-cholesterol (FC), the functional group to which a D-glucose molecule can be attached via the catalytic action of HP0421 protein is the only 3β-OH group in the pregnenolone (PN) framework (Fig. 2). The spot of glucosyl pregnenolone corresponding to the CGL spot detected in the TLC analysis must, in sum, be a 3β-(α-D-glucosyl)-pregnenolone. In addition, the spot of glucosyl pregnenolone corresponding to the CAG spot is guessed to be a 3β-(6-*O*-tetradecanoyl-α-D-glucosyl)-pregnenolone, and the spot of glucosyl pregnenolone corresponding to the CPG spot is guessed to be a 3β-(6-*O*-phosphatidyl-α-D-glucosyl)-pregnenolone.

2.2 Dehydroepiandrosterone and *Helicobacter pylori*

As with pregnenolone, the structure at the carbon-17 position of dehydroepiandrosterone framework also differs from that at the same carbon position of free-cholesterol framework. *Helicobacter pylori*, however, absorbed the exogenous dehydroepiandrosterone into the membranes and induced the glucosylation of this androgen. Though the TLC analysis detected the three spots of glucosyl dehydroepiandrosterones, the detection level of the glucosyl dehydroepiandrosterone corresponding to the CGL was remarkably lower than the detection levels of the other glucosyl dehydroepiandrosterones corresponding to the CAG and CPG.

Our previous study has demonstrated that the detection level of CGL, a basic structure of glucosyl cholesterols, in the membrane lipid compositions of *Helicobacter pylori* undergoing the long-term cultures reduces via the conversion to both CAG and CPG that are produced by modifying the CGL molecule with an acyl group and a phosphatidyl group, respectively, and thereby the detection levels of CAG and CPG increase in the membrane lipid compositions of organism (Shimomura et al., 2004). Our findings as to the assimilation of this androgen, in sum, suggest that *Helicobacter pylori* promptly converts the 3β-(α-D-glucosyl)-dehydroepiandrosterone, which is a fundamental structure of the glucosyl dehydroepiandrosterones, to those modified by an acyl group or a phosphatidyl group. However, the transferases that attach an acyl group or a phosphatidyl group to the CGL molecule have still not been identified in *Helicobacter pylori*. Investigations into the CGL acyltransferase and CGL phosphatidyltransferase will be, therefore, required to elucidate the anabolic pathway in glucosyl cholesterols and glucosyl steroid hormones.

2.3 Epiandrosterone and *Helicobacter pylori*

The only structural difference between dehydroepiandrosterone and epiandrosterone is in the part of double bond between the carbon-5 position and the carbon-6 position in the steroid molecule: dehydroepiandrosterone has the double bond between those carbon positions, while epiandrosterone lacks its double bond. The TLC analysis detected the three spots of glucosyl epiandrosterones in the membrane lipid compositions into which *Helicobacter pylori* assimilated this androgen, but the detection level of the glucosyl epiandrosterone corresponding to the CGL was remarkably lower than the detection levels of the other glucosyl epiandrosterones corresponding to the CAG and CPG, as with the case of dehydroepiandrosterone. These results also suggest that *Helicobacter pylori* promptly converts the 3β-(α-D-glucosyl)-epiandrosterone to those modified by an acyl group or a phosphatidyl group.

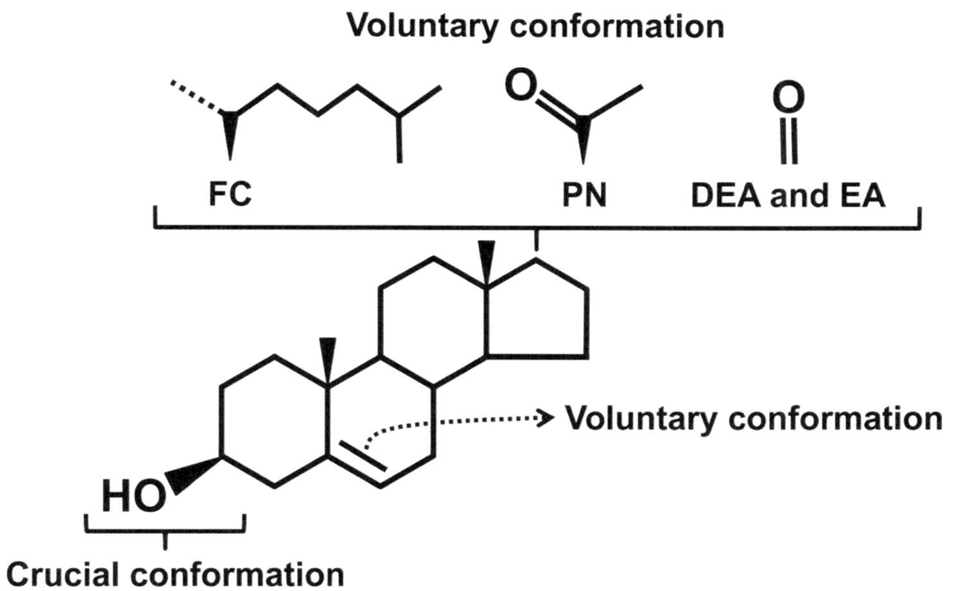

Fig. 2. The 3β-OH: a crucial conformation for steroid glucosylation by *Helicobacter pylori*

These findings from our recent study show that *Helicobacter pylori* glucosylates not only free-cholesterol, but also various 3β-OH steroid hormones. The only common structure among pregnenolone (PN), dehydroepiandrosterone (DEA), epiandrosterone (EA), and free-cholesterol (FC) is a 3β-OH group in the steroid framework (Fig. 2). This, thus, indicates that

the 3β-OH of steroids is a crucial conformation required for the steroid glucosylation by *Helicobacter pylori*. Further conformation analyses will be required to identify the chemical structures of glucosyl steroid hormones in more detail.
Our group has demonstrated the first report to describe the capability of *Helicobacter pylori* to glucosylate steroid hormones (Hosoda et al., 2009). In addition, no earlier studies have reported that the glucosyl sex hormones were detected in eukaryotes, prokaryotes, and/or environments. Further investigations will be necessary to analyze the hormonal actions or biological activities of these glucosyl sex hormones produced by *Helicobacter pylori*.

3. The 3-OH steroids and *Helicobacter pylori*

The three female hormones, namely, estrone (E1), estradiol (E2), and estriol (E3) possess a flat hydroxyl group (3-OH) at the carbon-3 position of the steroid framework. Our recent studies have revealed that these 3-OH steroid hormones have the different influences on the viability of *Helicobacter pylori*. This paragraph describes the relationship between the 3-OH steroid hormones and *Helicobacter pylori*.

3.1 Estrone and *Helicobacter pylori*

When *Helicobacter pylori* (10^5 CFU/ml) was cultured for 24 hours with estrone at the 50 μM concentration in a serum-free medium (10 ml) with continuous shaking under microaerobic conditions, the membranes of organism efficiently absorbed the estrone (Hosoda et al., 2009). These findings indicate that *Helicobacter pylori* aggressively uses as the membrane lipid components not only 3β-OH steroids (including free-cholesterol), but also 3-OH steroid estrone. However, the organism has failed to induce the glucosylation of estrone absorbed into the membranes. In combination with the results of glucosylation observed in the 3β-OH steroid hormones, they strongly indicate that *Helicobacter pylori* recognizes only the 3β-OH conformation of steroid molecule and glucosylates only the 3β-OH steroids with or without the other structural differences.

3.2 Estradiol and *Helicobacter pylori*

Our group has recently clarified the inhibitory effect of estradiol on the growth of *Helicobacter pylori*. When *Helicobacter pylori* (10^5 CFU/ml) was cultured for 24 hours with estradiol at the 50 and 100 μM concentrations in a serum-free medium (3 ml) with continuous shaking under microaerobic conditions, the estradiol at these concentrations made the division and proliferation of *Helicobacter pylori* stagnate: the levels of colony-forming unit (CFU), which indicates the number of living bacterial cells in the meaning of the wide sense, at that time maintained the baseline CFU level (10^5 CFU/ml) immediately after the culture initiation (Hosoda et al., 2011). Estradiol has been, in sum, found to exhibit the bacteriostatic action to *Helicobacter pylori*. This estrogen seems to act to *Helicobacter pylori* by attaching to the cell surface of the organism, since it is contained in the membrane lipids purified from the *Helicobacter pylori* incubated in the presence of estradiol. Incidentally, estrone has no influence on the growth of *Helicobacter pylori*, and the proliferation capability of the organism even in the presence of estrone at the 100 μM concentration is comparable to that of the organism in the absence of its estrogen.
Earlier investigations (including our own) have shown that *Helicobacter pylori* morphologically converts from a bacillary form to a coccoid form when the organism

exposed to various stresses such as excessive oxygen, alkaline pH, or long-term culture (Benaïssa et al., 1996; Catrenich & Makin, 1991; Donelli et al., 1998; Shimomura et al., 2004). For many years, there is a controversy as to whether the coccoid-converted *Helicobacter pylori* cells are maintaining a viable state. Cells that had changed to a coccoid form lack the ability to form colonies on an agar plate, which it makes very difficult to accurately determine the CFU in coccoid-converted *Helicobacter pylori*. Our group has, therefore, examined whether estradiol confers the bacteriostatic action to *Helicobacter pylori* by promoting the induction of coccoid-conversion in the bacterial cells. Though the cell morphologies of *Helicobacter pylori* were observed with a differential interference microscope after the organisms (10^5 CFU/ml) were incubated for 24 hours with estradiol at the 100 μM concentration in a serum-free medium (3 ml) with continuous shaking under microaerobic conditions, the coccoid *Helicobacter pylori* cells were unobserved. This indicates that estradiol inhibits the proliferation of *Helicobacter pylori* via a certain bacteriostatic mechanism but not the induction of coccoid-conversion against the bacterial cells.

Epidemiological studies and animal models have suggested that female hormones, particularly estrogens, play a protective role in gastric cancer (Campbell-Thompson et al., 1999; Freedman et al., 2007; Furukawa et al., 1982; Ketkar et al., 1978; Sipponen & Correa, 2002). *Helicobacter pylori* infection is also one of the risk factors in developing of gastric cancer in humans. Recent study by others has demonstrated that estradiol somehow protects against the development of *Helicobacter pylori*-induced gastric cancer in a mouse model (Ohtani et al., 2007). The bacteriostatic action of estradiol may play some role in mechanisms preventing the development of *Helicobacter pylori*-induced gastric cancer. Further investigations will be necessary to elucidate the relationship between estradiol and *Helicobacter pylori in vivo*.

3.3 Estriol and *Helicobacter pylori*

When *Helicobacter pylori* (10^5 CFU/ml) was cultured for 24 hours with estriol at the 50 and 100 μM concentrations in a serum-free medium (10 ml) with continuous shaking under microaerobic conditions, estriol had no influence on the growth of *Helicobacter pylori*, and the CFU levels of the organism cultured in the presence of estriol (both 50 μM and 100 μM) were comparable to the control CFU level (10^8 CFU/ml) of the organism cultured in the absence of estriol. In addition, this estrogen was undetectable in the membrane lipid compositions of the organism in the TLC analysis. *Helicobacter pylori* has, thus, failed to use as the membrane lipid component estriol.

4. Membrane distribution of steroids assimilated by *Helicobacter pylori*

In general, Gram-negative bacteria including *Helicobacter pylori* have two membranes that are composed of the phospholipid bilayer, namely an inner membrane and an outer membrane. The phospholipid components constituting both the inner and outer membranes are phosphatidylethanolamine, phosphatidylglycerol and cardiolipin. The outside lipid layer of the outer membrane also contains as the major glycolipid component a lipopolysaccharide (LPS) (Rietschel et al., 1994). LPS is composed of an *O*-polysaccharide chain, an outer core saccharide, an inner core saccharide, and a lipid A regions. The lipid A is composed of two phosphorylated glucosamine molecules linked by β (1→6)-glycosidic bond and plural fatty acid molecules (5 to 7 molecules) attached to the glucosamine molecules, and is buried in the outside lipid layer of the outer membrane. Meanwhile, the *O*-polysaccharide chain region has direct contact with the outside of the bacterial cells and maintains the membrane permeability against exogenous lipophilic compounds. The outer core saccharide and the inner core saccharide regions are located between *O*-polysaccharide chain region and lipid A region.

In addition to LPS, *Helicobacter pylori* retains the glucosyl cholesterols (CGL, CAG and CPG) as another glycolipid components into the membranes when the organism assimilated exogenous free-cholesterol. Our previous study has demonstrated that the percentage of total glucosyl cholesterols is greater than 20% in the total lipids (except for LPS) composing the *Helicobacter pylori* membranes (Shimomura et al., 2004). Glycerophospholipids, such as phosphatidylethanolamine and phosphatidylglycerol, have been known in Gram-negative bacteria to be in both the inner membrane and the outer membrane. No earlier reports have, however, investigated the localization of glucosyl cholesterols (CGL, CAG and CPG) in *Helicobacter pylori* membranes.

To elucidate the membrane distribution of glucosyl cholesterols in *Helicobacter pylori*, we have divided the two membranes into the inner membrane fraction and the outer membrane fraction via sucrose-gradient centrifugation method, purified the lipids from each membrane fraction by the Folch method, and analyzed the lipid compositions obtained from these membrane fractions by thin-layer chromatography (TLC) (Shimomura et al., 2009). The TLC analysis detected the spot of free-cholesterol itself at a similar density in both the inner membrane fraction and the outer membrane fraction obtained from *Helicobacter pylori* ingested free-cholesterol from the medium. In contrast, the glucosyl cholesterols (CGL, CAG and CPG) produced via the absorption of free-cholesterol were detected at clearly higher levels in the outer membrane fraction than in the inner membrane fraction. In sum, the steroid itself was distributed into both the inner membrane and the outer membrane, whereas the glucosyl steroids were distributed into the outer membrane rather than into the inner membrane. We have also fractionated the inner membrane and the outer membrane of *Helicobacter pylori* that was cultured in the presence of estrone, and analyzed the lipids purified from each membrane fraction by TLC. As with the free-cholesterol itself, the spot of estrone absorbed by *Helicobacter pylori* was also detected at a similar density in both the outer and inner membrane fractions.

These findings indicate that *Helicobacter pylori* assimilates exogenous steroids into the outer and inner membranes and uses the glucosylated steroids as major lipid components constituting the outer membrane. This membrane distribution of steroids also suggests a possibility that *Helicobacter pylori* possesses a certain membrane transport system for the steroids: the steroids absorbed into *Helicobacter pylori* are shifted from the outer membrane to the inner membrane, and thereafter, the steroids glucosylated in the inner membrane are transported to the outer membrane. There is, however, no evidence that HP0421 protein catalyzing the α-glucosylation of steroids is distributed into the inner membrane of *Helicobacter pylori*. Therefore, it is important to ascertain the localization of HP0421 protein in the *Helicobacter pylori* membranes. In addition, further investigations will be necessary to clarify whether *Helicobacter pylori* possesses such a steroidal membrane transport system.

5. The physiological role of steroid assimilation in *Helicobacter pylori*

Though *Helicobacter pylori* aggressively assimilates various exogenous steroids into the membrane lipid compositions, the organism divides and proliferates even in the absence of steroids as well as the other bacterial species that have no ability to assimilate the exogenous steroids into the membranes. Our recent study has elucidated why *Helicobacter pylori*

physiologically requires steroids to survive (Shimomura et al., 2009). This paragraph describes an importance of steroid assimilation in maintaining the viability of *Helicobacter pylori*.
Phosphatidylcholine, the most prevalent phospholipid in mammals, is much higher in concentration than free-cholesterol in the blood plasma of humans; phosphatidylcholine exists at a concentration of approximately 144 mg/dl, whereas free-cholesterol exists at a concentration of approximately 60 mg/dl. The fundamental chemical structure of phosphatidylcholine is 1,2-diacyl-*sn*-glycero-3-phosphocholine (Fig. 3). In general, the carbon-1 (C1) position in the glycerol backbone of phosphatidylcholine carries a saturated fatty acid such as palmitic acid ($C_{16:0}$) or stearic acid ($C_{18:0}$), whereas the carbon-2 (C2) position in the glycerol backbone carries an unsaturated fatty acid such as oleic acid ($C_{18:1}$), linoleic acid ($C_{18:2}$), or arachidonic acid ($C_{20:4}$). Lyso-phosphatidylcholine (LPC) is a monoacyl-type phosphatidylcholine and generally lacks an unsaturated fatty acid at the carbon-2 (C2) position of the glycerol backbone. A number of investigations have demonstrated that unsaturated fatty acids and lyso-phosphatidylcholines have the potential to kill various microorganisms including *Helicobacter pylori* (Bruyn et al., 1996; Conley & Kabara, 1973; Constance et al., 1992; Kabara et al., 1972; Kanai & Kondo, 1979; Kanetsuna, 1985; Knapp & Melly, 1986; Kondo & Kanai, 1985; Nieman, 1954; Steel et al., 2002; Thompson et al., 1994). Thus, these individual lipophilic compounds constituting phosphatidylcholine act as antimicrobial agents against the various microorganisms. It remains unclear, however, whether the phosphatidylcholine itself also confers an antimicrobial action against the microorganisms.

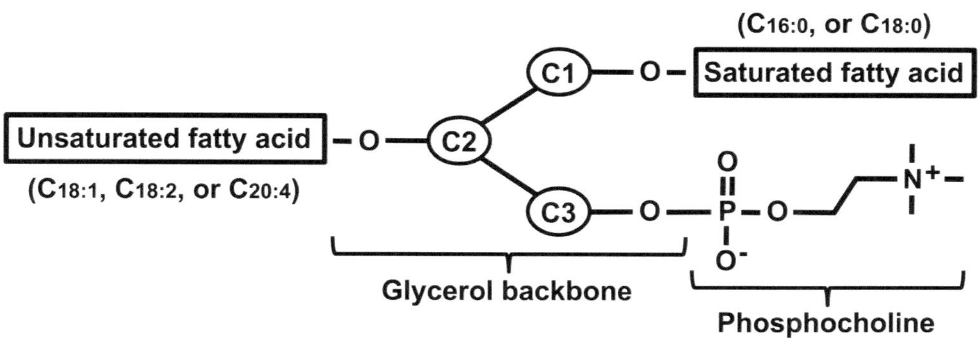

Fig. 3. The fundamental chemical structure of phosphatidylcholine

A previous study by others has shown that the concentration of phosphatidylcholine is 124.8 ± 62.6 μM in gastric juice from eight healthy volunteers (Berstad et al., 1992). We know that *Helicobacter pylori* colonizes the human gastric epithelium. In sum, this study indicates that *Helicobacter pylori* is surrounded by phosphatidylcholine *in vivo*. If phosphatidylcholine itself affects the survival of *Helicobacter pylori* that has failed to assimilate exogenous steroids such as free-cholesterol or steroid hormones, it may explain the importance of steroid assimilation in the organism. We have, therefore, investigated the antibacterial activity of phosphatidylcholine itself against *Helicobacter pylori* (Shimomura et al., 2009).

5.1 Antibacterial effects of phosphatidylcholine variants on the steroid-free *Helicobacter pylori*

When the steroid-free *Helicobacter pylori* (10^7 CFU/ml) that has no steroid in the membrane lipid compositions was incubated for 24 hours with various phosphatidylcholine variants carrying different fatty acid molecules at the carbon-2 position of the glycerol backbone in a serum-free medium (3 ml) with continuous shaking under microaerobic conditions, the phosphatidylcholine variants attaching either a linoleic acid ($C_{18:2}$) molecule or an arachidonic acid ($C_{20:4}$) molecule to the carbon-2 (C2) position in the glycerol backbone conferred an antibacterial action fatal to the steroid-free *Helicobacter pylori*. In contrast, the phosphatidylcholine variants attaching either an oleic acid ($C_{18:1}$) molecule or a palmitic acid ($C_{16:0}$) molecule to the carbon-2 (C2) position in the glycerol backbone had no influence on the viability of *Helicobacter pylori*.

To ascertain the antibacterial potencies of phosphatidylcholine-themselves, we have also investigated the antibacterial activity of compositional constituents of the two phosphatidylcholines that exhibited the anti-*Helicobacter pylori* action, a linoleic acid ($C_{18:2}$), an arachidonic acid ($C_{20:4}$), and a LPC (1-palmitoyl-*sn*-glycero-3-phosphocholine). When the steroid-free *Helicobacter pylori* (10^7 CFU/ml) was incubated for 24 hours with linoleic acid (10 μg/ml), arachidonic acid (10 μg/ml), or LPC (10 μg/ml) in the serum-free medium (3 ml) containing a 0.2% dMβCD (2,6-di-*O*-methyl-β-cyclodextrin) with continuous shaking under microaerobic conditions, the two fatty acids and LPC had no influence on the viability of the steroid-free organism. The dMβCD has, thus, completely counteracted the antibacterial action of these lipophilic compounds against the steroid-free *Helicobacter pylori*. Incidentally, the linoleic acid (10 μg/ml), arachidonic acid (10 μg/ml), and LPC (10 μg/ml) in the absence of dMβCD confer the antibacterial action fatal to the steroid-free *Helicobacter pylori*. Intriguingly, the dMβCD had no influence on the anti-*Helicobacter pylori* action of the phosphatidylcholine variants carrying either a linoleic acid molecule or an arachidonic acid molecule at the carbon-2 position of the glycerol backbone, and these two phosphatidylcholine variants (concentrations ranging from 10 μg/ml to 100 μg/ml) conferred the bactericidal action to the steroid-free *Helicobacter pylori* even in the presence of the 0.2% dMβCD, as with had being done in the absence of dMβCD.

The dMβCD is a cyclic oligomer consisting of seven 2,6-di-*O*-methyl-α-D-glucose molecules linked by α (1→4)-glycosidic bonds and has the ability to solubilize lipophilic compounds through the formation of molecular inclusion complexes (Ohtani et al., 1989). To examine whether dMβCD inhibits the adsorption of unsaturated fatty acids, or phosphatidylcholines onto the steroid-free *Helicobacter pylori* cells, we carried out the following experiments. The heat-killed *Helicobacter pylori* cells that have no steroid in the membranes were incubated for 24 hours with a linoleic acid (100 μg/ml), an arachidonic acid (100 μg/ml), or phosphatidylcholine variants (100 μg/ml), to which either a linoleic acid molecule or an arachidonic acid molecule is attached as the acyl group, in the serum-free medium containing a 0.2% dMβCD with continuous shaking at 37°C, and thereafter the membrane lipids were purified from the heat-killed cells recovered via the Folch method and analyzed by TLC. The membrane lipids obtained from the heat-killed cells incubated in the absence of dMβCD contained tremendous amounts of linoleic acid and arachidonic acid, whereas the membrane lipids obtained from the heat-killed cells incubated in the presence of dMβCD (0.2%) contained negligible amounts of those fatty acids. Surprisingly, the phosphatidylcholines contained in the membrane lipids of the heat-killed cells incubated in the presence of dMβCD (0.2%) were larger amount than those contained in the membrane lipids of the heat-killed cells incubated in the absence of dMβCD. In sum, dMβCD has inhibited the binding of the unsaturated fatty acids to the membranes of *Helicobacter pylori* but promoted the binding of the phosphatidylcholines to the membranes of the organism.

These results indicate that dMβCD obstructs the hydrophobic interaction between the unsaturated fatty acids and the *Helicobacter pylori* membranes by solubilizing those fatty acids, and thereby protects the organism from the bactericidal action of the unsaturated fatty acids, and probably LPC (Fig. 4). It is unclear why dMβCD promotes the adsorption of the two phosphatidylcholines onto the *Helicobacter pylori* membranes. These findings, however, indicate that the anti-*Helicobacter pylori* action originates in the potencies of phosphatidylcholine-themselves and that the unsaturated fatty acids (linoleic acid and arachidonic acid), and the LPC (1-palmitoyl-*sn*-glycero-3-phosphocholine), which result from the hydrolysis of the phosphatidylcholines, do not contribute to this action. We have, thus, elucidated the bactericidal activity of phosphatidylcholine (PC) variants carrying either a linoleic acid molecule or an arachidonic acid molecule at the carbon-2 position of the glycerol backbone against the steroid-free *Helicobacter pylori*.

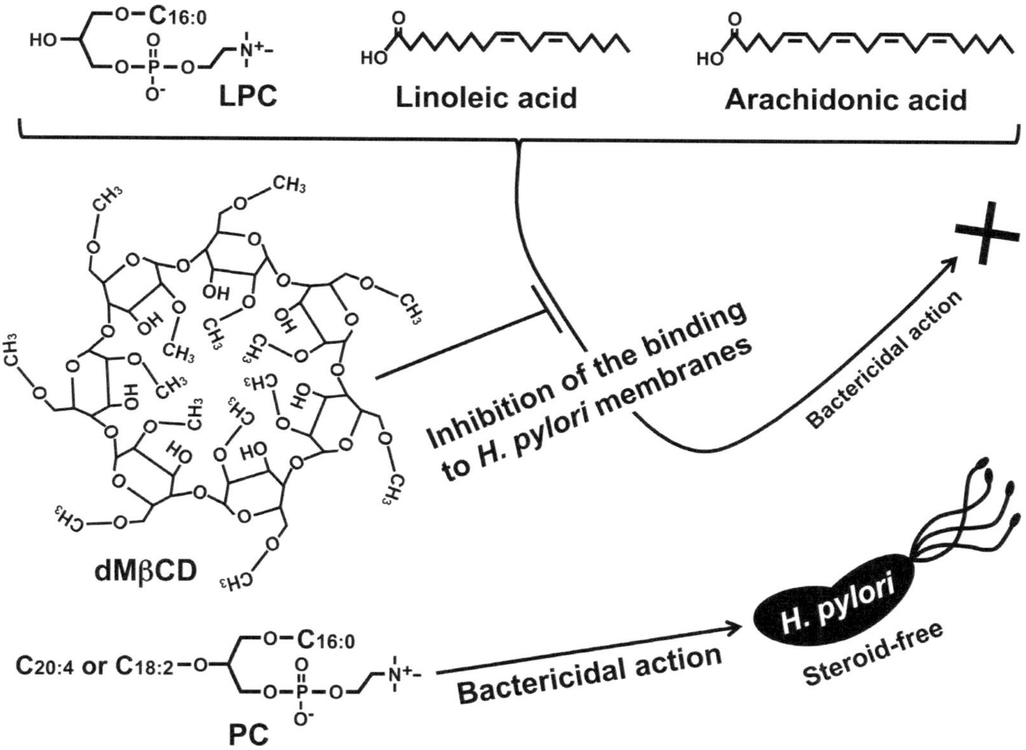

Fig. 4. The role of 2,6-di-*O*-methyl-β-cyclodextrin (dMβCD) on the anti-*Helicobacter pylori* action of lipophilic compounds

5.2 Bacteriolysis in the steroid-free *Helicobacter pylori* caused by the cell adsorption of phosphatidylcholines

To examine the antibacterial mechanism of phosphatidylcholine variants carrying either a linoleic acid molecule or an arachidonic acid molecule at the carbon-2 position of the glycerol backbone, we performed the following experiments. After the steroid-free *Helicobacter pylori* (10^8 CFU/ml) was incubated for 8 hours with each phosphatidylcholine

(100 μg/ml) in a serum-free medium (3 ml) with continuous shaking under microaerobic conditions, the supernatant recovered was subjected to the purification of proteins by an anion-exchange chromatography, and the proteins purified were analyzed by a sodium dodecyl sulfate-polyacrylamide gel electrophoresis (SDS-PAGE). A number of protein bands with tremendous high densities were detected in the supernatant obtained from the steroid-free *Helicobacter pylori* incubated with the phosphatidylcholines, in the SDS-PAGE analysis. Among those protein bands detected, the band for flavodoxin (FldA) protein was also contained. As FldA is an electron acceptor of the oxidoreductase that catalyzes acetyl-CoA synthesis in *Helicobacter pylori* cell (Hughes et al., 1995), we can assume that FldA is the intracellular protein. These results, in sum, indicate that the phosphatidylcholine variants attaching either a linoleic acid or an arachidonic acid as the acyl group to the carbon-2 position in the glycerol backbone exert deleterious effect on the cell membranes of steroid-free *Helicobacter pylori* and induce the bacterial cell lysis, resulting in abundant leakage of intracellular proteins (especially FldA protein) to outside of the bacterial cells. Incidentally, the SDS-PAGE analysis detected only negligible amount of proteins in the supernatant obtained from the steroid-free *Helicobacter pylori* incubated without either the phosphatidylcholines.

5.3 Acquirement of phosphatidylcholine resistance in *Helicobacter pylori* conferred by assimilating steroid

We next investigated whether the *Helicobacter pylori* with the assimilated steroid succumbs to the bactericidal action of the phosphatidylcholines, as with the steroid-free organism. When the steroid-free *Helicobacter pylori* is cultured for 24 hours in the serum-free medium containing free-cholesterol (50 μM concentration) with continuous shaking under microaerobic conditions, the organism recovered retains both free-cholesterol itself and glucosyl cholesterols (CGL, CAG and CPG) in the membranes. We, therefore, examined the anti-*Helicobacter pylori* action of the two phosphatidylcholine variants possessing the antibacterial action fatal to the steroid-free *Helicobacter pylori* by using the organism retaining the assimilated free-cholesterol that was prepared via the above culture procedure. When *Helicobacter pylori* (10^7 CFU/ml) with the assimilated free-cholesterol was incubated at various time points in a serum-free medium (3 ml) with shaking under microaerobic conditions in the presence or absence of each phosphatidylcholine (100 μg/ml), which carries either a linoleic acid molecule or an arachidonic acid molecule at the carbon-2 position of the glycerol backbone, the *Helicobacter pylori* did not succumb to the antibacterial effects of the two phosphatidylcholine variants: the time-dependent growth-decline curve of *Helicobacter pylori* with each phosphatidylcholine roughly corresponded to the time-dependent growth-decline curve of the organism without either the two phosphatidylcholines, when the CFU values ($\log_{10}$ CFU/ml: vertical axis) and the incubation times (hour: horizontal axis) were plotted in a graph. *Helicobacter pylori* that had assimilated free-cholesterol (FC) has been, thus, found to resist the bactericidal action of phosphatidylcholine variants carrying either a linoleic acid molecule or an arachidonic acid molecule at the carbon-2 position of the glycerol backbone.

As described above, *Helicobacter pylori* retains free-cholesterol in the form of glucosyl cholesterols (CGL, CAG and CPG). This raises the question as to whether the glucosyl cholesterols are more important rather than the free-cholesterol itself in the expression of phosphatidylcholine resistance in *Helicobacter pylori*. To resolve this question, we examined

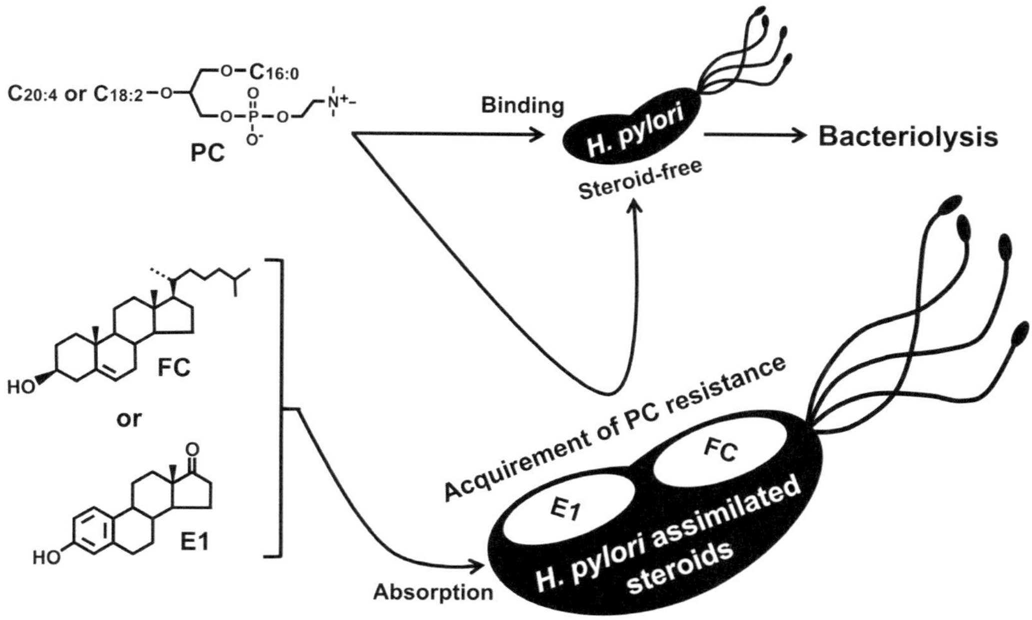

Fig. 5. The expression of phosphatidylcholine (PC) resistance in *Helicobacter pylori* with the assimilated steroids

the phosphatidylcholine resistance in *Helicobacter pylori* with another assimilated steroid. We have shown that *Helicobacter pylori* efficiently absorbs and retains the female hormone estrone into the membranes, but fails to glucosylate the estrogen (Hosoda et al., 2009). In addition, we have also found that other female hormone estriol is not absorbed into the membranes of *Helicobacter pylori*. Therefore, we decided to use estrone and estriol as steroid tools that are not glucosylated by *Helicobacter pylori*. After the steroid-free *Helicobacter pylori* was cultured for 24 hours with estrone (50 μM concentration) in a serum-free medium with continuous shaking under microaerobic conditions, the recovered organism (10^7 CFU/ml) that had assimilated estrone without glucosylation in the membranes was incubated for further 24 hours with each phosphatidylcholine (100 μg/ml), which carries either a linoleic acid molecule or an arachidonic acid molecule at the carbon-2 position of the glycerol backbone, in a serum-free medium (3 ml) with continuous shaking under the same conditions. As with the *Helicobacter pylori* that assimilated free-cholesterol into the membranes, the organism with the assimilated estrone also resisted the bactericidal action of the two phosphatidylcholine variants, and the CFU was maintained to a high level ($> 10^6$ CFU/ml) comparable to the control CFU (10^7 CFU/ml) of *Helicobacter pylori* incubated for 24 hours without either the phosphatidylcholines. *Helicobacter pylori* has, in sum, expressed phosphatidylcholine resistance even when assimilated estrone (E1) without glucosylating it. In addition, this finding indicates that the glucosylation of steroid is so far not important in conferring resistance to the bactericidal action of phosphatidylcholine upon *Helicobacter pylori*, although the glucosylation of steroid is essential for *Helicobacter pylori* to evade the host immune systems. In contrast, the *Helicobacter pylori* treated for 24 hours with estriol (50 μM concentration) succumbed to the bactericidal action of the two phosphatidylcholine variants as with the steroid-free organism, and the CFU level reduced from 10^7 CFU/ml to <

10^3 CFU/ml, when the estriol-treated organism was incubated for 24 hours in the serum-free medium containing the respective phosphatidylcholine variants (100 μg/ml) to which either a linoleic acid or an arachidonic acid is attached as the acyl group. These results, together with our findings on the free-cholesterol assimilation in *Helicobacter pylori*, indicate that bacteria of this species acquire a resistance against the bacteriolytic activity of phosphatidylcholine by assimilating the exogenous steroids into the membranes (Fig. 5).
Phosphatidylcholine is not a single molecule, but a family of variants with different fatty acid compositions attached to the glycerol backbone of the phosphatidylcholine (Fig. 3). The predominant phosphatidylcholine in human serum has been known to carry a palmitic acid ($C_{16:0}$) molecule and a linoleic acid ($C_{18:2}$) molecule, and recently, the predominant phosphatidylcholine in the human gastric mucus has also been shown to carry the same two fatty acids (Orihara et al., 2001). One of the two phosphatidylcholines investigated as to the anti-*Helicobacter pylori* effect by our group is exactly its variant carrying a palmitic acid molecule and a linoleic acid molecule: 2-linoleoyl-1-palmitoyl-*sn*-3-phosphocholine. In sum, the phosphatidylcholine attaching a palmitic acid and a linoleic acid to the carbon-1 position and to the carbon-2 position in the glycerol backbone is the most prevalent phosphatidylcholine in humans. *Helicobacter pylori* colonizes the human gastric epithelium and inhabits the human stomach for many years. On this basis, we can assume that *Helicobacter pylori* is constantly exposed to various phosphatidylcholine variants, particularly the phosphatidylcholine carrying a palmitic acid molecule and a linoleic acid molecule. Our recent study, in sum, indicates that the steroid assimilation in *Helicobacter pylori* plays an important role in reinforcing the membrane lipid barrier and conferring resistance to the bacteriolytic action of hydrophobic compounds such as phosphatidylcholine.

6. The 3=O steroids and *Helicobacter pylori*

Testosterone, androstenedione and progesterone possess an oxo (3=O) group at the carbon-3 position of the steroid framework. Our recent studies have revealed that *Helicobacter pylori* cannot use as the membrane lipid components these 3=O steroids and rather succumbs to the antibacterial action of certain 3=O steroids. This paragraph describes the 3=O steroids as bactericidal agents to *Helicobacter pylori*.

6.1 Testosterone and *Helicobacter pylori*

Like estriol, testosterone also was not utilized as the membrane lipid component of *Helicobacter pylori*: the TLC analysis did not detect testosterone in the membrane lipid compositions of *Helicobacter pylori* cultured for 24 hours with this androgen at the 50 μM concentration (Hosoda et al., 2009). Testosterone did not, therefore, contribute to the phosphatidylcholine resistance upon *Helicobacter pylori* (Shimomura et al., 2009). In addition, this 3=O steroid at the 50 μM concentration hardly affected the growth of *Helicobacter pylori*.

6.2 Androstenedione and *Helicobacter pylori*

When *Helicobacter pylori* (10^5 CFU/ml) was cultured for 24 hours in the serum-free medium (3 ml) containing androstenedione at concentrations ranging from 10 to 100 μM with continuous shaking under microaerobic conditions, this 3=O steroid exhibited inhibitory effect on the growth of *Helicobacter pylori* at concentrations grater than 50 μM. Androstenedione was, however, relatively low potency in inhibiting the growth of *Helicobacter pylori*. The decrease in CFU (10^4 CFU/ml) of *Helicobacter pylori* cultured with androstenedione at the 100 μM concentration was slight compared to the baseline CFU (10^5 CFU/ml) immediately after the culture initiation (Hosoda et al., 2011).

6.3 Progesterone and *Helicobacter pylori*

Of the three 3=O steroid hormones (testosterone, androstenedione, and progesterone) investigated, the progesterone has demonstrated the most effective anti-*Helicobacter pylori* action. Progesterone efficiently inhibited the growth of *Helicobacter pylori* by a manner dependent on the greater doses added into the medium, and the CFU of the organism in the presence of progesterone at the 100 μM concentration was below the limits of detection (< 10 CFU/ml), when *Helicobacter pylori* (10^6 CFU/ml) was cultured for 24 hours in the serum-free medium (3 ml) containing progesterone at concentrations ranging from 10 to 100 μM with continuous shaking under microaerobic conditions (Hosoda et al., 2011).

6.4 Progesterone derivatives and *Helicobacter pylori*

We have discovered the effective anti-*Helicobacter pylori* action of progesterone. Progesterone has at least two derivatives, namely, 17α-hydroxyprogesterone and 17α-hydroxyprogesterone caproate. The derivatives, 17α-hydroxyprogesterone and 17α-hydroxyprogesterone caproate are modified by a hydroxyl group and an acyl group (caproic acid), respectively, at the carbon-17 position of the progesterone framework. 17α-hydroxylprogesterone is a natural progesterone derivative, while 17α-hydroxyprogesterone caproate is a synthetic progesterone derivative. Noting this, we have examined the anti-*Helicobacter pylori* action of these progesterone derivatives. When *Helicobacter pylori* (10^6 CFU/ml) was cultured for 24 hours in a serum-free medium (3 ml) containing 17α-hydroxyprogesterone with continuous shaking under microaerobic conditions, surprisingly, this natural progesterone derivative had no influence on the growth of *Helicobacter pylori*: even in the presence of 17α-hydroxyprogesterone at the 100 μM concentration, the CFU was comparable to the control CFU (10^8 CFU/ml) of *Helicobacter pylori* cultured for 24 hours without steroid. In contrast, 17α-hydroxyprogesterone caproate had a stronger anti-*Helicobacter pylori* action than progesterone, and the CFU was below the limits of detection (< 10 CFU/ml), when the organism (10^6 CFU/ml) was cultured for 24 hours with 17α-hydroxyprogesterone caproate at the 10 μM concentration in a serum-free medium with continuous shaking under microaerobic conditions. Incidentally, caproic acid ($C_{6:0}$), a constituent of 17α-hydroxyprogesterone caproate, did not affect the viability of *Helicobacter pylori* even when added into the bacterial cell suspension at a 100 μM concentration (Hosoda et al., 2011). These findings suggest that the acylation at the carbon-17 position in the progesterone framework plays an important role in reinforcing the anti-*Helicobacter pylori* action of progesterone.

6.5 Antibacterial effects of progesterone and its derivative on *Helicobacter pylori*

To ascertain the antibacterial potencies of progesterone and 17α-hydroxyprogesterone caproate, we investigated the time-dependent antibacterial effects of these two gestagens on *Helicobacter pylori* (Fig. 6A). When *Helicobacter pylori* (approximately 10^7 CFU/ml) was incubated with progesterone (100 μM) or 17α-hydroxyprogesterone caproate (100 μM) in a serum-free medium (3 ml) at various time points with shaking under microaerobic conditions, the CFUs of the organism incubated with progesterone (PS) moved along a

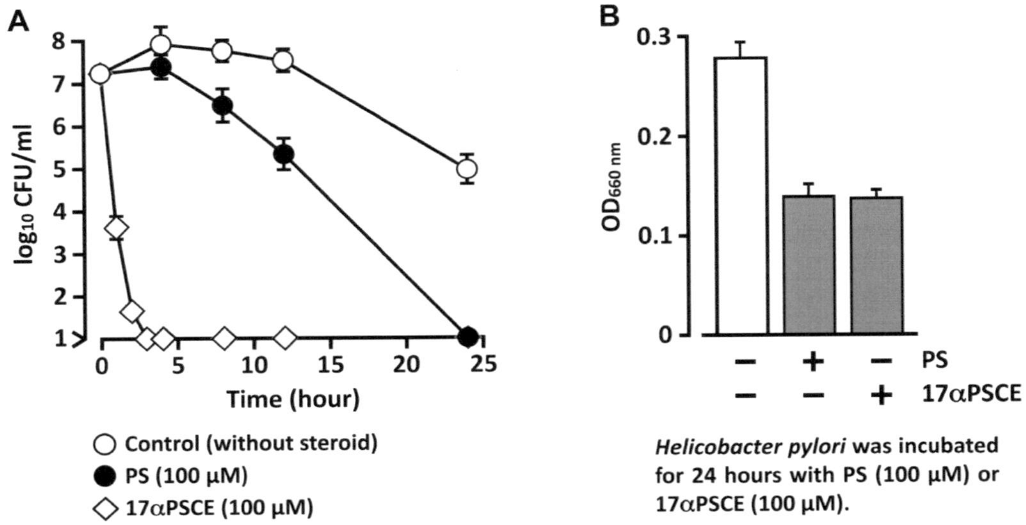

Fig. 6. Antibacterial effects of progesterone (PS) and 17α-hydroxyprogesterone caproate (17αPSCE) on *Helicobacter pylori*

gently-sloping curve, falling below the limits of detection (< 10 CFU/ml) by 24 hours after the start of incubation. In contrast, the CFUs of *Helicobacter pylori* incubated with 17α-hydroxyprogesterone caproate (17αPSCE) dropped off sharply, falling the limits of detection within 4 hours after the start of incubation. In sum, 17α-hydroxyprogesterone caproate (17αPSCE) has been found to be much more prompt in conferring the antibacterial action fatal to *Helicobacter pylori* than progesterone (PS).

6.6 Bacteriolysis in *Helicobacter pylori* caused by the cell surface binding of progesterone and its derivative

To clarify the antibacterial mechanism of progesterone and 17α-hydroxyprogesterone caproate against *Helicobacter pylori*, we measured an optical density ($OD_{660\ nm}$) in the bacterial cell suspensions after *Helicobacter pylori* (10^8 CFU/ml) was incubated for 24 hours with progesterone (100 μM) or 17α-hydroxyprogesterone caproate (100 μM) in a serum-free medium (3 ml) with continuous shaking under microaerobic conditions. The decline of $OD_{660\ nm}$ means that the bacterial cells in suspension had been lysed via certain physical or chemical actions. As it turned out, the $OD_{660\ nm}$ of the bacterial cell suspension incubated with progesterone or 17α-hydroxyprogesterone caproate declined to half value of that of the control cell suspension of *Helicobacter pylori* incubated for 24 hours in the absence of steroid (Fig. 6B).

To confirm the cell lysis of *Helicobacter pylori*, we examined the bacterial morphologies using a differential interference microscope (Fig. 7). When *Helicobacter pylori* (10^7 CFU/ml) was incubated for 24 hours in a serum-free medium in the presence or absence of the two 3=O steroids, the control cell suspension of *Helicobacter pylori* incubated without the steroids harbored the organisms in both mixed rod and coccoid forms. In contrast, the cell suspension of the *Helicobacter pylori* incubated with progesterone (100 μM) or 17α-hydroxyprogesterone caproate (100 μM) harbored hardly any organisms, although objects such as cellular debris were observed. These results, together with the findings from the measurement of $OD_{660\,nm}$ in the bacterial cell suspension, suggest that *Helicobacter pylori* cells are lysed by a certain action of progesterone (PS) and 17α-hydroxyprogesterone caproate (17αPSCE).

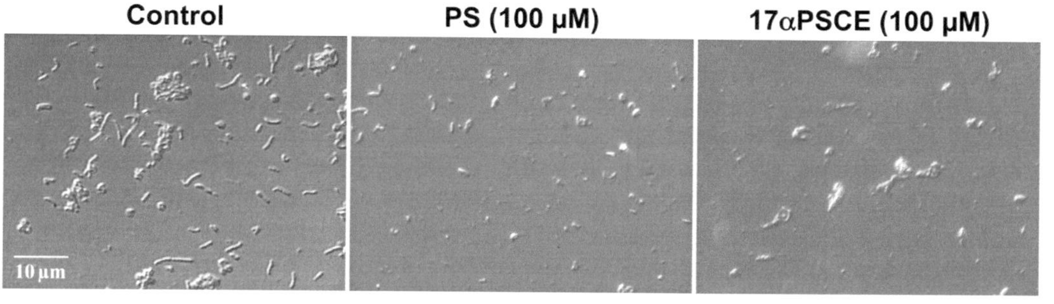

Fig. 7. Cell lysis on *Helicobacter pylori* induced by progesterone (PS) and 17α-hydroxyprogesterone caproate (17αPSCE)

Next, we carried out a series of experiments to examine whether progesterone and 17α-hydroxyprogesterone caproate induce the cell lysis of *Helicobacter pylori* via membrane injury. After *Helicobacter pylori* (10^9 CFU/ml) was incubated for 5 hours with progesterone (100 μM) or 17α-hydroxyprogesterone caproate (100 μM) using phosphate-buffered saline (PBS: 10 ml), in place of the serum-free medium, with continuous shaking under microaerobic conditions, the proteins in the bacterial cell supernatant were analyzed by SDS-PAGE. The protein bands detected in the cell supernatant of *Helicobacter pylori* incubated with progesterone or 17α-hydroxyprogesterone caproate were considerably denser than the protein bands detected in the control cell supernatant of *Helicobacter pylori* incubated for 5 hours without steroid. A band for flavodoxin (FldA), an intracellular protein, was also found among the other protein bands. Though progesterone conferred the remarkable antibacterial effect to *Helicobacter pylori* suspended into the PBS, the potency of progesterone to decrease the CFU of *Helicobacter pylori* was somewhat lower than that of 17α-hydroxyprogesterone caproate. In addition, the control CFU of *Helicobacter pylori* suspended into PBS without steroid was also decreased, but the decrease magnitude in the CFU was slight. The amount of FldA protein detected in the bacterial cell supernatant correlated closely with the decreases of CFU: the FldA protein band became more noticeable when the CFU decreased by a greater magnitude. In sum, a large amount of FldA protein has leaked from the *Helicobacter pylori* cells to outside, when the organism was exposed to progesterone and 17α-hydroxyprogesterone caproate. These results indicate that progesterone and 17α-hydroxyprogesterone caproate injure the membranes of *Helicobacter pylori* and thereby induce the cell lysis more promptly than autolysis (Hosoda et al., 2011).

6.7 Antibacterial effects of progesterone and its derivative on other Gram-positive and Gram-negative bacteria

To estimate the antibacterial effects of progesterone and 17α-hydroxyprogesterone caproate against other representative Gram-positive and Gram-negative bacteria, we have determined the minimum inhibitory concentrations (MICs) of these 3=O steroids by the following method. Progesterone or 17α-hydroxyprogesterone caproate was serially diluted 2-fold with a dimethyl sulfoxide (DMSO) solution and added to agar plates of serum-free medium. Bacterial cell suspension (10 μl) adjusted to approximately 10^7 CFU/ml was dotted onto agar plates containing progesterone or 17α-hydroxyprogesterone caproate (from 1.6 μM to 100 μM) and cultured for 1 week under microaerobic conditions. The MICs (μM) of progesterone and 17α-hydroxyprogesterone caproate for the four *Helicobacter pylori* strains (NCTC 11638, ATCC 43504, the clinical isolates A-13 and A-19), *Escherichia coli* strain NIH JC-2, *Pseudomonas aeruginosa* strain ATCC 10145, *Staphylococcus aureus* strain FDA 209D, and *Staphylococcus epiderimidis* strain sp-al-1 were determined by confirming the growth of colonies from the organisms on the agar plates. As it turned out, the MICs of progesterone and 17α-hydroxyprogesterone caproate for the four *Helicobacter pylori* strains were 50 μM and 3.1 μM, respectively (Table 1). Intriguingly, progesterone and 17α-hydroxyprogesterone caproate had no influence on the growth of the other four bacterial species, namely, *Escherichia coli, Pseudomonas aeruginosa, Staphylococcus aureus*, and *Staphylococcus epiderimidis*: all four species grew even in the presence of progesterone or 17α-hydroxyprogesterone caproate at 100 μM (the highest concentration examined). The antibacterial spectra of progesterone and 17α-hydroxyprogesterone caproate have, thus, been remarkably narrow. The four bacterial species, *Escherichia coli, Pseudomonas aeruginosa, Staphylococcus aureus*, and *Staphylococcus epiderimidis* have no capability to incorporate exogenous steroids into the membranes. Given the unique feature of *Helicobacter pylori* as an aggressive assimilator of exogenous steroids, we can assume that progesterone and 17α-hydroxyprogesterone caproate attacked *Helicobacter pylori* without targeting the other four bacterial species.

Bacterial species	MIC (μM)	
	PS	17αPSCE
Helicobacter pylori	**50**	**3.1**
Escherichia coli	**> 100**	**> 100**
Pseudomonas aeruginosa	**> 100**	**> 100**
Staphylococcus aureus	**> 100**	**> 100**
Staphylococcus epiderimidis	**> 100**	**> 100**

Table 1. MICs of progesterone (PS) and 17α-hydroxyprogesterone caproate (17αPSCE) for various bacterial species

7. Investigation of the steroid-binding site on *Helicobacter pylori*

As described above, we have demonstrated the relationship between *Helicobacter pylori* and steroids. Certain steroids such as free-cholesterol and estrone have been found to be beneficial for the survival of *Helicobacter pylori*. Conversely, other steroids such as estradiol and progesterone have been found to impair the viability of *Helicobacter pylori*. From these findings, in sum, *Helicobacter pylori* seems to bind various steroids to the identical regions on the cell surface. In light of this, we hypothesized that progesterone and free-cholesterol act to steroid-binding sites existing on the *Helicobacter pylori* cell surface. To verify this hypothesis, we carried out the following experiments (Hosoda et al., 2011). After a 24-hour preculture of *Helicobacter pylori* (10^6 CFU/ml) with progesterone (5 μM or 10 μM) in a serum-free medium (30 ml), the *Helicobacter pylori* cells (10^8 CFU/ml) recovered were incubated for 4 hours in a serum-free medium (30 ml) containing free-cholesterol fixed-beads (free-cholesterol concentration: 250 μM). Thereafter, the amount of free-cholesterol absorbed into the *Helicobacter pylori* cells was quantified via the ferric chloride-sulfuric acid reagent method. The amount of free-cholesterol per CFU obviously tended to reduce by preculturing *Helicobacter pylori* with progesterone. These results suggest that progesterone strongly binds to the *Helicobacter pylori* cell surface and thereby obstructs the free-cholesterol absorption of *Helicobacter pylori* by inhibiting the cell surface binding of free-cholesterol. Incidentally, progesterone had no influence on the viability of *Helicobacter pylori* at the 5 and 10 μM concentrations: the CFUs of the *Helicobacter pylori* cultured for 24 hours with progesterone were similar to the control CFU (10^8 CFU/ml) of the *Helicobacter pylori* cultured for 24 hours without progesterone.

Helicobacter pylori glucosylates the absorbed free-cholesterol and synthesizes glucosyl cholesterols (CGL, CAG and CPG). With this in mind, we decided to examine the influence of progesterone on the glucosylation of free-cholesterol. After a 24-hour preculture of *Helicobacter pylori* (10^6 CFU/ml) in the presence or absence of progesterone (10 μM) in a serum-free medium (30 ml), the *Helicobacter pylori* cells (10^8 CFU/ml) recovered were incubated for 4 hours with free-cholesterol fixed-beads (free-cholesterol concentration: 250 μM) in a serum-free medium (30 ml), and the membrane lipids were purified to analyze the glucosyl cholesterol levels in the membrane lipid compositions by TLC. The TLC analysis detected the glucosyl cholesterols (CGL, CAG and CPG) in the membrane lipids of *Helicobacter pylori* precultured with progesterone, although no free-cholesterol was found to have accumulated within the lipids. Meanwhile, the glucosyl cholesterol levels detected in the membrane lipids of *Helicobacter pylori* precultured with progesterone were similar to the glucosyl cholesterol levels detected in the membrane lipids of *Helicobacter pylori* precultured without progesterone. Progesterone has been found to exert no inhibitory effects on the enzymes involved in the glucosyl cholesterol synthesis.

Next, we examined whether free-cholesterol conversely inhibits the anti-*Helicobacter pylori* action of progesterone. When the *Helicobacter pylori* (10^6 CFU/ml) was cultured for 24 hours with free-cholesterol fixed-beads at various volumes (free-cholesterol concentration: 30 to 90 μM) in a serum-free medium (15 ml) containing progesterone (30 μM), the free-cholesterol did not inhibit the anti-*Helicobacter pylori* action of progesterone: the CFU increase was not observed in any concentrations of free-cholesterol, and the CFU levels hardly altered from the control CFU (10^6 CFU/ml) of *Helicobacter pylori* cultured for 24 hours with progesterone in the absence of free-cholesterol fixed-beads. These results, at least, indicate that free-cholesterol does not competitively inhibit the anti-*Helicobacter pylori* action of progesterone. This compelled us, in sum, to examine the inhibitory effect of a high concentration of free-cholesterol on the anti-*Helicobacter pylori* action of progesterone. When the *Helicobacter pylori* (10^6 CFU/ml) was cultured for 24 hours with progesterone at concentrations ranging from 10 to 30 μM in a serum-free medium (15 ml) containing free-cholesterol fixed-beads (free-cholesterol concentration: 500 μM) or simple-beads (the volumes similar to the free-cholesterol fixed-bead volumes), free-cholesterol at the highest concentration (500 μM) had a noticeable influence on the anti-*Helicobacter pylori* action of the

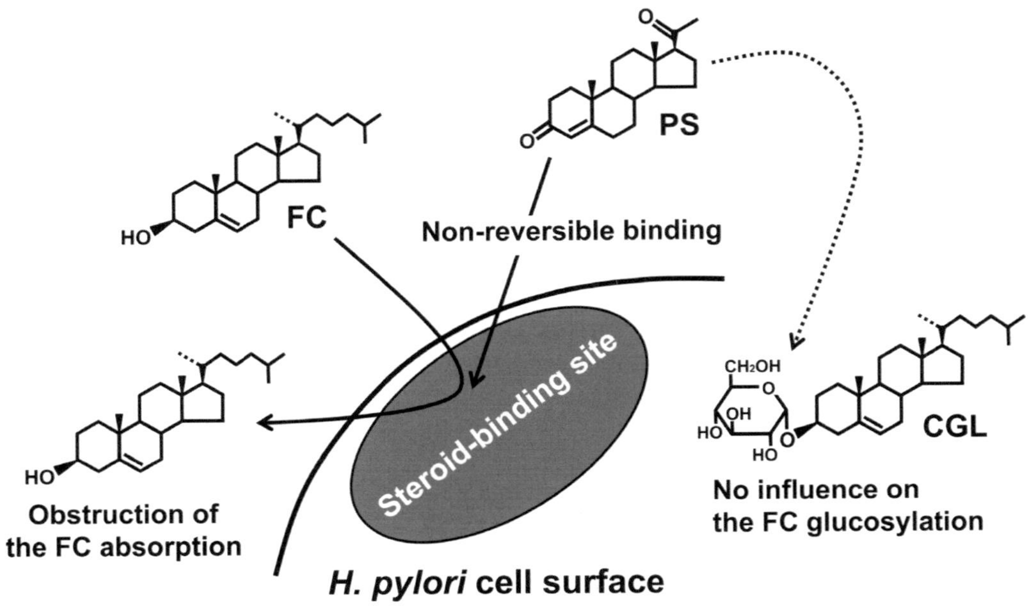

Fig. 8. The obstruction of free-cholesterol (FC) absorption in *Helicobacter pylori* by progesterone (PS)

progesterone: the growth-inhibitory curve of *Helicobacter pylori* cultured with progesterone in the presence of free-cholesterol fixed-beads shifted from the control growth-inhibitory curve of *Helicobacter pylori* cultured with progesterone in the presence of simple-beads to the right side, when the CFU values ($\log_{10}$ CFU/ml: vertical axis) and the progesterone concentrations (μM: horizontal axis) were plotted in a graph. These results indicate that free-cholesterol noncompetitively inhibits the anti-*Helicobacter pylori* action of progesterone. In combination with the results of the inhibitory effect of progesterone on the binding of free-cholesterol onto the *Helicobacter pylori* cells, they also strongly suggest that progesterone non-reversibly binds to the *Helicobacter pylori* cells and thereby induces the cell lysis, and/or inhibits the free-cholesterol absorption of the organism.

Our recent study has shown that progesterone inhibits the free-cholesterol absorption of *Helicobacter pylori*, and conversely, that a relatively high concentration of free-cholesterol inhibits the anti-*Helicobacter pylori* action of progesterone. Progesterone and free-cholesterol, in sum, seem to bind to identical sites on the *Helicobacter pylori* cell surfaces and thereby obstruct each other's effects (Fig. 8). This suggests that *Helicobacter pylori* may express a certain component, such as a steroid-binding protein, on the cell surface. Further investigations will be required to elucidate whether such a steroid-binding protein does indeed exist in *Helicobacter pylori*.

8. Conclusion

Our current basal research has revealed the following relationship between *Helicobacter pylori* and steroid hormones: pregnenolone (PN), dehydroepiandrosterone (DEA), epiandrosterone (EA), and estrone (E1) are absorbed into the membranes of *Helicobacter pylori* and play an important role to reinforcing the membrane lipid barrier, and thereby

Helicobacter pylori acquires the phosphatidylcholine resistance. Conversely, estradiol, androstenedione, and progesterone are harmful for the survival of *Helicobacter pylori*, and especially progesterone (PS) exhibit more effective antibacterial action to *Helicobacter pylori* than the other steroid hormones (Fig. 9). In addition, we have discovered that the acylation at the carbon-17 position of progesterone framework considerably augments the anti-*Helicobacter pylori* action of progesterone and that the hydroxylation at the same carbon position of progesterone framework conversely cancels out this action of progesterone. In sum, 17α-hydroxyprogesterone caproate (17αPSCE) exhibits much stronger anti-*Helicobacter pylori* action than progesterone, whereas 17α-hydroxyprogesterone has no anti-*Helicobacter pylori* action. These findings are expected to contribute to the development of a novel antibacterial steroidal medicine that targets *Helicobacter pylori* as an aggressive assimilator of exogenous steroids. Particularly, progesterone may be useful as a fundamental structure for designing new anti-*Helicobacter pylori* steroidal agents.

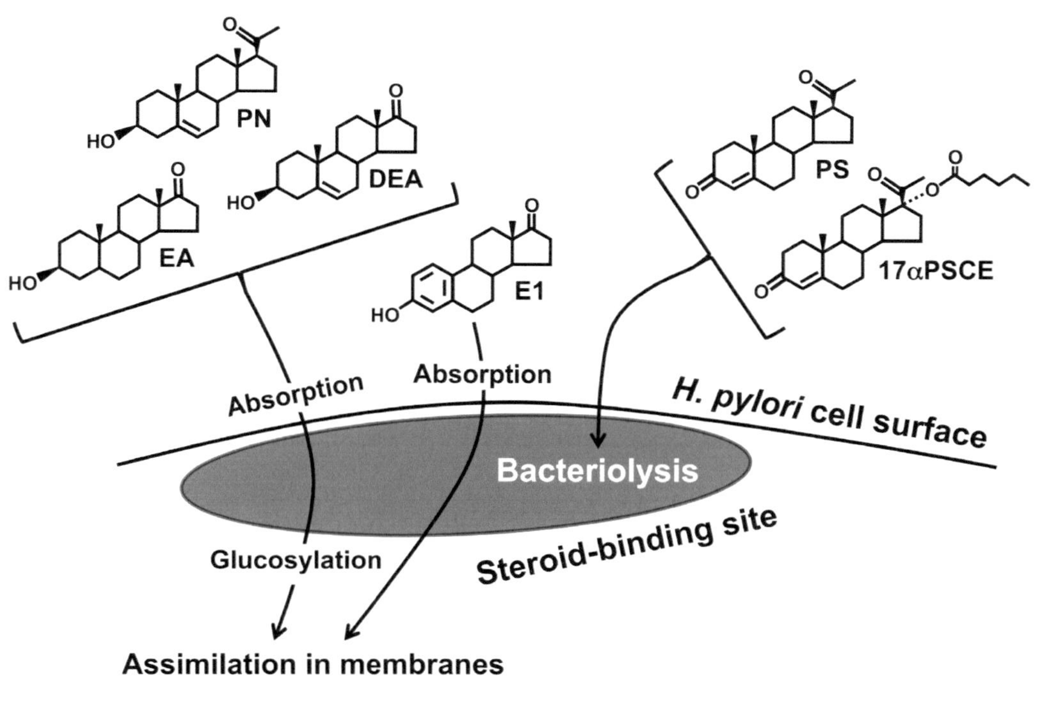

Fig. 9. The relationship between *Helicobacter pylori* and steroid hormones

9. Acknowledgment

A part of this publication was subsidized by JKA through its promotion funds from KEIRIN RACE.

10. References

Benaïssa, M. Babin, P. Quellard, N. Pezennec, L. Cenatiempo, Y. & Fauchere, J., L. (1996). Changes in *Helicobacter pylori* ultrastructure and antigens during conversion from the bacillary to the coccoid form. *Infect. Immune.*, Vol. 64, No. 6, pp. 2331-2335, ISSN 0019-9567

Ben-Menachem, G. Kubler-Kielb, J. Coxon, B. Yergey, A. & Schneerson, R. (2003). A newly discovered cholesteryl galactoside from *Borrelia burgdorferi*. *Proc. Natl. Acad. Sci. USA*, Vol. 100, No. 13, pp. 7193-7918, ISSN 0027-8424

Berstad, K. Berstad, A., Jr. Sjödahl, R. Weberg, R. & Berstad, A. (1992). Eosinophil cationic protein and phospholipase A_2 activity in human gastric juice with emphasis on *Helicobacter pylori* status and effects of antacids. *Scand. J. Gastroenterol.*, Vol. 27, No. 12, pp. 1011-1017, ISSN 0036-5521

Bruyn, E., E., D. Steel, H., C. Rensburg van, C., E., J. & Anderson, R. (1996). The riminophenazines, clofazimine and B669, inhibit potassium transport in gram-positive bacteria by a lysophospholipid-dependent mechanibm. *J. Antimicrob. Chemother.*, Vol. 38, No. 3, pp. 349-362, ISSN 0305-7453

Campbell-Thompson, M. Lauwers, G., Y. Reyher, K., K. Cromwell, J. & Shiverick, K., T. (1999). 17beta-estradiol modulates gastroduodenal preneoplastic alterations in rats exposed to the carcinogen. *Endocrinology*, Vol. 140, No. 10, pp. 4886-4894, ISSN 0013-7227

Cantrenich, C., E. & Makin, K., M. (1991). Characterization of the morphologic conversion of *Helicobacter pylori* from bacillary to coccid forms. *Scand. J. Gastroenterol. Suppl.*, Vol. 181, pp. 58-64, ISSN 0085-5928

Conley, A.J. & Kabara, J.J. (1973). Antimicrobial action of esters of polyhydric alcohols. *Antimicrob. Agents Ch.*, Vol. 4, No. 5, pp. 501-506, ISSN 0066-4804

Constance, E. van Rensburg, J. Joone, G., K. Osullivan, J., F. & Anderson, R. (1992). Antimicrobial activities of clofazimine and B669 are mediated by lysophospholipids. *Antimicrod. Agents Ch.*, Vol. 36, No. 12, pp. 2729-2735, ISSN 0066-4804

Donelli, G. Matarrese, P. Florentini, C. Dainelli, B. Taraborelli, T. Di-Campli, E. Di-Bartolomeo, S. & Cellini, L. (1998). The effect of oxygen on the growth and cell morphology of *Helicobacter pylori*. *FEMS Microbiol. Lett.*, Vol. 168, No. 1, pp. 9-15, ISSN 0378-1097

Folch, J. Lee, M. & Stanley, G., H., S. (1957). A simple method for the isolation and purification of total lipids from animal tissues. J. Biol. Chem. Vol. 226, No. 1, pp. 497-509, ISSN 0021-9258

Forman, D. & The Eurogast Study Group. (1993). An international association between *Helicobacter pylori* infection and gastric cancer. *Lancet*, Vol. 341, No. 8857, pp. 1359-1363, ISSN 0140-6736

Freedman, N., D. Chow, W., H. Gao, Y., T. Shu, X., O. Ji, B., T. Yang, G. Lubin, J., H. Li, H., L. Rothman, N. Zheng, W. & Abnet, C., C. (2007). Menstrual and reproductive factors and gastric cancer risk in a large prospective study of women. *Gut*, Vol. 56, No. 12, pp. 1671-1677, ISSN 0017-5749

Fukase, K. Kato, M. Kikuchi, S. Inoue, K. Uemura, N. Okamoto, S. Terano, S. Amagai, K. Hayashi, S. Asaka, M. & Japan Gast Study Group. (2008). Effect of eradication of *Helicobacter pylori* on incidence of metachronous gastric carcinoma after endoscopic resection of early gastric cancer: an open-label, randomised controlled trial. *Lancet*, Vol. 372, No. 9636, pp. 392-397, ISSN 0140-6736

Furukawa, H. Iwanaga, T. Koyama, H. & Taniguti, H. (1982). Effect of sex hormones on carcinogenesis in the stomach of rats. *Cancer Res.*, Vol. 42, No. 12, (December 1982), pp. 5181-5182, ISSN 0008-5472

Graham, D., Y. (1991). *Helicobacter pylori*: its epidemiology and its role in duodenal ulcer disease. *J. Gastroenterol. Hepatol.*, Vol. 6, No. 2, pp. 105-113, ISSN 0815-9319

Haque, M. Hirai, Y. Yokota, K. Mori, N. Jahan, I. Ito, H. Hotta, H. Yano, I. Kanemasa, Y. & Oguma, K. (1996). Lipid profile of *Helicobacter* spp.: presence of cholesteryl glucoside as a characteristic feature. *J. Bacteriol.*, Vol. 178, No. 7, pp. 2065-2070, ISSN 0021-9193

Haque M. Hirai, Y. Yokota, K. & Oguma, K. (1995). Steryl glucosides: a characteristic feature of the *Helicobacter* spp.?. *J. Bacteriol.*, Vol. 177, No. 18, pp. 5334-5337, ISSN 0021-9193

Hirai, Y. Haque, M. Yoshida, T. Yokota, K. Yasuda, T. & Oguma, K. (1995). Unique cholsteryl glucosides in *Helicobacter pylori*: composition and structural analysis. *J. Bacteriol.*, Vol. 177, No. 18, pp. 5327-5333, ISSN 0021-9193

Hosoda, K. Shimomura, H. Hayashi, S. Yokota, K. & Hirai, Y. (2011). Steroid hormones as bactericidal agents to *Helicobacter pylori*. *FEMS Microbiol. Lett.*, Vol. 318, No. 1, pp. 68-75, ISSN 0378-1097

Hosoda, K. Shimomura, H. Hayashi, S. Yokota, K. Oguma, K. & Hirai, Y. (2009). Anabolic utilization of steroid hormones in *Helicobacter pylori*. *FEMS Microbiol. Lett.*, Vol. 297, No. 2, pp. 173-179, ISSN 0378-1097

Hughes, N., J. Chalk, P., A. Clayton, C., L. & Kelly, D., J. (1995). Identification of carboxylation enzymes and characterization of a novel four-subunit pyruvate:flavodoxin oxidoreductase from *Helicobacter pylori*. *J. Bacteriol.*, Vol. 177, No. 14, pp. 3953-3959, ISSN 0021-9193

Javitt, N., B. Lee, Y., C. Shimizu, C. Fuda, H. & Strott C., A. (2001). Cholesterol and hydroxycholesterol sulfotransferase: identification, distinction from dehydroepiandrosterone sulfotransferase, and differential tissue expression. *Endocrinology*, Vol. 142, No. 7, pp. 2978-2984, ISSN 0013-7227

Kabara, J., J. Sweiczkowski, D., M. Conley, A., J. & Truant, J., P. (1972). Fatty acids and derivatives as antimicrobial agents. *Antimicrob. Agents Ch.*, Vol. 2, No. 1, pp. 23-28, ISSN 0066-4804

Kanai, K. & Kondo, E. (1979). Antibacterial and cytotoxic aspects of long-chain fatty acids as cell surface: selected topics. *Jpn. J. Med. Sci. Biol.*, Vol. 32, No. 3, pp. 135-174, ISSN 0021-5112

Kanetsuna, F. (1985). Bactericidal effect of Fatty acids on mycobacteria, with particular reference to the suggested mechanism of intracellular killing. *Microbiol. Immunol.*, Vol. 29, No. 2, pp. 127-141, ISSN 0385-5600

Ketkar, M. Reznik, G. & Green, U. (1978). Carcinogenic effect of N-methyl-N'-nitro-N-nitrosoguanidine (MNNG) in European hamsters. *Cancer Lett.*, Vol. 4, No. 4, pp. 241-244, ISSN 0304-3835

Kim, Y., K. Wang, Y. Liu, Z., M. & Kolattukudy, P., E. (2002). Identification of a hard surface contact-induced gene in *Colletotrichum gloeosporioides* conidia as a sterol glucosyl transferase, a novel fungal virulence factor. *Plant J.*, Vol. 30, No. 2, pp. 177-187, ISSN 0960-7412

Knapp, H., R. & Melly, M., A. (1986). Bactericidal effect of polyunsaturated fatty acids. *J. Infect. Dis.*, Vol. 154, No. 1, pp. 84-94, ISSN 0022-1899

Kondo, E. & Kanai, K. (1985). Mechanism of bactericidal activity of lyzolecithin and its biological implication. *Jpn. J. Med. Sci. Biol.*, Vol. 38, No. 4, pp. 181-194, ISSN 0021-5112

Kominea, A. Konstantinopoulos, P., A. Kapranos, N. Vondoros, G. Gkermpesi, M. Andricopoulos, P. Artelaris, S. Savva, S. Varakis, I. Sotiropoulou-Bonikou, G. & Papavassiliou, A., G. (2004). Androgen receptor (AR) expression is an independent unfavorable prognostic factor in gastric cancer. *J. Cancer Res. Clin. Oncol.*, Vol. 130, No. 5, pp. 253-258, ISSN 0171-5216

Lebrun, A., H. Wunder, C. Hildebrand, J. Churin, Y. Zähringer, U. Lindner, B. Meyer T., F. Heinz, E. & Warnecke, D. (2006). Cloning of a cholesterol-alpha-glucosyltransferase from *Helicobacter pylori*. *J. Biol. Chem.*, Vol. 281, No. 38, pp. 27765-27772, ISSN 0021-9258

Livermore, B., P. Bey, R., F. & Johnson, R, .C. (1978). Lipid metabolism of *Borrelia hermsi*. *Infect. Immune.* Vol. 20, No. 1, pp. 215-220, ISSN 0019-9567

Matsuyama, S. Ohkura, Y. Eguchi, H. Kobayashi, Y. Akagi, K. Uchida, K. Nakachi, K. Gustafsson, J., A. & Hayashi, S. (2002). Estrogen receptor beta is expressed in human stomach adenocarcinoma. *J. Cancer Res. Clin. Oncol.*, Vol. 128, No. 6, pp. 219-324, ISSN 0171-5216

Mayberry, W., R. & Smith, P., F. (1983). Structures and properties of acyl diglucosylcholesterol and galactofuranosyl diacylglycerol from *Acholeplasma axanthum*. *Biochim. Biophys. Acta.*, Vol. 752, No. 3, pp. 434-443, ISSN 0006-3002

Miki, Y. Nakata, T. Suzuki, T. Darnel, A., D. Moriya, T. Kaneko, C. Hidaka, K. Shiotsu, Y. Kusaka, H. & Sasano, H. (2002). Systematic distribution of steroid sulfatase and estrogen sulfotransferase in human adult and fetal tissues. *J. Clin. Endocrinol. Metab.*, Vol. 87, No. 12, pp. 5760-5768, ISSN 0021-972X

Nieman, C. (1954). Influence of trace amount of fatty acids on the growth of microorganisms. *Bacteriol. Rev.*, Vol. 18, No. 2., pp. 147-163, ISSN 1098-5557

Ohtani, M. Garcia, A. Rogers, A., B. Ge, Z. Taylor, N., S. Xu, S. Watanabe, K. Marini, R., P. Whary, M., T. Wang, T., C. Fox, J., G. (2007). Protective role of 17beta-estradiol against the development of *Helicobacter pylori*-induced gastric cancer in INS-GAS mice. *Carcinogenesis*, Vol. 28, No. 12, pp. 2597-2604, ISSN 0143-3334

Ohtani, Y. Irie, T. Uekama, K. Fukunaga, K. & Pitha, J. (1989). Differential effects of alpha-, beta-, and gamma-cyclodextrins on human erythrocytes. *Eur. J. Biochem.*, Vol. 186, No. 1-2, pp. 17-22, ISSN 0014-2956

Oku, M. Warnecke, D. Noda, T. Müller, F. Heinz, E. Mukaiyama H. Kato, N. & Sakai, Y. (2003). Peroxisome degradation requires catalytically active sterol glucosyltransferase with a GRAM domain. *EMBO J.*, Vol. 22, No. 13, pp. 3231-3241, ISSN 0261-4189

Orihara, T. Wakabayashi, H. Nakaya, A. Fukuta, K. Makimoto, S. Naganuma, K. Entani, A. & Watanabe, A. (2001). Effect of *Helicobacter pylori* eradication on gastric mucosal phospholipid content and its fatty acid composition. *J. Gastroenterol. Hepatol.*, Vol. 16, No. 3, pp. 269-275, ISSN 0815-9319

Patel, K., R. Smith, P., F. & Mayberry, W., R. (1978). Comparison of lipids from *Spiroplasma citri* and corn stunt *spiroplasma. J. Bacteriol.*, Vol. 136, No. 2, pp. 829-831, ISSN 0021-9193

Peek, R., M. Jr. & Blaser, M., J. (2002). *Helicobacter pylori* and gastrointestinal tract adenocarcinomas. *Nat. Rev. Cancer*, Vol. 2, No. 1, pp. 28-37, ISSN 1474-175X

Peek, R., M., Jr. & Crabtree, J., E. (2006). *Helicobacter* infection and gastric neoplasia. *J. Pathol.*, Vol. 208, No. 2, pp. 233-248, ISSN 0022-3417

Peng, L. Kawagoe, Y. Hogan, P. & Delmer, D. (2002). Sitosterol-beta-glucoside as primer for cellulose synthesis in plants. *Science*, Vol. 295, No. 5552, pp. 147-150, ISSN 0036-8075

Rietschel, E., T. Kirikae, T. Schade, F., U. Mamat, U. Schmidt, G. Loppnow, H. Ulmer, A., J. Zähringer, U. Seydel, U. Padova, F., D. Schreier, M. & Brade, H. (1994). Bacterial endotoxin: molecular relationship of structure to activity and function. *FASEB J.*, Vol. 8, No. 2, pp. 217-225, ISSN 0892-6638

Schröder, N., W. Schombel, U. Heine, H. Gobel, U., B. Zähringer, U. & Schumann, R., R. (2003). Acylated cholesteryl galactoside as a novel immunogenic motif in *Borrelia burgdorferi sensu stricto. J. Biol. Chem.*, Vol. 278, No. 36, pp. 33645-33653, ISSN 0021-9258

Shimomura, H. Hosoda, K. Hayashi, S. Yokota, K. Oguma, K. & Hirai, Y. (2009). Steroids mediates resistance to the bactericidal effect of phosphatidylcholines against *Helicobacter pylori. FEMS Microbiol. Lett.*, Vol. 301, No. 1, pp. 84-94, ISSN 0378-1097

Shimomura, H. Hayashi, S. Yokota, K. Oguma, K. & Hirai, Y. (2004). Alteration in the composition of cholesteryl glucosides and other lipids in *Helicobacter pylori* undergoing morphological change from spiral to coccoid form. *FEMS Microbiol. Lett.*, Vol. 237, No. 2, pp. 407-413, ISSN 0378-1097

Sipponen, P. & Correa, P. (2002). Delayed rise in incidence of gastric cancer in females results in unique sex ratio (M/F) pattern: etiologic hypothesis. *Gastric Cancer*, Vol. 5, No. 4, pp. 213-219, ISSN

Smith, P., F. (1971). Biosynthesis of cholesteryl glucoside by *Mycoplasma gallinarum. J. Bacteriol.*, Vol. 108, No. 3, pp. 986-991, ISSN 0021-9193

Steel, H., C. Cockeran, R. & Anderson, R. (2002). Platelet-activating factor and lyso-PAF possess direct antimicrobial properties *in vitro. APMIS*, Vol. 110, No. 2, pp. 158-164, ISSN 1600-0463

Stübs, G. Fingerle, V. Wilske, B. Gobel, U., B. Zähringer, U. Schumann, R., R. & Schröder N., W. (2009). Acylated cholesteryl galactosides are specific antigens of *Borrelia* causing lyme disease and frequency induce antibodies in late stages of disease. *J. Biol. Chem.*, Vol. 284, No. 20, pp. 13326-13334, ISSN 0021-9258

Stolte, M. Bayerdorffer, E. Morgner, A. Alpen, B. Wundish, T. Thiede, C. & Neubauer, A. (2002). *Helicobacter* and gastric MALT lymphoma. *Gut*, Vol. 50, pp. III19-III24, ISSN 0017-5749

Takano, N. Iizuka, N. Hazama, S. Yoshino, S. Tangoku, A. & Oka, M. (2002). Expression of estrogen receptor-alpha and -beta mRNAs in human gastric cancer. *Cancer Lett.*, Vol. 176, No. 2, pp. 129-135, ISSN 0304-3835

Takeyama, J. Suzuki, T. Hirasawa, G. Muramatsu, Y. Nagura, H. Iinuma, K. Nakamura, J. Kimura, K., I. Yoshihama, M. Harada, N. Andersson, S. & Sasano, H. (2000). 17beta-hydroxysteroid dehydrogenase type 1 and 2 expression in the human fetus. *J. Clin. Endocrinol. Metab.*, Vol. 85, No. 1, pp. 410-416, ISSN 0021-972X

Thompson, L. Cockayne, A. & Spiller R., C. (1994). Inhibitory effect of polyunsaturated fatty acids on the growth of *Helicobacter pylori*: a possible explanation of the effect of diet on peptic ulceration. *Gut*, Vol. 35, No. 11, pp. 1557-1561, ISSN 1468-3288

Turgeon, D. Carrier, J., S. Levesque, E. Hum, D., W. & Belanger, A. (2001). Relative enzymatic activity, protein stability, and tissue distribution of human steroid-metabolizing UGT2B subfamily members. *Endocrinology*, Vol. 142, No. 2, pp. 778-787, ISSN 0013-7227

Uemura, N. Okamoto, S. Yamamoto, S. Matsumura, M. Yamaguchi, S. Yamakido, M. Taniyama, K. Sasaki N. & Schlemper R., J. (2001). *Helicobacter pylori* infection and the development of gastric cancer. *N. Engl. J. Med.*, Vol. 345, No. 11, pp. 829-832, ISSN 0028-4793

Warnecke, D., C. & Heinz, E. (1994). Purification of a membrane-bound UDP-glucose:sterol beta-D-glucosyltransferase based on its solubility in diethyl ether. *Plant Physiol.*, Vol. 105, No. 4, pp. 1067-1073, ISSN 0032-0889

Warnecke, D., C. Baltrusch, M. Buck, F. Wolter, F., P. & Heinz, E. (1997). UDP-glucose:sterol glucosyltransferase: cloning and functional expression in *Escherichia coli*. *Plant Mol. Biol.*, Vol. 35, No. 5, pp. 597-603, ISSN 0167-4412

Warnecke, D. Erdmann, R. Fahl, A. Hube, B. Müller, F. Zank, T. Zähringer, U. & Heinz, E. (1999). Cloning and functional expression of *UGT* gene encoding sterol glucosyltransferase from *Saccharomyces cerevisiae, Candida albicans, Pichia pastoris,* and *Dictyostelium discoideum*. *J. Biol. Chem.*, Vol. 274, No. 19, pp. 13048-13059, ISSN 0021-9258

Warren, J., R. & Marshall, B. (1983). Unidentified curved bacilli on gastric epithelium in active chronic gastritis. *Lancet*, Vol. 1, No. 8336, pp. 1273-1275, ISSN 0140-6736

Wotherspoon, A., C. Ortiz-Hidalgo, C. Falzon, M., R. & Isaacson, P., G. (1991). *Helicobacter pylori*-associared gastritis and primary B-cell gastric lymphoma. *Lancet*, Vol. 338, No. 8776, pp. 1175-1176, ISSN 014-6736

Wunder, C. Churin, Y. Winau, F. Warnecke, D. Vieth, M. Lindner, B. Zähringer, U. Mollenkopf, H., J. Heinz E. & Meyer, T., F. (2006). Cholesterol glucosylation promotes immune evasion by *Helicobacter pylori*. *Nat. Med.*, Vol. 12, No .9, pp. 1030-1038, ISSN 1078-8956

Wyatt, J., I. & Dixon, M., F. (1988). Chronic gastritis-a pathogenetic approach. *J. Pathol.*, Vol. 152, No. 2, pp. 113-124, ISSN 0022-3417

6

Steroid Hormones and Ovarian Cancer

Erin R. King and Kwong-Kwok Wong
The University of Texas MD Anderson Cancer Center, Houston, TX, United States of America

1. Introduction

Globally, ovarian cancer is the 6th most common malignancy in developed countries, responsible for 100,300 new cases and 64,500 deaths annually (Jemal et al., 2011). Approximately 90% of ovarian cancers arise within the ovarian surface epithelium (OSE) or the fallopian tube surface epithelium; the remainder of ovarian malignancies develops from other ovarian tissues (sex cord-stromal, germ cell, or mixed cell tumors). The overall prognosis for epithelial ovarian carcinoma (EOC) is poor: Diagnosis is typically late-stage due to the lack of effective screening methods and vague presenting symptoms, with 5-year survival at 40% for stage III and 20% for stage IV patients (Heintz et al., 2006). Despite excellent initial activity, the standard treatment consisting of cytoreductive surgery followed by platinum- and taxane-based chemotherapy often fails with a recurrence rate of over 80% in stage III and IV disease. Therefore, novel therapeutic approaches are needed to improve the outcomes in this population.

Research efforts have yielded insight into the etiology, signaling mechanisms, and progression of ovarian cancer, yet much remains poorly understood. Physiologically, steroid hormones are intimately involved in ovulation, reproduction, and function of normal OSE cells. There is growing evidence that estrogen, progesterone, and other hormones also play a role in the development and progression of ovarian cancer (Leung & Choi, 2007). "Incessant ovulation" with repetitive injury and repair of OSE and subsequent cumulative DNA damage is one of the hypothesized risk factors for ovarian cancer (Fathalla, 1971), yet this does not explain the occurrence of the majority of ovarian carcinomas well after the reproductive years (Berek & Hacker, 2010). Interestingly, although oral contraceptives (OCs), increasing parity, and prolonged breastfeeding all decrease cumulative risk (Gwinn et al., 1990; Risch et al., 1994), progestin-only contraceptives offer just as much protective benefit as estrogen-containing OCs without prohibiting ovulation (Risch, 1998). Another hypothesis for the development of ovarian cancer, the "gonadotropin hypothesis," stipulates that gonadotropins contribute to ovarian carcinogenesis through follicle stimulating hormone (FSH)- and luteinizing hormone (LH)-mediated excess stimulation of ovarian tissue. This hypothesis is consistent with the protective effect of OCs, and the observation that the majority of cases of epithelial ovarian cancer develop postmenopausally after a surge in gonadotropin levels. *In vitro,* gonadotropins such as FSH activate mitogenic pathways and stimulate ovarian epithelial cell proliferation (Choi et al., 2002). In addition to gonadotropins, excess androgens and estrogen have also been linked to the progression and possibly development of ovarian cancer. *In vivo* treatment of mice with estrogen significantly increases tumor growth (Armaiz-Pena et al., 2009). These observations suggest that in addition to regulation of the menstrual cycle, certain steroid hormones may promote the progression—and possibly development—of ovarian cancer, while others offer a protective benefit. The objectives of this chapter are to summarize the signaling mechanisms involved in normal human OSE and its neoplastic counterparts, to highlight the effects of these steroid hormones on ovarian cancer cell growth, and to discuss the current clinical trials utilizing anti-hormonal approaches in ovarian cancer patients.

2. Steroid hormone signaling in normal ovarian surface epithelium and ovarian cancer

2.1 Steroid signaling in normal ovarian surface epithelium

Human ovarian surface epithelium is formed by a single layer of squamous to cuboidal cells covering the outermost layer of the ovary. While the exact function of OSE is unclear, with each ovulatory cycle, the OSE undergoes damage and repair. This damage incites an inflammatory response, the sequelae of which have been implicated in neoplastic transformation to tumor cells (Murdoch & Martinchick, 2004; Ness et al., 2000). Although steroid synthesis takes place elsewhere in the ovary, both normal and malignant OSE display estrogen, progesterone, and androgen receptors (Karlan et al., 1995; Lau et al., 1999; Li et al., 2003), and take part in steroid signaling. OSE also have FSH and LH receptors, though *in vitro* studies suggest these stimulate cellular growth and proliferation rather than steroidogenesis in OSE (Choi et al., 2004; Ji et al., 2004).

2.1.1 Estrogen and progesterone signaling in normal ovarian surface epithelium

Though the purpose of steroid signaling within the OSE remains uncertain, the effects of these steroids have been characterized *in vivo* and *in vitro*. The estrogen receptor (ER) and progesterone receptor (PR) are intracellular nuclear hormone receptors, which upon localization to the nucleus prompt transcriptional activity. Furthermore, the estrogen receptor participates in pathway crosstalk with known mitogenic pathways which have been associated with tumor progression and drug resistance, including transforming growth factor-Beta (TGF-β), human epidermal growth factor receptor 2 (HER-2/neu), and the insulin-like growth factor (IGF) receptors (Arpino et al., 2008; Band & Laiho, 2011; Fagan & Yee, 2008). In OSE, low doses of estrogen cause proliferation of ovarian surface epithelial cells *in vitro*, which involves the interleukin-6 (IL-6)/signal transducer and activator of transcription 3 (STAT-3) pathway (Syed et al., 2002). Others, however, have documented no effect at low doses of estrogen (Choi et al., 2001b; Karlan et al., 1995), or an inhibitory effect at high doses in OSE (Wright et al., 2005). *In vivo*, estrogen exposure causes rabbit OSE cell proliferation and an increase in the number of papillae but does not result in spontaneous development of tumors (Bai et al., 2000). In comparing normal OSE to ovarian carcinoma cell lines, Lau et al. (1999) found loss of ERα, PR, and androgen receptor (AR) mRNA in neoplastic cells compared to OSE, suggesting this loss may contribute to neoplastic transformation. Though the role of ERβ in Lau's work was uncertain, others assert that the ERβ receptor subtype promotes apoptosis in OSE (Bardin et al., 2004).

While estrogen has an unclear effect on cellular proliferation in OSE, progestins have a consistent effect of inhibiting cell growth and inflammation, and promoting apoptosis (Ivarsson et al., 2001; Karlan et al., 1995; Rae et al., 2004a). *In vivo*, macaques treated with progestin exhibited upregulation of apoptosis in OSE cells (Rodriguez et al., 1998). Though the exact mechanism by which progesterone exhibits growth-inhibitory effects is not fully-understood, Syed and Ho (2003) demonstrated involvement of the caspase 8 Fas/FasL pathway in progesterone-mediated apoptosis in OSE.

Culturing OSE *in vitro* with the inflammatory mediator IL-1 results in upregulation of several inflammation-associated genes, specifically *HSD11B1,* which plays a role in conversion of cortisone to cortisol (Rae et al., 2004b). With well-documented anti-inflammatory effects, cortisol prohibits downstream inflammatory signaling and may therefore exhibit a protective effect on the OSE. Together with the anti-inflammatory and growth-inhibitory effects of progesterone, glucocorticoids and progestin may serve to protect the OSE from inflammatory damage resulting from ovulation (Rae & Hillier, 2005).

2.1.2 Gonadotropin signaling in normal ovarian surface epithelium

The gonadotropins FSH and LH are members of a glycoprotein hormone family which also include thyroid stimulating hormone (TSH) and human placental chorionic gonadotropin (hCG). Gonadotropin receptors belong to the G protein-coupled receptor family (GPCR), which harbor seven transmembrane domains and upon their activation convert guanosine diphosphate (GDP) to guanosine triphosphate (GTP). This subsequently results in downstream activation of the phosphatidylinositol-3-kinase (PI3K) pathway; a pathway whose involvement in oncogenesis has been well-characterized. The type I isoform of gonadotropin-releasing hormone (GnRH) and its receptor are found on OSE, and interestingly, GnRH analogs appear to inhibit growth of OSE and ovarian cancer cells *in vitro* (Kang et al., 2000). The GnRH type II isoform also has growth inhibitory effects *in vitro.* (Choi et al., 2001a). While the exact mechanism of growth inhibition is not fully-understood, it is discussed in more detail later in the chapter.

Synthesized in the anterior pituitary, the gonadotropins FSH and LH regulate the menstrual cycle: FSH stimulates follicular growth and the FSH receptor (FSHR) is expressed mainly in granulosa cells, while LH triggers ovulation and the LH receptor (LHR) is expressed mostly in theca but also by granulosa cells. FSHRs and LHRs are found in both OSE and ovarian cancer cells (Minegishi et al., 2000; Parrott et al., 2001). Leung and Choi (2007) characterized the signaling pathway of FSHR in preneoplastic immortalized OSE, and found that Extracellular-Related Signaling Kinase 1/2 (ERK 1/2), *c-myc,* and HER2/neu were upregulated, and cell growth was accelerated in response to FSHR overexpression. Epidermal growth factor receptor (EGFR) is also upregulated via the ERK 1/2 and PI3K/Akt pathways in immortalized OSE treated with gonadotropins (Choi et al., 2005). Others have similarly confirmed increased proliferation in OSE in response to FSH and LH administration (Choi et al., 2002; Syed et al., 2001). *In vitro,* treatment with FSH results in upregulation oncogenic genes and downregulation of tumor suppressor genes *RB1, BRCA1,* and *BS69* (Ji et al., 2004).

2.2 Steroid signaling in ovarian cancer

Steroid hormone signaling in ovarian cancer involves complex pathways which are not yet fully understood. Figure 1 depicts some of the established routes of signaling in EOC.

2.2.1 The role of estrogen in ovarian cancer

Although the influence of exogenous estrogen in OSE is ambiguous, it most certainly triggers proliferation and cellular growth in ovarian cancer cells (Choi et al., 2001b). This is

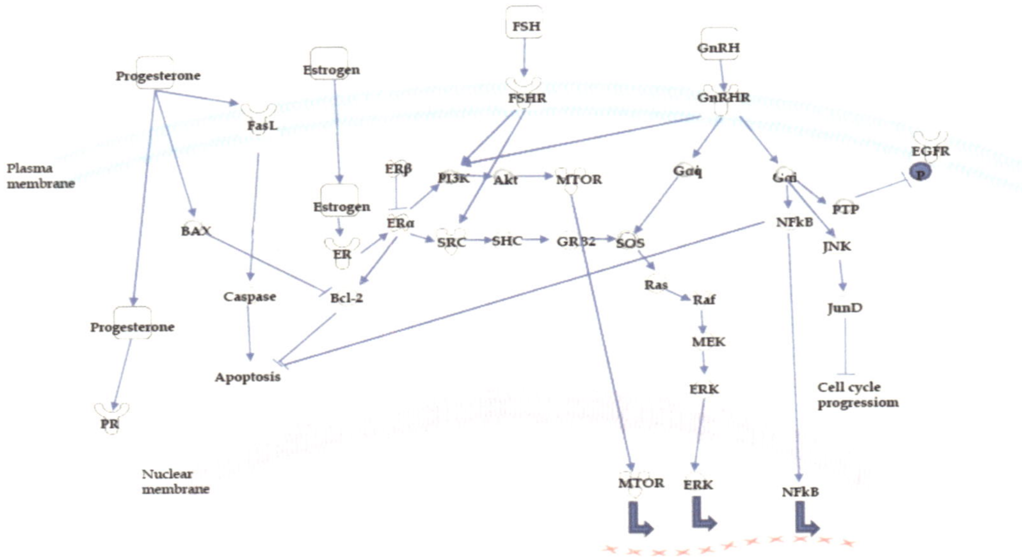

Fig. 1. Steroid hormone signaling in ovarian cancer.

accomplished in part through activation of the PI3K/Akt pathway and the transcription factor *c*-myc (Chien et al., 1994), and via estrogen receptor crosstalk with other pathways such as IGF-1, TGF-α, and EGFR (Simpson et al., 1998; Wimalasena et al., 1993). Estrogen also inhibits apoptosis via bcl-2, an anti-apoptotic protein (Choi et al., 2001b), and increases invasive capacity via upregulation of ezrin (Song et al., 2005), fibulin-1 (Galtier-Dereure et al., 1992), cathepsin D (Galtier-Dereure et al., 1992), and kallikreins (Yousef et al., 2003). In ovarian cancer cell lines treated with 17-B-estradiol, pro-angiogenic hypoxia-inducible factor-1 (HIF-1) expression was increased, the effect of which was abrogated by the Akt inhibitor snf and via Akt short-interfering RNA (siRNA) (Hua et al., 2009).

Both ER subtypes α and β are expressed in EOC. It has been suggested that ERα is mainly responsible for proliferation in the ovary, while ERβ modulates differentiation (Britt & Findlay, 2002). This is supported by the fact that ERβ is abundant in OSE and benign tumors, and ERα is mainly found in malignant ovarian tumors (Brandenberger et al., 1998; Hillier et al., 1998). An increased ERα: ERβ ratio has also been observed in ovarian cancer (Cunat et al., 2004), with an increase in ERα and inverse decrease in ERβ expression throughout tumor progression (Brandenberger et al., 1998). Overexpression of ERβ in an ovarian cancer cell line decreased proliferation by 50%.

In vivo studies support the role of 17-β-estradiol in accelerating tumor growth. Using a transgenic mouse model, Laviolette et al. (2010) showed that treatment of tumors with 17-β-estradiol resulted in the earlier onset of tumors, decreased survival time, and papillary histology, while treatment with progesterone resulted in no difference. Armaiz-Pena et al. (2009) similarly showed that treatment with 17-β-estradiol increased ovarian tumor growth, and inoculation with tumor cells during the proestrus when estrogen levels are high significantly increased tumor burden, compared to inoculation during the estrus phase. Furthermore, treatment with 17-β-estradiol resulted in increased vascular endothelial growth factor (VEGF), increased cell adhesion in ER positive cells, increased migratory potential, and mitogen-activated protein kinase (MAPK) upregulation.

Correspondingly, the estrogen antagonist tamoxifen abrogates the estrogen effect in epithelial ovarian cancer cell lines, and is surprisingly effective in both ER-positive and ER-negative and platinum-resistant ovarian carcinomas (Mabuchi et al., 2004; Markman et al., 1996). In ER-negative ovarian carcinomas, tamoxifen functions independently of estrogen via ERK, c-Jun N-terminal protein kinase (JNK), and p38 (Mabuchi et al., 2004).

2.2.2 The role of progesterone in ovarian cancer

Progesterone decreases cellular proliferation *in vitro* via multiple pathways. Blumenthal et al. (2003) demonstrated that progesterone activated the cyclin-dependent (CDK) pathway and promoted a more differentiated cell type. In the ovarian cancer cell line SKOV3, progesterone inhibited invasion and suppressed urokinase plasminogen activator (UPA), thereby decreasing the metastatic potential of cells (McDonnel & Murdoch, 2001). As in OSE cells, progesterone induces apoptosis via caspases and the FasL pathway (Syed & Ho, 2003), and enhances tumor necrosis factor-related apoptosis-inducing ligand (TRAIL)-induced cell death (Syed et al., 2007). Recent evidence supports that progesterone also causes apoptosis by upregulating the proapoptotic gene expression of p53 and BAX, and decreasing antiapoptotic gene expression of BCL-2 in ovarian cancer cells, thereby preventing oxidative damage (Nguyen & Syed, 2010).

In vivo, treatment of athymic mice with progesterone suppressed tumorigenesis after inoculation with the ovarian cancer cell line SKOV3 and increased survival (McDonnel et al., 2005). Furthermore, progesterone treatment in athymic nude mice inoculated with platinum-resistant SKOV3 enhanced platinum activity and sensitivity (Murdoch et al., 2008). However, the actions of progesterone in ovarian carcinomas is complex, and clinical trials utilizing progesterone have not proved as promising as *in vivo* and *in vitro* observations. In part, this may be due to the action of progesterone receptor membrane component 1 (PGRMC1), which recently *in vitro* was found to promote ovarian tumor cell proliferation, while its depletion slows cellular growth (Peluso et al., 2008). *In vivo,* PGRMC1-depleted mice had fewer and smaller tumors, again supporting the pro-oncogenic nature of PGRMC1 (Peluso et al., 2009).

As is the case with estrogen receptors, different progesterone receptor isoforms exist, including isoforms A and B. Akahira et al. examined the expression of PRA and PRB in the normal ovary, and in benign, borderline, and malignant ovarian tumors (2002). Using immunohistochemistry and RT-PCR in normal and malignant tissue and cell lines, they found that PRA receptor expression declined ($p<0.05$) during the transition from benign to borderline to malignant tissues, whereas there was no significant difference in PRB expression. They suggest that downregulation of PRA is associated with the development of ovarian cancer.

2.2.3 The role of gonadotropins in ovarian cancer

An alternative theory to the incessant ovulation hypothesis is that excessive gonadotropin stimulation leads to the development of ovarian cancer. Early animal models simulated hypogonadism, which prevented development of ovarian tumors in mice (Marchant, 1961). Oral contraceptives, which are proven to reduce the risk of EOC, also provide negative feedback on the gonadotropin axis and reduce circulating gonadotropins, which further supports this hypothesis. Additionally, the peak incidence of ovarian cancer occurs postmenopausally, with a temporal relationship to an increase in circulating gonadotropins (Choi et al., 2007).

Similar to estrogen, FSH promotes ovarian cancer cell growth *in vitro*. One way this occurs is through inhibition of apoptosis through activation of survivin via the PI3K/Akt pathway, and downregulation of the programmed cell death gene 6 (PCDG6) and death receptor 5 (DR5) (Huang et al., 2010). Promotion of cell growth through FSH also occurs through activation of the MAPK, PI3K/Akt pathways (Choi et al., 2002). Overexpression of the FSH receptor promotes well-established oncogenic signaling pathways including upregulation of EGFR (Choi et al., 2004), and angiogenesis promotion via VEGF upregulation (Schiffenbauer et al., 1997; Wang et al., 2002). In ovarian cancer cell lines, both FSH and LH exploit the PI3K/Akt pathway to upregulate cyxlooxygenase (COX)-1 and COX-2, resulting in increased cell motility and invasion (Lau et al., 2010). The FSH receptor (FSHR) is also prominent in ovarian carcinomas—Ji et al reported higher levels of the FSHR in cancerous ovarian tissue compared to normal controls (2004). The role of LH is controversial; in one study, LHR mRNA expression decreased in the transition from benign to malignant ovarian lesions (Lu et al., 2000). LH also appears to abrogate the proliferative effects of FSH (Zheng et al., 2000), but also has been reported to stimulate growth of OSE and contribute to tumor progression (Tashiro et al., 2003).

In vivo, treatment of rats with gonadotropins increased OSE proliferation (Stewart et al., 2004); similarly, mice treated with gonadotropins experienced increased ovarian cellular proliferation and decreased apoptosis (Burdette et al., 2006). Mice displaying hypergonadotropism from overexpression of FSH develop multicystic hemorrhagic ovaries, while overexpression of LH resulted in the formation of granulosa cell tumors (Kumar et al., 1999; Risma et al., 1995). However, it is important to note that these tumors formed in stromal or granulosa cells—not epithelial cells—and to date, no evidence exists establishing that gonadotropins can initiate malignant transformation of the ovarian epithelium.

2.2.4 The role of androgens in ovarian cancer

The role of androgens in promoting growth, tumorigenesis, and tumor progression in prostate cancer is well-established. In ovarian cancer cell lines, androgens 5α-dihydrotestosterone (DHT) and testosterone also cause cell proliferation which is mediated by upregulation of interleukin-6 (IL-6) (Syed et al., 2001; Syed et al., 2002). Levine and Boyd (2001) found that androgen receptor allele length influenced age at diagnosis with ovarian cancer; those patients with a shorter AR allele length were diagnosed 7 years earlier than those with normal allele length. *In vitro*, androgens decrease TGF-β receptors levels, which provides a mechanism for ovarian cancer cells to evade the growth inhibitory effects of TGF-β (Evangelou et al., 2000). Shi et al. (2011) examined the role of DHT, testosterone, and dehydroepiandrosterone (DHEA) in breast and ovarian cancer cell lines, and found that DHT but not the other androgens induced the degradation of the tumor suppressor p27 in both cell lines. Furthermore, in ovarian carcinoma cell lines, testosterone and androstenedione were found to increase cell viability, and induce telomerase activity which was blocked by PI3K inhibitors (Nourbakhsh et al., 2010). Sheach et al. (2009) found that the ovarian cancer cell lines OVCAR3 and OSEC2 expressed the androgen receptor, and treatment with androgen upregulated 121 genes, including G-protein-related genes Rab25 and Rab35. Level of gene expression correlated with tumor grade as well.

2.2.5 The role of GnRH in ovarian cancer

Two of twelve vertebrate GnRH isoforms exist in humans: GnRHI and GnRHII. GnRHI and its receptor are present in 80% of biopsies of ovarian carcinomas (Emons et al., 1989). While

GnRH functions in a paracrine manner systemically, there is evidence that GnRH functions in an autocrine manner in epithelial ovarian cancer, with GnRHI and GnRHII mRNA identified in both ovarian carcinoma and OSE (Choi et al., 2001a; Kang et al., 2000). Although the traditional gonadotropin GnRH signaling pathway involves $G_{\alpha q}$, protein kinase C, and MAP kinases, the autocrine mechanism of GnRH-related signaling in ovarian carcinomas differs (So et al., 2008). Interestingly, it appears that GnRH receptors in ovarian malignancy function via the pertussis toxin-sensitive protein $G_{\alpha i}$, and activate protein phosphatase (Imai et al., 2006). This alternate pathway is responsible for the antiproliferative effects of GnRH in ovarian carcinomas; however, the antiapoptotic function of GnRHI remains controversial. GnRHI and its agonists exert an inhibitory effect in ovarian cancer *in vitro* and *in vivo,* reducing cell growth and inducing cell cycle arrest in G_0/G_1 (Kim et al., 1999). However, GnRH agonists are in fact protective *against* apoptosis in ovarian cancer cell lines treated with doxorubicin (Sugiyama et al., 2005). Somewhat paradoxically, there is also emerging evidence that GnRH promotes tumor cell migration, metastasis, and invasion. *In vitro,* GnRHII enhances Akt pathway activation, and increased nuclear beta-catenin accumulation. This was reversed with siRNA targeting the GnRH receptor, and with treatment of cells with a PI3K/Akt inhibitor. GnRH treatment also increases type I matrix metalloproteinase (MT-1MMP) levels, thereby increasing cells' invasiveness and metastatic potential which increases cell migration and invasion during tumor progression through activation of Rho GTPases and accumulation of p120 catenin, with reversible effects upon inhibition of p120 (Cheung et al., 2010). *In vivo,* mice treated with a GnRH agonist displayed increased tumor weight (Romero et al., 2009). Thus, while GnRH and its agonists work via $G_{\alpha i}$ to decrease cellular growth and proliferation, it also enhances other pathways which promote cellular migration and invasion, essentially increasing metastatic potential.

3. Endogenous steroid hormones and ovarian cancer

3.1 Endogenous hormones

Population-based studies have supported the *in vitro* findings that progestins harbor protective effects against ovarian cancer. Conditions in which excess progesterone is present decrease cumulative risk of developing EOC, including multiple gestations, multiparity with an additional 10% decrease in risk with each birth, and breastfeeding (Lambe et al., 1999; Risch et al., 1994). While these findings support the incessant ovulation hypothesis by sparing the epithelium from monthly ovulations and repetitive damage, there is also evidence that progesterone independently increases the magnitude of benefit by promoting cellular apoptosis (Rodriguez et al., 1998).

3.2 Hormone receptors

Much effort has been directed at correlating hormone receptor status and outcomes in ovarian cancer. Geisler et al. (1996) examined estrogen and progesterone receptor status as prognostic indicators in patients with optimally cytoreduced stage IIIC serous carcinoma of ovary. Out of 96 patients, those with an estrogen receptor level <10 fmol/mg had better mean survival (41 vs 34 mos) than patients with higher levels of ER, whereas there was no correlation between PR status and survival. Others have found opposing results: One study examined ER mRNA expression in 35 stage III-IV ovarian carcinoma patients receiving neoadjuvant chemotherapy, and in multivariate analysis found that elevated baseline ER mRNA levels predicted prolonged progression-free survival (p=0.041) and overall survival (p=0.01), independently of pathological grade and age (Zamagni et al., 2009). Another group examined hormone receptor status in older and younger patients with advanced papillary serous ovarian carcinoma (Liu et al., 2009). They reported a higher percentage of ER-positivity and PR-negativity in older patients, while both groups were largely Her2/neu receptor-negative. Although there was no significant association between receptor status and survival, for the younger cohort, those who expressed both ER and PR receptor types had better overall survival (OS) (p=0.056) at 51 months, compared to 35 months in those not expressing both receptors. In a large cohort of Danish patients with ovarian cancer, Hogdall et al (2007) examined the prognostic value of ER and PR status via immunohistochemistry and microarray analysis in 582 women with EOC and 191 patients with serous borderline ovarian tumors. They noted that ER positivity increased with stage (p=0.0003), PR positivity increased with increasing grade (p=0.0006), and tissue ER and/or PR expression greater than 10% pointed to a more favorable prognostic outcome.

Estrogen receptor subtypes have also received attention in predicting ovarian cancer outcome. Halon et al. (2011b) examined ERβ via immunohisto- and immunocytochemistry in 43 patients pre-chemotherapy and 30 patients post-chemotherapy with stage III ovarian cancer. They determined that patients with higher initial ERβ expression (>30% of cells) enjoyed longer OS and progression-free survival (PFS) (p=0.0016, p=0.032, respectively). Similarly, Halon et al. (2011a) looked at ERα expression in the same group of patients and found that loss of ERα expression predicted significantly shorter OS and PFS.

Another group (Yue et al., 2010) also examined steroid receptors as possible prognostic markers in EOC. They described the steroid and xenobiotic receptor (SXR, also known as the pregnane X receptor), which regulates gene transcription and triggers proliferation of ovarian cancer cells *in vitro* and *in vivo* and induces drug resistance (Gupta et al., 2008). In 141 cases of EOC, SXR immunostaining was correlated with older patient age, clear cell histology, higher grade, and ER- and PR-positive tissues. SXR expression correlated with a higher likelihood of recurrence, and worse disease-free and overall survival. However, ER and PR status were not associated with disease-free survival (DFS) or OS.

3.3 Circulating hormones

In general, there is no documented consistent association between circulating hormone levels and the risk of developing EOC. Studies have addressed serum FSH and LH, and have not found any relationship between serum levels and ovarian cancer incidence (Akhmedkhanov et al., 2001; Arslan et al., 2003). Although there is no known association between the development of EOC and LH levels, high LH levels have been observed in BRCA1 mutation carriers compared to controls without BRCA1 mutations, which may comprise part of the BRCA1 phenotype (Jernstrom et al., 2005). While serum circulating levels of gonadotropins are nonpredictive, high levels of gonadotropins in ovarian cysts and peritoneal fluid are associated with malignancy. In comparing patients with and without malignant ovarian neoplasms, there was no difference in serum levels of LH or FSH, but ovarian cyst fluid levels of LH and FSH were elevated in serous ovarian carcinomas compared to benign tumors (Kramer et al., 1998). Similarly, peritoneal fluid aspirates contained elevated levels of FSH and LH in ovarian carcinoma versus benign tumors (Chudecka-Glaz et al., 2004; Halperin et al., 2003). One recent study actually found that in 67 patients with ovarian cancer versus controls, increased circulating levels of FSH were correlated with a reduced prediagnostic risk of EOC, which argues against the excess gonadotropin hypothesis in ovarian carcinogenesis (McSorley et al., 2009).

In a large European study, 192 ovarian cancer cases and 346 matched controls were compared for serum levels of testosterone, androstenedione, dehydroepiandrostenedione, and sex hormone binding globulin (SHBG) (Rinaldi et al., 2007). Free testosterone levels were inversely related to risk of EOC (p=0.01) in postmenopausal women, whereas free testosterone was positively associated with EOC risk in women under age 55, though this was not statistically significant. Other circulating androgens were not associated with risk.

In a nested case-control study of 31 cases of ovarian cancer and 63 controls, FSH and LH were measured (Helzlsouer et al., 1995). Mean FSH was lower in the cases (p=0.04) compared to controls, and LH was also lower but the difference was not statistically significant. The risk of ovarian cancer increased with higher androstenedione levels (p=0.03) and higher DHEA levels (p=0.02). Lukanova et al. (2003) followed by evaluating pre-diagnostic levels of serum testosterone, DHEA-sulfate, estrone, and SHBG in a case-control study nested within three cohorts, including 132 patients with primary EOC matched with 2 controls per case. There was no apparent association between any of the five hormone levels and ovarian carcinoma risk. Increased levels of circulating androstenedione in premenopausal patients did increase overall risk, but the low number of subjects in that subgroup precluded a definitive association.

In nonepithelial ovarian cancer (NEOC), circulating levels of steroid hormones may provide information about risk of NEOC development (Chen et al., 2010). In a case-control study within the Finnish Maternity Cohort, serum specimens were obtained from women with a singleton pregnancy that preceded their diagnosis of NEOC: 41 women had sex cord stromal tumors (SCST), and 21 had germ cell tumors (GCT). Doubling of testosterone, androstenedione, and 17-hydroxyprogesterone were associated with a two-fold increased risk of SCST compared to matched controls, a trend which remained after exclusion of women with a 2-, 4-, or 6-year time lag between blood donation and SCST diagnosis.

4. Exogenous hormones and ovarian cancer

4.1 Infertility treatment and risk of ovarian cancer

The relationship between infertility and steroid hormones is a controversial one. Many initially speculated that exogenous treatment with FSH and LH in infertility patients would lead to subsequent epithelial proliferation and tumorigenesis. In a case-control study, Whittemore et al. (1992) concluded that infertility patients who used infertility medications were at an increased risk of EOC compared to infertile women not using infertility medications. Since that time, however, other studies have emerged refuting that theory, and in fact it seems that infertility itself rather than gonadotropin use is an inherent risk for ovarian cancer (Ness et al., 2000; Tworoger et al., 2007). Brinton et al. reported on the relationship between ovarian cancer and infertility in a retrospective cohort study of 12,193 subjects (2004a). There were 45 identified cases of ovarian carcinoma, and infertility patients had a significantly elevated risk when compared to the general population, with a higher rate for primary versus secondary infertility, and the highest rate for those patients with endometriosis (Relative Risk or Hazard Ratio: RR=2.72 for patients with primary infertility and endometriosis). Examining the same patient cohort, they also reported on the risk of ovarian cancer with ovulation-stimulating drugs (Brinton et al., 2004b). They concluded a "slight but insignificant elevation in risk associated with drug usage among certain subgroups," including those using clomiphene citrate, which warrants continued surveillance.

4.2 Hormone replacement therapy

The topic of hormone replacement therapy (HRT) use and ovarian cancer risk has sparked much debate and controversy. Several large cohort studies deserve mention.

In a large study as part of the Cancer Prevention Study II Nutrition Cohort, a group of 54,436 postmenopausal women were followed starting in 1992 (Hildebrand et al., 2010). Over 15 years of follow-up, 297 incident cases of EOC were identified. Relative to never users, estrogen-only HRT was associated with a twofold higher relative risk (RR=2.07) of ovarian cancer, each 5-year increment of use was associated with a 25% higher risk, and greater than or equal to 20 years with a threefold higher risk (RR=2.89). Neither current nor former combination estrogen and progesterone use was associated with an increased ovarian cancer risk.

The UK Million Women Study enrolled 948,576 women and followed them for an average of 5.3 years for incident ovarian cancer (Beral et al., 2007). They identified 2273 cases of ovarian cancer, with 1591 associated deaths, and reported that current users of HRT were significantly more likely to develop (RR=1.2, p=0.0002) and die (RR=1.23, p=0.0006) from EOC versus never users. As in other studies, risk increased with duration of use, but interestingly did not differ by type of HRT used, and past users were not at an increased risk.

In a large prospective study, Rodriguez et al. (2001) examined the effects of postmenopausal estrogen use and risk of ovarian cancer. Of 211,581 women prospectively enrolled in the American Cancer Society's Prevention Study II, 944 ovarian cancer deaths were recorded over 14 years. Ovarian cancer mortality in women using estrogen replacement therapy (ERT) was higher than never users (RR=1.51), and risk was slightly but not significantly increased in former ERT users (RR=1.16). They noted that duration of use was correlated to risk, baseline current use for ≥10 years resulted in an RR of 2.20, versus former use for ≥10 years which resulted in a decreased but still elevated relative risk of 1.59. Risk did, however, decrease with increasing time since last use. The increased risk of ovarian cancer mortality persisted for up to 29 years.

Another large prospective cohort involved 329 women who developed ovarian cancer from a pool of 44,241 women in the Breast Cancer Detection Demonstration Project (Lacey et al., 2002). After adjustment for age and OC use, ever use of ERT was the only form of HRT associated with ovarian cancer (RR=1.6), in a dose dependent manner with RR for 10-19 years at 1.8 and more than 20 years at 3.2 ($p<0.001$). The addition of progesterone in an estrogen-progesterone regimen after estrogen-only use was still associated with an elevated risk (RR=1.5), but was not significant for estrogen-progesterone use only (RR=1.1). Women who used estrogen-only therapy for greater than 10 years were at a significantly increased risk of ovarian cancer, whereas estrogen-progestin only users were not at an increased risk.

Data from the Women's Health Initiative also merits mention (Anderson et al., 2003). This was a randomized, double-blind, placebo-controlled trial with 16,608 postmenopausal women given a daily tablet of estrogen-progesterone versus placebo. They identified 32 cases of ovarian cancer, and the hazard ratio for HRT use was 1.58, suggesting that continuous combination therapy may increase EOC risk.

In the clear cell and endometrioid non-serous subtypes of epithelial ovarian cancer, endometriosis is a known precursor lesion to the development of these malignancies. Correspondingly, there have been reports that HRT use is more strongly associated with clear cell and endometrioid histologic subtypes than serous EOC (Riman, 2003; Risch, 2002).

In light of these large cohort studies and the lack of definitive molecular evidence that steroid hormones initiate carcinogenesis, it is most likely that exogenous hormones hasten and perhaps fuel pre-existing lesions. As Risch points out, given the long latency between HRT use and development of these neoplasms, it is unlikely that these agents cause malignant transformation (2002).

4.3 Oral contraceptives and BRCA carriers

Whereas hormone replacement therapy may increase risk of ovarian carcinoma, oral contraceptive use diminishes the risk of EOC. Use over five years decreases risk by up to 50% lasting 10 to 15 years (Gwinn, 1985; Gwinn et al., 1990). While the exact protective mechanism is unknown, it is hypothesized that the apoptotic effects of progesterone are responsible for this effect. In a case-control study of 546 women with ovarian cancer and 4228 controls, women who had used OCs had a 40% reduction in risk compared to those who had never used them, with a protective effect lasting for 15 years (The Centers for Disease Control, 1987). BRCA mutation carriers harbor an especially high lifetime risk of development of EOC, ranging from 40 to 45% in BRCA1 carriers and 15-20% amongst BRCA2 mutation carriers (Narod et al., 2002). Studies support the use of OCs in high-risk women. Narod et al. particularly addressed this subgroup, and conducted a cohort study on 207 women with hereditary ovarian cancer, with 161 of their sisters serving as controls (1998). Lifetime history of oral contraceptive use was obtained, and the investigators found a decreased odds ratio of 0.5 for ovarian cancer associated with oral contraceptive use, with adjustment for age and parity. As in prior studies, the risk decreased with increasing duration of use, with a 60% reduction in risk with use for 6 or more years. In specifically examining BRCA mutation status, OR for OC use and development of EOC for BRCA1 carriers was 0.5, and was 0.4 for BRCA2 mutation carriers. A subsequent study in 1311 matched pairs of women with BRCA1 and BRCA2 mutations, however, revealed a modest increase in breast cancers in BRCA1 mutation carriers (OR=1.2) compared to controls, whereas there was no increased risk for BRCA2 mutation carriers (OR=0.94) (Narod et al., 2002). While oral contraceptives undoubtedly provide benefit in ovarian cancer prevention and are recommended in young BRCA mutation carriers, there is a minimal increased risk of breast cancer which must be weighed against the benefits.

5. Clinical trials with hormonally-targeted therapeutics in ovarian cancer

Several clinical trials in ovarian cancer have examined the utility of hormonal therapy in ovarian carcinoma, including antiestrogens (tamoxifen, fulvestrant), aromatase inhibitors (letrozole), progestins and progesterone receptor antagonists (medroxyprogesterone acetate, megestrol acetate, mifepristone), GnRH agonists (leuprolide acetate, triptorelin, goserelin), and antiandrogens (flutamide). Virtually all the trials examine these agents in the recurrent setting or in combination with other therapies; rarely are they studied as a component of up-front therapy. Given the overall low response rate to chemotherapy in recurrent ovarian cancer, most hormonal agents have a modest effect, with tamoxifen used the most frequently. Hormone-directed therapy is particularly popular in the setting of "chemical recurrence," in other words a rising CA-125 without clinical or radiographic evidence of disease. In this situation, clinicians are reluctant to initiate cytotoxic chemotherapy as early initiation does not prolong OS (Rustin et al., 2010), while patients often experience anxiety waiting for full return of their disease. With much more acceptable side effects than cytotoxic chemotherapy, hormonal therapeutics offer some activity and are generally well-tolerated. Not surprisingly, levels of endocrine receptor expression correlate positively with response; however, even patients without high receptor expression may enjoy clinical benefit.

5.1 Estrogen antagonists

5.1.1 Selective estrogen receptor modulators

Tamoxifen is a selective estrogen receptor modulator (SERM) with mixed estrogen agonist and antagonist activity. In the endometrium, it acts in an agonistic manner and has been associated with endometrial carcinoma (Bland et al., 2009); in the breast it is an antagonist. Use in ovarian carcinoma is generally restricted to the setting of recurrence or maintenance, with modest effects. Nonetheless, it is an attractive option for patients with biochemical recurrence and a rising CA-125 in the absence of obvious radiologic disease or symptoms. In this situation, early treatment offers no advantage and unnecessary toxicity, yet watchful waiting often causes patient anxiety. In this regard, tamoxifen may offer some activity while maintaining a favorable side effect profile.

Markman et al. explored this particular patient group in a retrospective review of patients with recurrent small-volume disease who received tamoxifen prior to initiation of cytotoxic chemotherapy (2004). Of 56 patients, the median duration of treatment was 3 months, but 42% of patients remained on tamoxifen for over 6 months, and 19% were still on tamoxifen at 9 months. They concluded that while tamoxifen is a reasonable treatment option, it is unknown whether the delay in chemotherapy resulted from the tamoxifen itself or the natural history of the patients' disease.

In a prospective trial, the Gynecologic Oncology Group (GOG) examined 105 patients with stage III or IV epithelial ovarian cancer whose disease recurred or persisted after surgery and were treated with tamoxifen 20 mg twice daily (Hatch et al., 1991). They reported an 18% response rate: 10% of patients had a complete response (CR) with a median duration of 7.4 months, while 8% experienced a partial response (PR), and 38% of patients had short-term disease stabilization. Median duration for PR or stable disease (SD) was 3 months. Of those with a complete response, 89% had elevated ER levels, versus 59% in SD or PR groups. Markman et al. (1996) followed with an ancillary report on the group, examining those patients with platinum-refractory disease. They reported an objective response rate of 13% in patients with platinum-resistant ovarian cancer, and a median duration of response of 4.4 months. The Mid-Atlantic Oncology Program (MAOP) conducted three separate phase II trials in patients with refractory ovarian carcinoma, and treated patients with either high-dose megestrol acetate, high-dose tamoxifen, or aminoglutethimide (Ahlgren et al., 1993). Of 30 patients who received high-dose megestrol acetate (800 mg/day for 30 days, then 400 mg/day thereafter), there were no identified responses. Among 29 patients treated with tamoxifen (80 mg /day for 30 days, then 40 mg/day thereafter), 17% responded, and two of those responses exceeded five years. Finally, aminoglutethimide was administered at a dose of 1g/day to 15 patients, and no responses were observed.

A more recent trial explored the role of tamoxifen versus thalidomide and its effects on VEGF expression in a randomized phase III trial in 138 women with stage III or IV EOC, primary peritoneal cancer, or fallopian tube carcinoma who were disease-free following first line chemotherapy and experienced a "biochemical" recurrence only as defined by rising CA-125 (Hurteau et al., 2010). Thalidomide was not superior to tamoxifen on interim analysis, with a similar risk of progression, higher toxicity, and an increased risk of death, and the trial was closed. VEGF expression was also not a prognostic factor in determining response.

Tamoxifen has also been explored in combination with cytotoxic agents. In a phase II trial, 50 patients with recurrent or progressive ovarian cancer after platinum-based chemotherapy received either 100 mg/m^2 cisplatin or 400 mg/m^2 carboplatin q3 weeks with tamoxifen 80 mg/day for 30 days followed by 40 mg/day thereafter (Benedetti Panici et al., 2001). Overall response rate was 50% with a 30% CR and 20% PR, with a higher response rate (64%) in the platinum-sensitive group compared to platinum-resistant cases (39%). Toxicity included nausea and vomiting, neuropathy, nephrotoxicity, and bone marrow suppression. While encouraging, it is difficult to interpret the effects of tamoxifen without a comparison group of platinum-alone, or platinum plus paclitaxel as is often used for recurrent platinum-sensitive disease.

In combination with the EGFR inhibitor gefitinib, tamoxifen was administered to 56 patients with platinum- and taxane-refractory EOC, peritoneal cancer, or fallopian tube cancer (Wagner et al., 2007). Sixteen patients had stable disease, although there were no tumor responses and in 10% the medications were discontinued secondary to adverse events, the most common of which were rash and diarrhea. Median time to progression was 58 days, with a median survival of 253 days. The investigators concluded that the drug combination was not efficacious.

5.1.2 Aromatase inhibitors

Letrozole is a non-steroidal aromatase inhibitor. It competitively and reversibly binds to aromatase and thereby prevents conversion of androgens to estrogen. In the setting of relapsed ovarian cancer, aromatase inhibitors can achieve a response in 35.7% of patients and stable disease in 20-42% of patients (Li et al., 2008). In a phase II setting, Smyth et al. (2007) investigated letrozole 2.5 mg orally daily in previously-treated patients with ER+ ovarian carcinoma. Of 42 patients, 17% had CA-125 response (defined as a decrease >50%), and 26% had not progressed (defined as doubling of CA-125). In terms of radiologic response, 9% of patients had a partial response, and 42% had stable disease at 12 weeks. Progression free survival of greater than 6 months was observed in 26% of patients. Response correlated to level of ER expression as defined by immunohistochemistry.

In another phase II trial examining patients with recurrent ovarian cancer, 50 patients received letrozole 2.5 mg daily (Bowman et al., 2002). Primary tumors were assessed for ER, PR, EGFR, erbB2, and HSP27 expression via immunohistochemistry. Though no PR or CR was observed, 10 patients experienced stable disease for at least 12 weeks. Those with stable disease exhibited significantly higher ER and PR levels, implying that endocrine receptor expression may help identify those patients most likely to benefit from treatment.

Walker et al (2007) aimed to explore estrogen-related gene expression and its predictive value in patient response to letrozole. Protein expression was measured via immunohistochemistry in tissue sections of tumors from patients treated with letrozole, and eight genes were significantly differentially expressed amongst patients who responded or had disease stabilization versus those who progressed. They concluded that these results might help identify those patients who would benefit most from endocrine therapy.

In 2010, Pan and Kao (2010) published a case report of two patients with endometrioid type histology. Both patients with advanced ER+ endometrioid ovarian carcinoma were treated with letrozole. The first patient had undergone optimal debulking, followed by completion of carboplatin and paclitaxel, had residual disease on second look surgery, and was subsequently disease-free for 30 months with letrozole treatment. The second patient was on her third recurrence and also experienced a 30 month remission with letrozole.

5.1.3 Estrogen receptor antagonists

Fulvestrant is a pure estrogen receptor antagonist without agonistic effects on other tissues. It competitively binds the ER, blocking estrogen binding and causing degradation and internalization of the estrogen receptor. In a phase II trial of fulvestrant in 26 women with ER positive recurrent ovarian or primary peritoneal carcinoma, patients received 500 mg IM on day 1, 250 mg IM on day 15, and 250 mg IM on day 29 and every 28 days thereafter (Argenta et al., 2009). The group had been heavily pretreated, with a median of 5 chemotherapy regimens prior to enrollment. Half of women experienced disease stabilization, though there was only one complete response and one partial response. Median time to progression was 62 days, and the regimen was well tolerated.

5.2 Progesterone

Given its promising apoptotic effects *in vitro* and *in vivo*, clinical trials with progestins have been disappointing. Several trials have used megestrol acetate or medroxyprogesterone acetate in the recurrent setting. Zheng et al. provide a nice summary of 13 trials, with 432 patients total (2007). Complete response was observed in 10 patients (2.3%), with a partial response in 4.9% of patients and stable disease in 47 or 10.9% of patients. They note that of the ten patients, 6 of them were reported in one study which also noted an overall 45% response rate (Geisler, 1985). A higher dose regimen does not appear to provide any additional benefit: In a phase II trial of 800 mg/day for 1 month followed by 400 mg/day thereafter, patients did not experience an overall increased benefit from higher doses, with an overall response rate of 10% (Veenhof et al., 1994) and 3 thromboembolic events.

Interestingly, combination therapy with medroxyprogesterone acetate and ethinyl estradiol yielded a partial response rate of 17% and stable disease in 24% of 25 patients with recurrent EOC, all patients had ER+ tumors (Fromm et al., 1991). Surprisingly, combination of progestins with tamoxifen does not appear to provide any clinical benefit (Jakobsen et al., 1987); nor does combination with chemotherapy. Based on *in vitro* evidence that megestrol acetate may reverse P-glycoprotein-mediated drug resistance, a phase I trial investigating the combination of megestrol acetate and paclitaxel was initiated (Markman et al., 2000). In 44 patients with paclitaxel-resistant EOC, four patients exhibited a response. However, 32% of patients experienced peripheral neuropathy, four patients developed venous blood clots, and one patient suffered from a stroke. Given the relatively low level of activity and significant toxicity, the authors did not recommend further study of the treatment regimen.

Mifepristone is a progesterone antagonist, more commonly known for its abortifacent properties. Rocereto et al. (2000) conducted a phase II study of mifepristone in the treatment of recurrent of persistent EOC, fallopian tube, or primary peritoneal cancer. Patients with persistent or recurrent disease less than 1 year after chemotherapy were eligible, and received mifepristone 200 mg daily for 28 day cycles. Of 44 patients enrolled, 34 were evaluable and 9 (26.5%) of patients experienced a response (9% CR, 17.5% PR). Duration of response was 1 to 3 months, except in one patient who continues to respond after three years. The major cited toxicity was rash.

5.3 GnRH agonists

GnRH agonists, principally leuprolide acetate, triptorelin, and goserelin, have been investigated in recurrent ovarian cancer. Emons & Schulz reported on 245 published phase II trials in patients with recurrent disease, mostly platinum-refractory, treated with GnRH agonists: 9% had an objective remission and 26% experienced disease stabilization (2000). Compared to estrogen-directed endocrine therapy, responses are minimal and GnRH agonist therapy is generally not used in this setting anymore.

Initial studies with GnRH agonists were small, with 5 to 37 patients, and employed leuprolide acetate in the setting of recurrent EOC. Of 161 combined patients in 7 studies, there were 2 reported CRs, 15 PRs, and a disease stabilization rate of about 24% (So et al., 2008).

Triptorelin was the next generation GnRH agonist examined in EOC, and results were generally disappointing. In a large European Organisation for Research and Treatment of Cancer (EORTC) study, 74 patients with progressive ovarian cancer were treated with the LHRH agonist triptorelin via IM injections of 3.75 mg (on days 1, 8, and 28 followed by monthly injections thereafter) (Duffaud et al., 2001). There were no objective responses, and only 16% of patients experienced stable disease with a median PFS of 5 months for SD. Though the treatment was well-tolerated, the authors concluded that triptorelin exhibits only modest efficacy in this patient cohort. Emons et al. also conducted a large study, with the benefit of a prospective randomized double blind trial design (1996) in 135 patients with Stage III or IV EOC after cytoreduction. Patients received standard platinum-based chemotherapy and were randomized to placebo or triptorelin 3.75 mg IM. There was no difference in survival between the two groups.

Following triptorelin, cetrorelix—a GnRH antagonist—was found *in vitro* to have better activity in ovarian carcinoma, and was hypothesized to act directly on the GnRH receptors in the tumor as well as centrally (Yano et al., 1994). A phase II study utilized cetrorelix 10 mg subcutaneously daily in 17 patients with platinum-resistant recurrent EOC or mullerian carcinoma. Three patients had a PR of 9, 16, and 17 weeks, there was one grade 4 anaphylactic reaction, and two patients exhibited a 20% increase in cholesterol not requiring treatment. Stable disease was observed in 35% of patients for up to 62 months. They also examined LHRH receptor status, and two of the three responding patients were LHRH positive.

Goserelin, another GnRH agonist, was evaluated in combination with tamoxifen in a phase II trial for patients with recurrent advanced ovarian cancer (Hasan et al., 2005). Patients had received a median of 3 prior chemotherapy regimens, and 17 of 26 patients had platinum-resistant disease. Tamoxifen was prescribed at 20 mg orally daily, and goserelin was provided subcutaneously at 3.6 mg once monthly. The overall response rate was 50%, with one CR, 2 PRs, and 10 with SD. Median PFI was 4 months, while median OS was 13 months. The regimen was well-tolerated. Zidan et al. (2002) treated 15 patients with advanced recurrent disease with 3.6 mg of goserelin monthly; two of these patients had not received initial chemotherapy due to poor performance status. They reported one CR lasting 8 months, one PR lasting 14 months, and disease stabilization in 20% for a median of 7.5 months, and there was no significant toxicity. Most recently, a 2007 study considered the activity of goserelin 3.6 mg subcutaneously monthly and bicalutamide (an oral anti-androgen often used in prostate cancer) 50 mg orally daily in patients in their second or greater complete disease remission (Levine et al.). Of 35 patients, PFS for second disease remission was 11.4 months, and was 11.9 months for patients in their third or fourth disease remission. There was no association between androgen receptor expression and PFS. Toxicities included liver function abnormalities, fatigue, and hot flushes. They concluded that the combination did not prolong PFS in patients with second or greater disease remission.

Emons et al. recently reported on a novel compound, AEZS-108, which is composed of [D-Lys]LHRH linked to doxorubicin (2010). In a phase I dose escalation trial of 17 women with metastatic unresectable EOC, endometrial, or breast cancer and immunohistochemical LHRH positivity, a total of 6 patients exhibited responses, both in the highest dose group. Dose-limiting toxicities included leukopenia and neutropenia.

5.4 Antiandrogens in ovarian cancer

Few studies exist assessing the efficacy of antiandrogenic therapy in ovarian cancer. Flutamide, a nonsteroidal antiandrogen, has been studied in the phase II setting (Vassilomanolakis et al., 1997). In 24 patients with relapsed stage III or IV ovarian cancer, flutamide was given at a dose of 100 mg three times daily. There was one partial response lasting 3 months, and two patients with stable disease for 7 and 8 months. Reported toxicity was mild. Another trial utilized flutamide in 68 pretreated patients with EOC (median prior chemotherapy of two regimens), dosed at 750 mg/daily for at least 2 months (Tumolo et al., 1994). Of 68 patients, there was one complete and one partial response lasting 44 and 72 weeks, and 28% of patients experienced stable disease for a median of 24 weeks. Toxicities included nausea and vomiting in 34.5% of patients. The authors concluded that flutamide was ineffective in heavily pretreated patients, in light of the significant percentage of side effects.

5.5 Ongoing clinical trials with hormonally-targeted therapeutics in ovarian cancer

While there are many clinical trials open to ovarian carcinoma patients, there are not many currently investigating hormonally-directed agents. There is currently one phase II trial exploring tamoxifen in combination with the EGFR tyrosine kinase inhibitor ZD839 in patients with recurrent ovarian cancer refractory to platinum and taxane-based therapy (NCT00189358).

There are a few trials exploring the newer SERMs. One of the newer agents, arzoxifene, is a SERM with higher potency than raloxifene. A current study, NCT00003670, is examining arzoxifene in patients with metastatic refractory EOC or peritoneal cancer in the phase II setting, and aims to correlate response to serum estradiol, FSH, LH, and SHBG. Another SERM, toremifene citrate, has just finished assessment in the recurrent ovarian cancer population, but results have not yet been published (NCT00003865). Endoxifen, a tamoxifen-related compound with higher affinity for the estrogen receptor, is undergoing evaluation in the setting of hormone-receptor positive breast, solid, desmoid, or gynecologic tumors which have not responded to standard chemotherapy (NCT01273168).

Some studies with aromatase inhibitors have completed recruitment. One study with combination anastrozole and gefitinib, an EGFR inhibitor, has completed enrollment in a phase II trial for patients with relapsed ovarian cancer (NCT00181688). Exemestane has also been utilized in a phase II trial in patients with recurrent stage II to IV ovarian cancer (NCT00261027). The trial has completed enrollment, and initial results presented at the American Society of Clinical Oncology reported that in 24 patients, 36% experienced stable disease lasting a median duration of 23 weeks (Verma et al., 2006). One patient had stable disease lasting greater than 95 weeks.

Though there are no current trials investigating progesterone-based compounds and active disease, NCT00445887 is studying the use of oral levonorgestrel to prevent ovarian carcinoma in patients at high risk of developing EOC.

6. Granulosa cell tumors of the ovary

As aforementioned, while it is generally agreed upon that gonadotropins contribute to tumor progression in ovarian carcinoma, there is a lack of clear evidence that they can *initiate* carcinogenesis in EOC. Claims that gonadotropins may cause EOC are derived from *in vivo* studies, in which rodents treated with excess gonadotropins formed sex cord stromal tumors, specifically granulosa cell tumors. In α-inhibin deficient mice, which results in a lack of negative feedback on the gonadotropin axis and resultant excess gonadotropins, gonadal stromal tumors formed (Matzuk et al., 1992). However, the tumors failed to form in these α-inhibin deficient mice in the absence of gonadotropins (Kumar et al., 1996). Dorward et al. (2007) treated hypogonadotropic immunodeficient mice with grafted ovaries from prepubertal genetically susceptible mice with an LH analog or FSH, and found that LH-treated mice developed granulosa cell tumors, while FSH-treated mice did not.

The role of granulosa cells in the ovary is well-established: they convert androgens to estradiol via aromatase, and are stimulated to do so by FSH. They also produce progesterone during the later stages of the menstrual cycle. Similarly, steroid signaling in granulosa cells has been extensively studied *in vivo*. In granulosa cells, FSH activates several pathways, including ERK, MAPK, and PI3K (Hunzicker-Dunn & Maizels, 2006). Estrogen protects against FasL-mediated apoptosis in the G1 to S phase transition of the cell cycle (Quirk et al., 2006), and GnRH agonists stimulate apoptosis (Takekida et al., 2003). In malignant granulosa cell tumors (GCTs), ER2 is upregulated (Chu et al., 2000). Nearly all GCTs express progesterone receptors, while about 30% express estrogen receptors (Hardy et al., 2005).

Granulosa cell tumors comprise approximately 5% of all ovarian tumors (Schumer & Cannistra, 2003), and often present with symptoms associated with estrogen excess—such as vaginal bleeding or virilization in postmenopausal women, or precocious puberty in juveniles. Given their relative rarity, there is a paucity of clinical trials, but antihormonal therapy has had activity in recurrent disease. There have been reports of disease stabilization or response after administration of megestrol acetate, goserelin, leuprolide, and anastrozole (Fishman et al., 1996; Freeman & Modesitt, 2006; Malik & Slevin, 1991; Martikainen et al., 1989).

7. Conclusions

In summary, steroid signaling plays an important part in both normal ovarian surface epithelial cells and in malignant epithelial ovarian carcinoma. The pathways that promote growth and inhibit apoptosis in OSE are often exploited and upregulated in EOC, while protective components are downregulated, thereby allowing evasion of apoptosis as well as cellular migration and invasion. While estrogen and FSH promote cellular growth and tumor progression *in vitro* and *in vivo*, there is no definitive evidence that they can initiate ovarian carcinogenesis. Progesterone impressively enhances apoptosis, and is valuable in preventive efforts, yet treatment with progestins in ovarian cancer has not yielded equally impressive results in the clinical setting. The reasons for this remain unclear, and warrant further investigation into signaling pathways and receptor crosstalk mechanisms. Perhaps even more interesting, the GnRH signaling pathway appears to operate via dual and opposing mechanisms, inhibiting cell growth through one pathway yet increasing cellular migration and invasion through another. Efforts to exploit the growth inhibitory effects while curbing the invasive component may generate more effective GnRH analogs. Despite our growing knowledge surrounding steroid hormone signaling in OSE and EOC, much still remains unknown.

While serum levels of steroid hormones are generally not useful as disease markers in determining disease risk or prognosis, ovarian tumors undoubtedly contain elevated levels of gonadotropins. Whether or not these elevated levels are a byproduct of aberrant signaling pathways or a contributor to carcinogenesis remains to be determined. Tumor expression of estrogen and progesterone receptors does appear to correlate to treatment response in patients, though results regarding estrogen receptor expression and prognosis are mixed. Certainly, the shift in ERα: ERβ expression and loss of PRB in tumor progression merits further investigation, and indeed has triggered exploration into targeted therapy. Inhibiting these receptor subtypes may result in more robust, specific responses in disease. While fulvestrant is an ERα antagonist, attention has now turned towards developing ERβ agonists. Benzopyran-derived selective estrogen receptor beta-agonist-1 (SERBA-1) is a selective ERβ receptor agonist which has been studied in mice and prostate hyperplasia, with promising effects (Norman et al., 2006). Monoaryl-substituted salicylaldoximes also show high ERβ affinity and are interesting new compounds (Bertini et al., 2011).

The role of exogenous hormones in ovarian cancer also remains unclear. As Risch suggests, at best HRT may accelerate the proliferation of pre-existing malignancy (Risch, 2002). Despite the completion of multiple large cohort studies, confounding and bias are likely responsible for ambiguous results. Still, the use of HRT is best avoided in women at high risk of developing EOC, such as BRCA mutation carriers, or women with a strong family history of ovarian cancer. Conversely, use of oral contraceptive prophylaxis is recommended for women with a high risk of EOC, to be weighed against a perhaps slightly elevated risk of breast cancer with extended use.

Hormonally-targeted therapeutics offer modest benefit for women with recurrent ovarian cancer, along with a much more tolerable side effect profile when compared to cytotoxic chemotherapy. In all fairness, clinical trials have not included hormone antagonists as first-line agents; they are most frequently studied in recurrent disease when even cytotoxic chemotherapy yields little benefit. It is possible that antihormonals may offer even more activity when used up front in combination with cytotoxic compounds, and this is an area warranting further investigation.

As is the case with emerging targeted therapies and resistance, inhibition of one pathway often results in upregulation of another, requiring combination with other therapeutics. Combination therapy of hormone antagonists with novel targeted agents offers exciting opportunities for overcoming resistance and improving patient outcomes. For example, the estrogen receptor pathway participates in crosstalk with multiple other mitogenic pathways, and concomitant inhibition of these pathways could produce a synergistic effect. Targeting other portions of the hormone receptors themselves has also evoked interest. Small molecule inhibitors target alternative binding sites on the estrogen and androgen receptor, which may result in improved selectivity or novel interactions (Shapiro et al., 2011). Likewise, while estrogen and progesterone receptor expression does correlate with response to antihormonal therapy, those patients without receptor expression also experience some benefit. Thus, better markers for response are needed. Post-translational modification of steroid receptors—particularly the estrogen receptor—include phosphorylation, ubiquitination, sumoylation, methylation, and palmitoylation, and affect receptor stability, localization, and perhaps drug resistance (Le Romancer et al., 2011).

Steroid hormones and their receptors participate in complex signaling which is not yet fully understood. Gaining insight into these interactions and downstream effectors is paramount to developing new targeted therapies and advancing the treatment of ovarian cancer.

8. Acknowledgements

We wish to acknowledge the HERA Women's Cancer Foundation, the Sara Brown Musselman Fund for Serous Ovarian Cancer Research, and the University of Texas MD Anderson Cancer Center Specialized Program of Research Excellence in Ovarian Cancer.

9. References

The Cancer and Steroid Hormone Study of the Centers for Disease Control and the National Institute of Child Health and Human Development. (1987). The reduction in risk of ovarian cancer associated with oral-contraceptive use. *N Engl J Med*, Vol. 316, No. 11, pp. 650-5, ISSN 0028-4793.

Ahlgren, J.D., Ellison, N.M., Gottlieb, R.J., et al. (1993). Hormonal palliation of chemoresistant ovarian cancer: three consecutive phase II trials of the Mid-Atlantic Oncology Program. *J Clin Oncol*, Vol. 11, No. 10, pp. 1957-68, ISSN 0732-183X.

Akahira, J., Suzuki, T., Ito, K., et al. (2002). Differential expression of progesterone receptor isoforms A and B in the normal ovary, and in benign, borderline, and malignant ovarian tumors. *Jpn J Cancer Res*, Vol. 93, No. 7, pp. 807-15, ISSN 0910-5050.

Akhmedkhanov, A., Toniolo, P., Zeleniuch-Jacquotte, A., et al. (2001). Luteinizing hormone, its beta-subunit variant, and epithelial ovarian cancer: the gonadotropin hypothesis revisited. *Am J Epidemiol*, Vol. 154, No. 1, pp. 43-9, ISSN 0002-9262.

Anderson, G.L., Judd, H.L., Kaunitz, A.M., et al. (2003). Effects of estrogen plus progestin on gynecologic cancers and associated diagnostic procedures: the Women's Health Initiative randomized trial. *JAMA*, Vol. 290, No. 13, pp. 1739-48, ISSN 1538-3598.

Argenta, P.A., Thomas, S.G., Judson, P.L., et al. (2009). A phase II study of fulvestrant in the treatment of multiply-recurrent epithelial ovarian cancer. *Gynecol Oncol*, Vol. 113, No. 2, pp. 205-9, ISSN 1095-6859.

Armaiz-Pena, G.N., Mangala, L.S., Spannuth, W.A., et al. (2009). Estrous cycle modulates ovarian carcinoma growth. *Clin Cancer Res*, Vol. 15, No. 9, pp. 2971-8, ISSN 1078-0432.

Arpino, G., Wiechmann, L., Osborne, C.K., et al. (2008). Crosstalk between the estrogen receptor and the HER tyrosine kinase receptor family: molecular mechanism and clinical implications for endocrine therapy resistance. *Endocr Rev*, Vol. 29, No. 2, pp. 217-33, ISSN 0163-769X.

Arslan, A.A., Zeleniuch-Jacquotte, A., Lundin, E., et al. (2003). Serum follicle-stimulating hormone and risk of epithelial ovarian cancer in postmenopausal women. *Cancer Epidemiol Biomarkers Prev*, Vol. 12, No. 12, pp. 1531-5, ISSN 1055-9965.

Bai, W., Oliveros-Saunders, B., Wang, Q., et al. (2000). Estrogen stimulation of ovarian surface epithelial cell proliferation. *In Vitro Cell Dev Biol Anim*, Vol. 36, No. 10, pp. 657-66, ISSN 1071-2690.

Band, A.M.&Laiho, M. (2011). Crosstalk of TGF-beta and Estrogen Receptor Signaling in Breast Cancer. *J Mammary Gland Biol Neoplasia*, Vol. 16, No. 2, pp. 109-15, ISSN 1573-7039.

Bardin, A., Hoffmann, P., Boulle, N., et al. (2004). Involvement of estrogen receptor beta in ovarian carcinogenesis. *Cancer Res*, Vol. 64, No. 16, pp. 5861-9, ISSN 0008-5472.

Benedetti Panici, P., Greggi, S., Amoroso, M., et al. (2001). A combination of platinum and tamoxifen in advanced ovarian cancer failing platinum-based chemotherapy: results of a Phase II study. *Int J Gynecol Cancer*, Vol. 11, No. 6, pp. 438-44, ISSN 1048-891X.

Beral, V., Bull, D., Green, J., et al. (2007). Ovarian cancer and hormone replacement therapy in the Million Women Study. *Lancet*, Vol. 369, No. 9574, pp. 1703-10, ISSN 1474-547X.

Berek, J.S. & Hacker, N.F. (2010). Berek and Hacker's Gynecologic Oncology, In: *Berek and Hacker's Gynecologic Oncology*, (Ed.), pp. Lippincott Williams & Wilkins, ISBN 978-0-7817-9512-8, 0-7817-9512-5, Philadelphia, PA.

Bertini, S., De Cupertinis, A., Granchi, C., et al. (2011). Selective and potent agonists for estrogen receptor beta derived from molecular refinements of salicylaldoximes. *Eur J Med Chem*, Vol. 46, No. 6, pp. 2453-62, ISSN 1768-3254.

Bland, A.E., Calingaert, B., Secord, A.A., et al. (2009). Relationship between tamoxifen use and high risk endometrial cancer histologic types. *Gynecol Oncol*, Vol. 112, No. 1, pp. 150-4, ISSN 1095-6859.

Blumenthal, M., Kardosh, A., Dubeau, L., et al. (2003). Suppression of the transformed phenotype and induction of differentiation-like characteristics in cultured ovarian tumor cells by chronic treatment with progesterone. *Mol Carcinog*, Vol. 38, No. 4, pp. 160-9, ISSN 0899-1987.

Bowman, A., Gabra, H., Langdon, S.P., et al. (2002). CA125 response is associated with estrogen receptor expression in a phase II trial of letrozole in ovarian cancer: identification of an endocrine-sensitive subgroup. *Clin Cancer Res*, Vol. 8, No. 7, pp. 2233-9, ISSN 1078-0432.

Brandenberger, A.W., Tee, M.K. & Jaffe, R.B. (1998). Estrogen receptor alpha (ER-alpha) and beta (ER-beta) mRNAs in normal ovary, ovarian serous cystadenocarcinoma and ovarian cancer cell lines: down-regulation of ER-beta in neoplastic tissues. *J Clin Endocrinol Metab*, Vol. 83, No. 3, pp. 1025-8, ISSN 0021-972X.

Brinton, L.A., Lamb, E.J., Moghissi, K.S., et al. (2004a). Ovarian cancer risk associated with varying causes of infertility. *Fertil Steril*, Vol. 82, No. 2, pp. 405-14, ISSN 0015-0282.

Brinton, L.A., Lamb, E.J., Moghissi, K.S., et al. (2004b). Ovarian cancer risk after the use of ovulation-stimulating drugs. *Obstet Gynecol*, Vol. 103, No. 6, pp. 1194-203, ISSN 0029-7844.

Britt, K.L. & Findlay, J.K. (2002). Estrogen actions in the ovary revisited. *J Endocrinol*, Vol. 175, No. 2, pp. 269-76, ISSN 0022-0795.

Burdette, J.E., Kurley, S.J., Kilen, S.M., et al. (2006). Gonadotropin-induced superovulation drives ovarian surface epithelia proliferation in CD1 mice. *Endocrinology*, Vol. 147, No. 5, pp. 2338-45, ISSN 0013-7227.

Chen, T., Surcel, H.M., Lundin, E., et al. (2010). Circulating sex steroids during pregnancy and maternal risk of non-epithelial ovarian cancer. *Cancer Epidemiol Biomarkers Prev*, Vol. 20, No. 2, pp. 324-36, ISSN 1538-7755.

Cheung, L.W., Leung, P.C. & Wong, A.S. (2010). Cadherin switching and activation of p120 catenin signaling are mediators of gonadotropin-releasing hormone to promote tumor cell migration and invasion in ovarian cancer. *Oncogene*, Vol. 29, No. 16, pp. 2427-40, ISSN 1476-5594.

Chien, C.H., Wang, F.F. & Hamilton, T.C. (1994). Transcriptional activation of c-myc proto-oncogene by estrogen in human ovarian cancer cells. *Mol Cell Endocrinol*, Vol. 99, No. 1, pp. 11-9, ISSN 0303-7207.

Choi, J.H., Choi, K.C., Auersperg, N., et al. (2004). Overexpression of follicle-stimulating hormone receptor activates oncogenic pathways in preneoplastic ovarian surface epithelial cells. *J Clin Endocrinol Metab*, Vol. 89, No. 11, pp. 5508-16, ISSN 0021-972X.

Choi, J.H., Choi, K.C., Auersperg, N., et al. (2005). Gonadotropins upregulate the epidermal growth factor receptor through activation of mitogen-activated protein kinases and phosphatidyl-inositol-3-kinase in human ovarian surface epithelial cells. *Endocr Relat Cancer*, Vol. 12, No. 2, pp. 407-21, ISSN 1351-0088.

Choi, J.H., Wong, A.S., Huang, H.F., et al. (2007). Gonadotropins and ovarian cancer. *Endocr Rev*, Vol. 28, No. 4, pp. 440-61, ISSN 0163-769X.

Choi, K.C., Auersperg, N. & Leung, P.C. (2001a). Expression and antiproliferative effect of a second form of gonadotropin-releasing hormone in normal and neoplastic ovarian surface epithelial cells. *J Clin Endocrinol Metab*, Vol. 86, No. 10, pp. 5075-8, ISSN 0021-972X.

Choi, K.C., Kang, S.K., Tai, C.J., et al. (2001b). Estradiol up-regulates antiapoptotic Bcl-2 messenger ribonucleic acid and protein in tumorigenic ovarian surface epithelium cells. *Endocrinology*, Vol. 142, No. 6, pp. 2351-60, ISSN 0013-7227.

Choi, K.C., Kang, S.K., Tai, C.J., et al. (2002). Follicle-stimulating hormone activates mitogen-activated protein kinase in preneoplastic and neoplastic ovarian surface epithelial cells. *J Clin Endocrinol Metab*, Vol. 87, No. 5, pp. 2245-53, ISSN 0021-972X.

Chu, S., Mamers, P., Burger, H.G., et al. (2000). Estrogen receptor isoform gene expression in ovarian stromal and epithelial tumors. *J Clin Endocrinol Metab*, Vol. 85, No. 3, pp. 1200-5, ISSN 0021-972X.

Chudecka-Glaz, A., Rzepka-Gorska, I.&Kosmowska, B. (2004). Gonadotropin (LH, FSH) levels in serum and cyst fluid in epithelial tumors of the ovary. *Arch Gynecol Obstet*, Vol. 270, No. 3, pp. 151-6, ISSN 0932-0067.

Cunat, S., Hoffmann, P. & Pujol, P. (2004). Estrogens and epithelial ovarian cancer. *Gynecol Oncol*, Vol. 94, No. 1, pp. 25-32, ISSN 0090-8258.

Dorward, A.M., Shultz, K.L. & Beamer, W.G. (2007). LH analog and dietary isoflavones support ovarian granulosa cell tumor development in a spontaneous mouse model. *Endocr Relat Cancer*, Vol. 14, No. 2, pp. 369-79, ISSN 1351-0088.

Duffaud, F., van der Burg, M.E., Namer, M., et al. (2001). D-TRP-6-LHRH (Triptorelin) is not effective in ovarian carcinoma: an EORTC Gynaecological Cancer Co-operative Group Study. *Anticancer Drugs*, Vol. 12, No. 2, pp. 159-62, ISSN 0959-4973.

Emons, G., Pahwa, G.S., Brack, C., et al. (1989). Gonadotropin releasing hormone binding sites in human epithelial ovarian carcinomata. *Eur J Cancer Clin Oncol*, Vol. 25, No. 2, pp. 215-21, ISSN 0277-5379.

Emons, G., Ortmann, O., Teichert, H.M., et al. (1996). Luteinizing hormone-releasing hormone agonist triptorelin in combination with cytotoxic chemotherapy in patients with advanced ovarian carcinoma. A prospective double blind randomized trial. Decapeptyl Ovarian Cancer Study Group. *Cancer*, Vol. 78, No. 7, pp. 1452-60, ISSN 0008-543X.

Emons, G. & Schulz, K.D. (2000). Primary and salvage therapy with LH-RH analogues in ovarian cancer. *Recent Results Cancer Res*, Vol. 153, No. pp. 83-94, ISSN 0080-0015.

Emons, G., Kaufmann, M., Gorchev, G., et al. (2010). Dose escalation and pharmacokinetic study of AEZS-108 (AN-152), an LHRH agonist linked to doxorubicin, in women with LHRH receptor-positive tumors. *Gynecol Oncol*, Vol. 119, No. 3, pp. 457-61, ISSN 1095-6859.

Evangelou, A., Jindal, S.K., Brown, T.J., et al. (2000). Down-regulation of transforming growth factor beta receptors by androgen in ovarian cancer cells. *Cancer Res*, Vol. 60, No. 4, pp. 929-35, ISSN 0008-5472.

Fagan, D.H. & Yee, D. (2008). Crosstalk between IGF1R and estrogen receptor signaling in breast cancer. *J Mammary Gland Biol Neoplasia*, Vol. 13, No. 4, pp. 423-9, ISSN 1573-7039.

Fathalla, M.F. (1971). Incessant ovulation--a factor in ovarian neoplasia? *Lancet*, Vol. 2, No. 7716, pp. 163, ISSN 0140-6736.

Fishman, A., Kudelka, A.P., Tresukosol, D., et al. (1996). Leuprolide acetate for treating refractory or persistent ovarian granulosa cell tumor. *J Reprod Med*, Vol. 41, No. 6, pp. 393-6, ISSN 0024-7758.

Freeman, S.A. & Modesitt, S.C. (2006). Anastrozole therapy in recurrent ovarian adult granulosa cell tumors: a report of 2 cases. *Gynecol Oncol*, Vol. 103, No. 2, pp. 755-8, ISSN 0090-8258.

Fromm, G.L., Freedman, R.S., Fritsche, H.A., et al. (1991). Sequentially administered ethinyl estradiol and medroxyprogesterone acetate in the treatment of refractory epithelial ovarian carcinoma in patients with positive estrogen receptors. *Cancer*, Vol. 68, No. 9, pp. 1885-9, ISSN 0008-543X.

Galtier-Dereure, F., Capony, F., Maudelonde, T., et al. (1992). Estradiol stimulates cell growth and secretion of procathepsin D and a 120-kilodalton protein in the human ovarian cancer cell line BG-1. *J Clin Endocrinol Metab*, Vol. 75, No. 6, pp. 1497-502, ISSN 0021-972X.

Geisler, H.E. (1985). The use of high-dose megestrol acetate in the treatment of ovarian adenocarcinoma. *Semin Oncol*, Vol. 12, No. 1 Suppl 1, pp. 20-2, ISSN 0093-7754.

Geisler, J.P., Wiemann, M.C., Miller, G.A., et al. (1996). Estrogen and progesterone receptor status as prognostic indicators in patients with optimally cytoreduced stage IIIc serous cystadenocarcinoma of the ovary. *Gynecol Oncol*, Vol. 60, No. 3, pp. 424-7, ISSN 0090-8258.

Gupta, D., Venkatesh, M., Wang, H., et al. (2008). Expanding the roles for pregnane X receptor in cancer: proliferation and drug resistance in ovarian cancer. *Clin Cancer Res*, Vol. 14, No. 17, pp. 5332-40, ISSN 1078-0432.

Gwinn, M.L. (1985). Oral contraceptives and breast, endometrial, and ovarian cancers. The Cancer and Steroid Hormone Study Group, Atlanta Georgia. *J Obstet Gynaecol (Lahore)*, Vol. 5 Suppl 2, No. pp. S83-7.

Gwinn, M.L., Lee, N.C., Rhodes, P.H., et al. (1990). Pregnancy, breast feeding, and oral contraceptives and the risk of epithelial ovarian cancer. *J Clin Epidemiol*, Vol. 43, No. 6, pp. 559-68, ISSN 0895-4356.

Halon, A., Materna, V., Drag-Zalesinska, M., et al. (2011a). Estrogen Receptor Alpha Expression in Ovarian Cancer Predicts Longer Overall Survival. *Pathol Oncol Res*, Vol. No. pp. ISSN 1532-2807.

Halon, A., Nowak-Markwitz, E., Maciejczyk, A., et al. (2011b). Loss of estrogen receptor beta expression correlates with shorter overall survival and lack of clinical response to chemotherapy in ovarian cancer patients. *Anticancer Res*, Vol. 31, No. 2, pp. 711-8, ISSN 1791-7530.

Halperin, R., Pansky, M., Vaknin, Z., et al. (2003). Luteinizing hormone in peritoneal and ovarian cyst fluids: a predictor of ovarian carcinoma. *Eur J Obstet Gynecol Reprod Biol*, Vol. 110, No. 2, pp. 207-10, ISSN 0301-2115.

Hardy, R.D., Bell, J.G., Nicely, C.J., et al. (2005). Hormonal treatment of a recurrent granulosa cell tumor of the ovary: case report and review of the literature. *Gynecol Oncol*, Vol. 96, No. 3, pp. 865-9, ISSN 0090-8258.

Hasan, J., Ton, N., Mullamitha, S., et al. (2005). Phase II trial of tamoxifen and goserelin in recurrent epithelial ovarian cancer. *Br J Cancer*, Vol. 93, No. 6, pp. 647-51, ISSN 0007-0920.

Hatch, K.D., Beecham, J.B., Blessing, J.A., et al. (1991). Responsiveness of patients with advanced ovarian carcinoma to tamoxifen. A Gynecologic Oncology Group study of second-line therapy in 105 patients. *Cancer*, Vol. 68, No. 2, pp. 269-71, ISSN 0008-543X.

Heintz, A.P., Odicino, F., Maisonneuve, P., et al. (2006). Carcinoma of the ovary. FIGO 26th Annual Report on the Results of Treatment in Gynecological Cancer. *Int J Gynaecol Obstet*, Vol. 95 Suppl 1, No. pp. S161-92, ISSN 0020-7292.

Helzlsouer, K.J., Alberg, A.J., Gordon, G.B., et al. (1995). Serum gonadotropins and steroid hormones and the development of ovarian cancer. *JAMA*, Vol. 274, No. 24, pp. 1926-30, ISSN 0098-7484.

Hildebrand, J.S., Gapstur, S.M., Feigelson, H.S., et al. (2010). Postmenopausal hormone use and incident ovarian cancer: Associations differ by regimen. *Int J Cancer*, Vol. 127, No. 12, pp. 2928-35, ISSN 1097-0215.

Hillier, S.G., Anderson, R.A., Williams, A.R., et al. (1998). Expression of oestrogen receptor alpha and beta in cultured human ovarian surface epithelial cells. *Mol Hum Reprod*, Vol. 4, No. 8, pp. 811-5, ISSN 1360-9947.

Hogdall, E.V., Christensen, L., Hogdall, C.K., et al. (2007). Prognostic value of estrogen receptor and progesterone receptor tumor expression in Danish ovarian cancer patients: from the 'MALOVA' ovarian cancer study. *Oncol Rep*, Vol. 18, No. 5, pp. 1051-9, ISSN 1021-335X.

Hua, K., Din, J., Cao, Q., et al. (2009). Estrogen and progestin regulate HIF-1alpha expression in ovarian cancer cell lines via the activation of Akt signaling transduction pathway. *Oncol Rep*, Vol. 21, No. 4, pp. 893-8, ISSN 1021-335X.

Huang, Y., Jin, H., Liu, Y., et al. (2010). FSH inhibits ovarian cancer cell apoptosis by up-regulating survivin and down-regulating PDCD6 and DR5. *Endocr Relat Cancer*, Vol. 18, No. 1, pp. 13-26, ISSN 1479-6821.

Hunzicker-Dunn, M.&Maizels, E.T. (2006). FSH signaling pathways in immature granulosa cells that regulate target gene expression: branching out from protein kinase A. *Cell Signal*, Vol. 18, No. 9, pp. 1351-9, ISSN 0898-6568.

Hurteau, J.A., Brady, M.F., Darcy, K.M., et al. (2010). Randomized phase III trial of tamoxifen versus thalidomide in women with biochemical-recurrent-only epithelial ovarian, fallopian tube or primary peritoneal carcinoma after a complete response to first-line platinum/taxane chemotherapy with an evaluation of serum vascular endothelial growth factor (VEGF): A Gynecologic Oncology Group Study. *Gynecol Oncol*, Vol. 119, No. 3, pp. 444-50, ISSN 1095-6859.

Imai, A., Sugiyama, M., Furui, T., et al. (2006). Gi protein-mediated translocation of serine/threonine phosphatase to the plasma membrane and apoptosis of ovarian cancer cell in response to gonadotropin-releasing hormone antagonist cetrorelix. *J Obstet Gynaecol*, Vol. 26, No. 1, pp. 37-41, ISSN 0144-3615.

Ivarsson, K., Sundfeldt, K., Brannstrom, M., et al. (2001). Production of steroids by human ovarian surface epithelial cells in culture: possible role of progesterone as growth inhibitor. *Gynecol Oncol*, Vol. 82, No. 1, pp. 116-21, ISSN 0090-8258.

Jakobsen, A., Bertelsen, K. & Sell, A. (1987). Cyclic hormonal treatment in ovarian cancer. A phase-II trial. *Eur J Cancer Clin Oncol*, Vol. 23, No. 7, pp. 915-6, ISSN 0277-5379.

Jemal, A., Bray, F., Center, M.M., et al. (2011). Global cancer statistics. *CA Cancer J Clin*, Vol. 61, No. 2, pp. 69-90, ISSN 1542-4863.

Jernstrom, H., Borg, K.&Olsson, H. (2005). High follicular phase luteinizing hormone levels in young healthy BRCA1 mutation carriers: implications for breast and ovarian cancer risk. *Mol Genet Metab*, Vol. 86, No. 1-2, pp. 320-7, ISSN 1096-7192.

Ji, Q., Liu, P.I., Chen, P.K., et al. (2004). Follicle stimulating hormone-induced growth promotion and gene expression profiles on ovarian surface epithelial cells. *Int J Cancer*, Vol. 112, No. 5, pp. 803-14, ISSN 0020-7136.

Kang, S.K., Cheng, K.W., Nathwani, P.S., et al. (2000). Autocrine role of gonadotropin-releasing hormone and its receptor in ovarian cancer cell growth. *Endocrine*, Vol. 13, No. 3, pp. 297-304, ISSN 1355-008X.

Karlan, B.Y., Jones, J., Greenwald, M., et al. (1995). Steroid hormone effects on the proliferation of human ovarian surface epithelium in vitro. *Am J Obstet Gynecol*, Vol. 173, No. 1, pp. 97-104, ISSN 0002-9378.

Kim, J.H., Park, D.C., Kim, J.W., et al. (1999). Antitumor effect of GnRH agonist in epithelial ovarian cancer. *Gynecol Oncol*, Vol. 74, No. 2, pp. 170-80, ISSN 0090-8258.

Kramer, S., Leeker, M. & Jager, W. (1998). Gonadotropin levels in ovarian cyst fluids: a predictor of malignancy? *Int J Biol Markers*, Vol. 13, No. 3, pp. 165-8, ISSN 0393-6155.

Kumar, T.R., Wang, Y. & Matzuk, M.M. (1996). Gonadotropins are essential modifier factors for gonadal tumor development in inhibin-deficient mice. *Endocrinology*, Vol. 137, No. 10, pp. 4210-6, ISSN 0013-7227.

Kumar, T.R., Palapattu, G., Wang, P., et al. (1999). Transgenic models to study gonadotropin function: the role of follicle-stimulating hormone in gonadal growth and tumorigenesis. *Mol Endocrinol*, Vol. 13, No. 6, pp. 851-65, ISSN 0888-8809.

Lacey, J.V., Jr., Mink, P.J., Lubin, J.H., et al. (2002). Menopausal hormone replacement therapy and risk of ovarian cancer. *JAMA*, Vol. 288, No. 3, pp. 334-41, ISSN 0098-7484.

Lambe, M., Wuu, J., Rossing, M.A., et al. (1999). Twinning and maternal risk of ovarian cancer. *Lancet*, Vol. 353, No. 9168, pp. 1941, ISSN 0140-6736.

Lau, K.M., Mok, S.C. & Ho, S.M. (1999). Expression of human estrogen receptor-alpha and -beta, progesterone receptor, and androgen receptor mRNA in normal and malignant ovarian epithelial cells. *Proc Natl Acad Sci U S A*, Vol. 96, No. 10, pp. 5722-7, ISSN 0027-8424.

Lau, M.T., Wong, A.S. & Leung, P.C. (2010). Gonadotropins induce tumor cell migration and invasion by increasing cyclooxygenases expression and prostaglandin E(2) production in human ovarian cancer cells. *Endocrinology*, Vol. 151, No. 7, pp. 2985-93, ISSN 1945-7170.

Laviolette, L.A., Garson, K., Macdonald, E.A., et al. (2010). 17beta-estradiol accelerates tumor onset and decreases survival in a transgenic mouse model of ovarian cancer. *Endocrinology*, Vol. 151, No. 3, pp. 929-38, ISSN 1945-7170.

Le Romancer, M., Poulard, C., Cohen, P., et al. (2011). Cracking the Estrogen Receptor's Posttranslational Code in Breast Tumors. *Endocr Rev*, Vol. No. pp. ISSN 1945-7189.

Leung, P.C. & Choi, J.H. (2007). Endocrine signaling in ovarian surface epithelium and cancer. *Human Reproduction Update*, Vol. 13, No. 2, pp. 143-162.

Levine, D., Park, K., Juretzka, M., et al. (2007). A phase II evaluation of goserelin and bicalutamide in patients with ovarian cancer in second or higher complete clinical disease remission. *Cancer*, Vol. 110, No. 11, pp. 2448-56, ISSN 0008-543X.

Levine, D.A. & Boyd, J. (2001). The androgen receptor and genetic susceptibility to ovarian cancer: results from a case series. *Cancer Res*, Vol. 61, No. 3, pp. 908-11, ISSN 0008-5472.

Li, A.J., Baldwin, R.L. & Karlan, B.Y. (2003). Estrogen and progesterone receptor subtype expression in normal and malignant ovarian epithelial cell cultures. *Am J Obstet Gynecol*, Vol. 189, No. 1, pp. 22-7, ISSN 0002-9378.

Li, Y.F., Hu, W., Fu, S.Q., et al. (2008). Aromatase inhibitors in ovarian cancer: is there a role? *Int J Gynecol Cancer*, Vol. 18, No. 4, pp. 600-14, ISSN 1525-1438.

Liu, J.F., Hirsch, M.S., Lee, H., et al. (2009). Prognosis and hormone receptor status in older and younger patients with advanced-stage papillary serous ovarian carcinoma. *Gynecol Oncol*, Vol. 115, No. 3, pp. 401-6, ISSN 1095-6859.

Lu, J.J., Zheng, Y., Kang, X., et al. (2000). Decreased luteinizing hormone receptor mRNA expression in human ovarian epithelial cancer. *Gynecol Oncol*, Vol. 79, No. 2, pp. 158-68, ISSN 0090-8258.

Lukanova, A., Lundin, E., Akhmedkhanov, A., et al. (2003). Circulating levels of sex steroid hormones and risk of ovarian cancer. *Int J Cancer*, Vol. 104, No. 5, pp. 636-42, ISSN 0020-7136.

Mabuchi, S., Ohmichi, M., Kimura, A., et al. (2004). Tamoxifen inhibits cell proliferation via mitogen-activated protein kinase cascades in human ovarian cancer cell lines in a manner not dependent on the expression of estrogen receptor or the sensitivity to cisplatin. *Endocrinology*, Vol. 145, No. 3, pp. 1302-13, ISSN 0013-7227.

Malik, S.T. & Slevin, M.L. (1991). Medroxyprogesterone acetate (MPA) in advanced granulosa cell tumours of the ovary--a new therapeutic approach? *Br J Cancer*, Vol. 63, No. 3, pp. 410-1, ISSN 0007-0920.

Marchant, J. (1961). The effect of hypophysectomy on the development of ovarian tumours in mice treated with dimethylbenzanthracene. *Br J Cancer*, Vol. 15, No. pp. 821-7, ISSN 0007-0920.

Markman, M., Iseminger, K.A., Hatch, K.D., et al. (1996). Tamoxifen in platinum-refractory ovarian cancer: a Gynecologic Oncology Group Ancillary Report. *Gynecol Oncol*, Vol. 62, No. 1, pp. 4-6, ISSN 0090-8258.

Markman, M., Kennedy, A., Webster, K., et al. (2000). Phase I trial of paclitaxel plus megestrol acetate in patients with paclitaxel-refractory ovarian cancer. *Clin Cancer Res*, Vol. 6, No. 11, pp. 4201-4, ISBN 1078-0432.

Markman, M., Webster, K., Zanotti, K., et al. (2004). Use of tamoxifen in asymptomatic patients with recurrent small-volume ovarian cancer. *Gynecol Oncol*, Vol. 93, No. 2, pp. 390-3, ISSN 0090-8258.

Martikainen, H., Penttinen, J., Huhtaniemi, I., et al. (1989). Gonadotropin-releasing hormone agonist analog therapy effective in ovarian granulosa cell malignancy. *Gynecol Oncol*, Vol. 35, No. 3, pp. 406-8, ISSN 0090-8258.

Matzuk, M.M., Finegold, M.J., Su, J.G., et al. (1992). Alpha-inhibin is a tumour-suppressor gene with gonadal specificity in mice. *Nature*, Vol. 360, No. 6402, pp. 313-9, ISSN 0028-0836.

McDonnel, A.C. & Murdoch, W.J. (2001). High-dose progesterone inhibition of urokinase secretion and invasive activity by SKOV-3 ovarian carcinoma cells: evidence for a receptor-independent nongenomic effect on the plasma membrane. *J Steroid Biochem Mol Biol*, Vol. 78, No. 2, pp. 185-91, ISSN 0960-0760.

McDonnel, A.C., Van Kirk, E.A., Isaak, D.D., et al. (2005). Effects of progesterone on ovarian tumorigenesis in xenografted mice. *Cancer Lett*, Vol. 221, No. 1, pp. 49-53, ISSN 0304-3835.

McSorley, M.A., Alberg, A.J., Allen, D.S., et al. (2009). Prediagnostic circulating follicle stimulating hormone concentrations and ovarian cancer risk. *Int J Cancer*, Vol. 125, No. 3, pp. 674-9, ISSN 1097-0215.

Minegishi, T., Kameda, T., Hirakawa, T., et al. (2000). Expression of gonadotropin and activin receptor messenger ribonucleic acid in human ovarian epithelial neoplasms. *Clin Cancer Res*, Vol. 6, No. 7, pp. 2764-70, ISSN 1078-0432.

Murdoch, W.J. & Martinchick, J.F. (2004). Oxidative damage to DNA of ovarian surface epithelial cells affected by ovulation: carcinogenic implication and chemoprevention. *Exp Biol Med (Maywood)*, Vol. 229, No. 6, pp. 546-52, ISSN 1535-3702.

Murdoch, W.J., Van Kirk, E.A., Isaak, D.D., et al. (2008). Progesterone facilitates cisplatin toxicity in epithelial ovarian cancer cells and xenografts. *Gynecol Oncol*, Vol. 110, No. 2, pp. 251-5, ISSN 1095-6859.

Narod, S.A., Risch, H., Moslehi, R., et al. (1998). Oral contraceptives and the risk of hereditary ovarian cancer. Hereditary Ovarian Cancer Clinical Study Group. *N Engl J Med*, Vol. 339, No. 7, pp. 424-8, ISSN 0028-4793.

Narod, S.A., Dube, M.P., Klijn, J., et al. (2002). Oral contraceptives and the risk of breast cancer in BRCA1 and BRCA2 mutation carriers. *J Natl Cancer Inst*, Vol. 94, No. 23, pp. 1773-9, ISSN 0027-8874.

Ness, R.B., Grisso, J.A., Cottreau, C., et al. (2000). Factors related to inflammation of the ovarian epithelium and risk of ovarian cancer. *Epidemiology*, Vol. 11, No. 2, pp. 111-7, ISSN 1044-3983.

Nguyen, H. & Syed, V. (2010). Progesterone inhibits growth and induces apoptosis in cancer cells through modulation of reactive oxygen species. *Gynecol Endocrinol*, Vol. No. pp. ISSN 1473-0766.

Norman, B.H., Dodge, J.A., Richardson, T.I., et al. (2006). Benzopyrans are selective estrogen receptor beta agonists with novel activity in models of benign prostatic hyperplasia. *J Med Chem*, Vol. 49, No. 21, pp. 6155-7, ISSN 0022-2623.

Nourbakhsh, M., Golestani, A., Zahrai, M., et al. (2010). Androgens stimulate telomerase expression, activity and phosphorylation in ovarian adenocarcinoma cells. *Mol Cell Endocrinol*, Vol. 330, No. 1-2, pp. 10-6, ISSN 1872-8057.

Pan, Y. & Kao, M.S. (2010). Endometrioid ovarian carcinoma benefits from aromatase inhibitors: case report and literature review. *Curr Oncol*, Vol. 17, No. 6, pp. 82-5, ISSN 1198-0052.

Parrott, J.A., Doraiswamy, V., Kim, G., et al. (2001). Expression and actions of both the follicle stimulating hormone receptor and the luteinizing hormone receptor in normal ovarian surface epithelium and ovarian cancer. *Mol Cell Endocrinol*, Vol. 172, No. 1-2, pp. 213-22, ISSN 0303-7207.

Peluso, J.J., Liu, X., Saunders, M.M., et al. (2008). Regulation of ovarian cancer cell viability and sensitivity to cisplatin by progesterone receptor membrane component-1. *J Clin Endocrinol Metab*, Vol. 93, No. 5, pp. 1592-9, ISSN 0021-972X.

Peluso, J.J., Gawkowska, A., Liu, X., et al. (2009). Progesterone receptor membrane component-1 regulates the development and Cisplatin sensitivity of human ovarian tumors in athymic nude mice. *Endocrinology*, Vol. 150, No. 11, pp. 4846-54, ISSN 1945-7170.

Quirk, S.M., Cowan, R.G. & Harman, R.M. (2006). The susceptibility of granulosa cells to apoptosis is influenced by oestradiol and the cell cycle. *J Endocrinol*, Vol. 189, No. 3, pp. 441-53, ISSN 0022-0795.

Rae, M.T., Niven, D., Critchley, H.O., et al. (2004a). Antiinflammatory steroid action in human ovarian surface epithelial cells. *J Clin Endocrinol Metab*, Vol. 89, No. 9, pp. 4538-44, ISSN 0021-972X.

Rae, M.T., Niven, D., Ross, A., et al. (2004b). Steroid signalling in human ovarian surface epithelial cells: the response to interleukin-1alpha determined by microarray analysis. *J Endocrinol*, Vol. 183, No. 1, pp. 19-28, ISSN 0022-0795.

Rae, M.T. & Hillier, S.G. (2005). Steroid signalling in the ovarian surface epithelium. *Trends Endocrinol Metab*, Vol. 16, No. 7, pp. 327-33, ISSN 1043-2760.

Riman, T. (2003). Hormone replacement therapy and epithelial ovarian cancer: is there and association? *J Br Menopause Soc*, Vol. 9, No. 2, pp. 61-8, ISSN 1362-1807.

Rinaldi, S., Dossus, L., Lukanova, A., et al. (2007). Endogenous androgens and risk of epithelial ovarian cancer: results from the European Prospective Investigation into Cancer and Nutrition (EPIC). *Cancer Epidemiol Biomarkers Prev*, Vol. 16, No. 1, pp. 23-9, ISSN 1055-9965.

Risch, H.A., Marrett, L.D. & Howe, G.R. (1994). Parity, contraception, infertility, and the risk of epithelial ovarian cancer. *Am J Epidemiol*, Vol. 140, No. 7, pp. 585-97, ISSN 0002-9262.

Risch, H.A. (1998). Hormonal etiology of epithelial ovarian cancer, with a hypothesis concerning the role of androgens and progesterone. *J Natl Cancer Inst*, Vol. 90, No. 23, pp. 1774-86, ISSN 0027-8874.

Risch, H.A. (2002). Hormone replacement therapy and the risk of ovarian cancer. *Gynecol Oncol*, Vol. 86, No. 2, pp. 115-7, ISSN 0090-8258.

Risma, K.A., Clay, C.M., Nett, T.M., et al. (1995). Targeted overexpression of luteinizing hormone in transgenic mice leads to infertility, polycystic ovaries, and ovarian tumors. *Proc Natl Acad Sci U S A*, Vol. 92, No. 5, pp. 1322-6, ISSN 0027-8424.

Rocereto, T.F., Saul, H.M., Aikins, J.A., Jr., et al. (2000). Phase II study of mifepristone (RU486) in refractory ovarian cancer. *Gynecol Oncol*, Vol. 77, No. 3, pp. 429-32, ISSN 0090-8258.

Rodriguez, C., Patel, A.V., Calle, E.E., et al. (2001). Estrogen replacement therapy and ovarian cancer mortality in a large prospective study of US women. *JAMA*, Vol. 285, No. 11, pp. 1460-5, ISSN 0098-7484.

Rodriguez, G.C., Walmer, D.K., Cline, M., et al. (1998). Effect of progestin on the ovarian epithelium of macaques: cancer prevention through apoptosis? *J Soc Gynecol Investig*, Vol. 5, No. 5, pp. 271-6, ISSN 1071-5576.

Romero, I.L., Gordon, I.O., Jagadeeswaran, S., et al. (2009). Effects of oral contraceptives or a gonadotropin-releasing hormone agonist on ovarian carcinogenesis in genetically engineered mice. *Cancer Prev Res (Phila)*, Vol. 2, No. 9, pp. 792-9, ISSN 1940-6215.

Rustin, G.J., van der Burg, M.E., Griffin, C.L., et al. (2010). Early versus delayed treatment of relapsed ovarian cancer (MRC OV05/EORTC 55955): a randomised trial. *Lancet*, Vol. 376, No. 9747, pp. 1155-63, ISSN 1474-547X.

Schiffenbauer, Y.S., Abramovitch, R., Meir, G., et al. (1997). Loss of ovarian function promotes angiogenesis in human ovarian carcinoma. *Proc Natl Acad Sci U S A*, Vol. 94, No. 24, pp. 13203-8, ISSN 0027-8424.

Schumer, S.T. & Cannistra, S.A. (2003). Granulosa cell tumor of the ovary. *J Clin Oncol*, Vol. 21, No. 6, pp. 1180-9, ISSN 0732-183X.

Shapiro, D.J., Mao, C. & Cherian, M.T. (2011). Small molecule inhibitors as probes for estrogen and androgen receptor action. *J Biol Chem*, Vol. 286, No. 6, pp. 4043-8, ISSN 1083-351X.

Sheach, L.A., Adeney, E.M., Kucukmetin, A., et al. (2009). Androgen-related expression of G-proteins in ovarian cancer. *Br J Cancer*, Vol. 101, No. 3, pp. 498-503, ISSN 1532-1827.

Shi, P., Zhang, Y., Tong, X., et al. (2011). Dihydrotestosterone induces p27 degradation via direct binding with SKP2 in ovarian and breast cancer. *Int J Mol Med*, Vol. 28, No. 1, pp. 109-14, ISSN 1791-244X.

Simpson, B.J., Langdon, S.P., Rabiasz, G.J., et al. (1998). Estrogen regulation of transforming growth factor-alpha in ovarian cancer. *J Steroid Biochem Mol Biol*, Vol. 64, No. 3-4, pp. 137-45, ISSN 0960-0760.

Smyth, J.F., Gourley, C., Walker, G., et al. (2007). Antiestrogen therapy is active in selected ovarian cancer cases: the use of letrozole in estrogen receptor-positive patients. *Clin Cancer Res*, Vol. 13, No. 12, pp. 3617-22, ISSN 1078-0432.

So, W.K., Cheng, J.C., Poon, S.L., et al. (2008). Gonadotropin-releasing hormone and ovarian cancer: a functional and mechanistic overview. *FEBS J*, Vol. 275, No. 22, pp. 5496-511, ISSN 1742-4658.

Song, J., Fadiel, A., Edusa, V., et al. (2005). Estradiol-induced ezrin overexpression in ovarian cancer: a new signaling domain for estrogen. *Cancer Lett*, Vol. 220, No. 1, pp. 57-65, ISSN 0304-3835.

Stewart, S.L., Querec, T.D., Gruver, B.N., et al. (2004). Gonadotropin and steroid hormones stimulate proliferation of the rat ovarian surface epithelium. *J Cell Physiol*, Vol. 198, No. 1, pp. 119-24, ISSN 0021-9541.

Sugiyama, M., Imai, A., Furui, T., et al. (2005). Gonadotropin-releasing hormone retards doxorubicin-induced apoptosis and serine/threonine phosphatase inhibition in ovarian cancer cells. *Oncol Rep*, Vol. 13, No. 5, pp. 813-7, ISSN 1021-335X.

Syed, V., Ulinski, G., Mok, S.C., et al. (2001). Expression of gonadotropin receptor and growth responses to key reproductive hormones in normal and malignant human ovarian surface epithelial cells. *Cancer Res*, Vol. 61, No. 18, pp. 6768-76, ISSN 0008-5472.

Syed, V., Ulinski, G., Mok, S.C., et al. (2002). Reproductive hormone-induced, STAT3-mediated interleukin 6 action in normal and malignant human ovarian surface epithelial cells. *J Natl Cancer Inst*, Vol. 94, No. 8, pp. 617-29, ISSN 0027-8874.

Syed, V.&Ho, S.M. (2003). Progesterone-induced apoptosis in immortalized normal and malignant human ovarian surface epithelial cells involves enhanced expression of FasL. *Oncogene*, Vol. 22, No. 44, pp. 6883-90, ISSN 0950-9232.

Syed, V., Mukherjee, K., Godoy-Tundidor, S., et al. (2007). Progesterone induces apoptosis in TRAIL-resistant ovarian cancer cells by circumventing c-FLIPL overexpression. *J Cell Biochem*, Vol. 102, No. 2, pp. 442-52, ISSN 0730-2312.

Takekida, S., Matsuo, H.&Maruo, T. (2003). GnRH agonist action on granulosa cells at varying follicular stages. *Mol Cell Endocrinol*, Vol. 202, No. 1-2, pp. 155-64, ISSN 0303-7207.

Tashiro, H., Katabuchi, H., Begum, M., et al. (2003). Roles of luteinizing hormone/chorionic gonadotropin receptor in anchorage-dependent and -independent growth in human ovarian surface epithelial cell lines. *Cancer Sci*, Vol. 94, No. 11, pp. 953-9, ISSN 1347-9032.

Tumolo, S., Rao, B.R., van der Burg, M.E., et al. (1994). Phase II trial of flutamide in advanced ovarian cancer: an EORTC Gynaecological Cancer Cooperative Group study. *Eur J Cancer*, Vol. 30A, No. 7, pp. 911-4, ISSN 0959-8049.

Tworoger, S.S., Fairfield, K.M., Colditz, G.A., et al. (2007). Association of oral contraceptive use, other contraceptive methods, and infertility with ovarian cancer risk. *Am J Epidemiol*, Vol. 166, No. 8, pp. 894-901, ISSN 0002-9262.

Vassilomanolakis, M., Koumakis, G., Barbounis, V., et al. (1997). A phase II study of flutamide in ovarian cancer. *Oncology*, Vol. 54, No. 3, pp. 199-202, ISSN 0030-2414.

Veenhof, C.H., van der Burg, M.E., Nooy, M., et al. (1994). Phase II study of high-dose megestrol acetate in patients with advanced ovarian carcinoma. *Eur J Cancer*, Vol. 30A, No. 5, pp. 697-8, ISSN 0959-8049.

Verma, S., Alhayki, M., Le, K., et al. (2006). Phase II study of exemestane (E) in refractory ovarian cancer (ROC) *Journal of Clinical Oncology, 2006 ASCO Annual Meeting Proceedings (Post-Meeting Edition).* Vol. 24, No. 18S, pp. 5026.

Wagner, U., du Bois, A., Pfisterer, J., et al. (2007). Gefitinib in combination with tamoxifen in patients with ovarian cancer refractory or resistant to platinum-taxane based therapy--a phase II trial of the AGO Ovarian Cancer Study Group (AGO-OVAR 2.6). *Gynecol Oncol*, Vol. 105, No. 1, pp. 132-7, ISSN 0090-8258.

Walker, G., MacLeod, K., Williams, A.R., et al. (2007). Estrogen-regulated gene expression predicts response to endocrine therapy in patients with ovarian cancer. *Gynecol Oncol*, Vol. 106, No. 3, pp. 461-8, ISSN 0090-8258.

Wang, J., Luo, F., Lu, J.J., et al. (2002). VEGF expression and enhanced production by gonadotropins in ovarian epithelial tumors. *Int J Cancer*, Vol. 97, No. 2, pp. 163-7, ISSN 0020-7136.

Whittemore, A.S., Harris, R. & Itnyre, J. (1992). Characteristics relating to ovarian cancer risk: collaborative analysis of 12 US case-control studies. II. Invasive epithelial ovarian cancers in white women. Collaborative Ovarian Cancer Group. *Am J Epidemiol*, Vol. 136, No. 10, pp. 1184-203, ISSN 0002-9262.

Wimalasena, J., Meehan, D., Dostal, R., et al. (1993). Growth factors interact with estradiol and gonadotropins in the regulation of ovarian cancer cell growth and growth factor receptors. *Oncol Res*, Vol. 5, No. 8, pp. 325-37, ISSN 0965-0407.

Wright, J.W., Stouffer, R.L. & Rodland, K.D. (2005). High-dose estrogen and clinical selective estrogen receptor modulators induce growth arrest, p21, and p53 in primate ovarian surface epithelial cells. *J Clin Endocrinol Metab*, Vol. 90, No. 6, pp. 3688-95, ISSN 0021-972X.

Yano, T., Pinski, J., Radulovic, S., et al. (1994). Inhibition of human epithelial ovarian cancer cell growth in vitro by agonistic and antagonistic analogues of luteinizing hormone-releasing hormone. *Proc Natl Acad Sci U S A*, Vol. 91, No. 5, pp. 1701-5, ISSN 0027-8424.

Yousef, G.M., Fracchioli, S., Scorilas, A., et al. (2003). Steroid hormone regulation and prognostic value of the human kallikrein gene 14 in ovarian cancer. *Am J Clin Pathol*, Vol. 119, No. 3, pp. 346-55, ISSN 0002-9173.

Yue, X., Akahira, J., Utsunomiya, H., et al. (2010). Steroid and Xenobiotic Receptor (SXR) as a possible prognostic marker in epithelial ovarian cancer. *Pathol Int*, Vol. 60, No. 5, pp. 400-6, ISSN 1440-1827.

Zamagni, C., Wirtz, R.M., De Iaco, P., et al. (2009). Oestrogen receptor 1 mRNA is a prognostic factor in ovarian cancer patients treated with neo-adjuvant chemotherapy: determination by array and kinetic PCR in fresh tissue biopsies. *Endocr Relat Cancer*, Vol. 16, No. 4, pp. 1241-9, ISSN 1479-6821.

Zheng, H., Kavanagh, J.J., Hu, W., et al. (2007). Hormonal therapy in ovarian cancer. *Int J Gynecol Cancer*, Vol. 17, No. 2, pp. 325-38, ISSN 1048-891X.

Zheng, W., Lu, J.J., Luo, F., et al. (2000). Ovarian epithelial tumor growth promotion by follicle-stimulating hormone and inhibition of the effect by luteinizing hormone. *Gynecol Oncol*, Vol. 76, No. 1, pp. 80-8, ISSN 0090-8258.

Zidan, J., Zohar, S., Mijiritzky, I., et al. (2002). Treating relapsed epithelial ovarian cancer with luteinizing hormone-releasing agonist (goserelin) after failure of chemotherapy. *Isr Med Assoc J*, Vol. 4, No. 8, pp. 597-9, ISSN 1565-1088.

7

Salivary Cortisol Can Reflect Adiposity and Insulin Sensitivity in Type 2 Diabetes

Yoko Matsuzawa[1,2], Kenichi Sakurai[1], Jun Saito[2], Masao Omura[2] and Tetsuo Nishikawa[2]

[1]*Clinical Cell Biology and Medicine, Graduate School of Medicine, Chiba University,*
[2]*Division of Endocrinology and Metabolism, Endocrinology and Diabetes Center, Department of Medicine, Yokohama Rosai Hospital, Japan*

1. Introduction

Glucocorticoids are well known to play an important role in the regulation of most essential physiological processes (Atanasov & Odermatt,2007). Patients with Cushing`s syndrome show central obesity with insulin resistance, caused by hypersecretion of cortisol (F) (Arnaldi et al.,2004). Obese patients with type 2 diabetes often have symptoms usually observed in patients with Cushing`s syndrome, and F levels might reflect the severity of complications and metabolic abnormalities in diabetes (Chiodini et al.,2007). High levels of F are associated with activation or dysregulation of the hypothalamic-pituitary-adrenal (HPA) axis and increased volume of the adrenal glands (Pasquali et al.,2006, Godoy-Matos et al.,2006).

Moreover, various metabolic abnormalities induced by enhanced glucocorticoid activity were found to be not only due to accelerated function of the HPA axis, but also by an impairment in 11β-hydroxysteroid dehydrogenase (11β-HSD) enzymes within the target cells (Godoy-Matos et at.,2006). 11β-HSD has two isoforms: 11β-HSD type 1 (11β-HSD1) mainly works as a reductase which converts inactive cortisone (E) to active cortisol (F) in F target tissues (Walker & Andrew,2006). 11β-HSD type 2 (11β-HSD2) is expressed in mineralocorticoid target tissues such as the distal nephron, colon, and salivary glands (Tannin et al.,1991, Draper & Stewart, 2005, Edwards et al., 1988), converting F to E to protect mineralocorticoid receptors from activation by F.

Animal models demonstrated that activation of 11β-HSD1 exhibited features of metabolic syndrome (Masuzaki et al.,2004, Morton et al.,2004). It was also reported that 11β-HSD1 is increased in subcutaneous adipose tissue in obese patients (Rask et al.,2002, Paulmyer-Lacroi et al.,2002), and higher 11β-HSD1 activity in adipose tissue is associated with features of metabolic syndrome in Caucasians and Pima Indians (Lindsay et al.,2003). Thus, it is suggested that F may play a crucial role in the regulation of adiposity in type 2 diabetes with obesity. On the other hand, the exact role of abnormal glucocorticoid metabolism in the pathogenesis of obesity has not fully been clarified yet. Salivary cortisol has been reported to be in closer agreement with the real adrenocortical function than serum cortisol concentration (Bolufer et al.,1989). Measurement of salivary cortisol was also reported to have several advantages, such as directly reflecting free cortisol level (Vining et al.,1983), and non-invasiveness for sampling (Chen et al.,1985). We, therefore, analyzed samples from serum, saliva, and 24h-collected urine from obese type 2 diabetic patients as well as healthy subjects in order to evaluate clinical usefulness of salivary cortisol accurately measured by liquid mass spectroscopy in obese patients with type 2 diabetes.

2. Subjects and methods

2.1 Subjects

Eighteen Japanese men without underlying diseases cooperated as the healthy subject group. As the patient group, 23 Japanese male patients with type 2 diabetes, admitted to the Department of Endocrinology and Metabolism in Yokohama Rosai Hospital between March 2006 and March 2007, who met the following conditions were selected:1) waist circumference of 85 cm or greater, 2) stage 1 or 2 diabetic nephropathy, 3) not treated with oral biguanide or thiazolidine derivatives, and 4)understanding the objective of this study and giving written consent. This study was approved by the research ethics committee of Yokohama Rosai Hospital.

2.2 Measurement of serum and salivary steroids

Five ml of blood and 1 ml of saliva were collected before breakfast and supper on the same day under regular conditions of daily life from the controls and patients. Furthermore, 5ml of blood and 1ml of saliva 2 hours after breakfast, lunch and supper, and 20 ml of 24-h accumulated urine were collected on the same day during hospitalization on 7 days after admission from the patient group. The diet consisted of 25kcal/kg for ideal body weight distributed in three meals.

Blood samples were immediately centrifuged, and the sera were stored at -30°C until measurement. Saliva and accumulated urine samples were stored with no processing at -30°C. Cortisol and cortisone in the samples were measured by liquid chromatography-tandem mass spectrometry (LC-MS/MS) (Teikoku Hormone Mfg.-Asuka Pharmaceutical Co., Tokyo, Japan).

2.3 Glucose clamp

Euglycemic-hyperinsulinemic glucose clamping was performed in 14 of the patient group using an artificial pancreas (STG-22, Nikkiso, Tokyo, Japan), following the method described previously (Bergman et al.,1985, Nishikawa et al.,1996). Average age, HbA1c and BMI of these patients were not significantly different from those of the whole cases in

	Diabetic subjects	Healthy Volunteers	P value
n	23	18	
Age (yr)	54.7±13.6	48.3±14.3	0.32
BMI(kg/m^2)	28.2± 5.4	22.1±2.0	<.001
Waist circumference (cm)	96.6±12.4	80.8±5.6	<.001
Duration of diabetes (yr)	7.0±4.7	—	—
HbA1c(%)	10.6±1.9	—	—

(data expressed as mean ±SD)

Table 1. Anthropometric measures and background of the subjects

patient group. In patients under drug treatment for diabetes, administration of sulfonylurea and a long-acting insulin preparation was suspended from the previous evening to avoid their influence on the test.

2.4 Statistical analysis

The subjects' backgrounds are presented as the means ± standard deviation, and the t-test was used to compare healthy subjects with patients. To analyze the correlation between 2 variables, Spearman's correlation coefficient was used, and a level of less than 5% was regarded as significant.

3. Results

3.1 Subject characteristics

The characteristics of the healthy and patient group, including age and BMI, are described in Table 1. The mean duration of illness was 7.0 ± 4.7 years in the patient group, and 14 (60.9%) and 8 (34.8%) patients were under treatment with insulin and oral drugs, respectively at the time of sample collection.

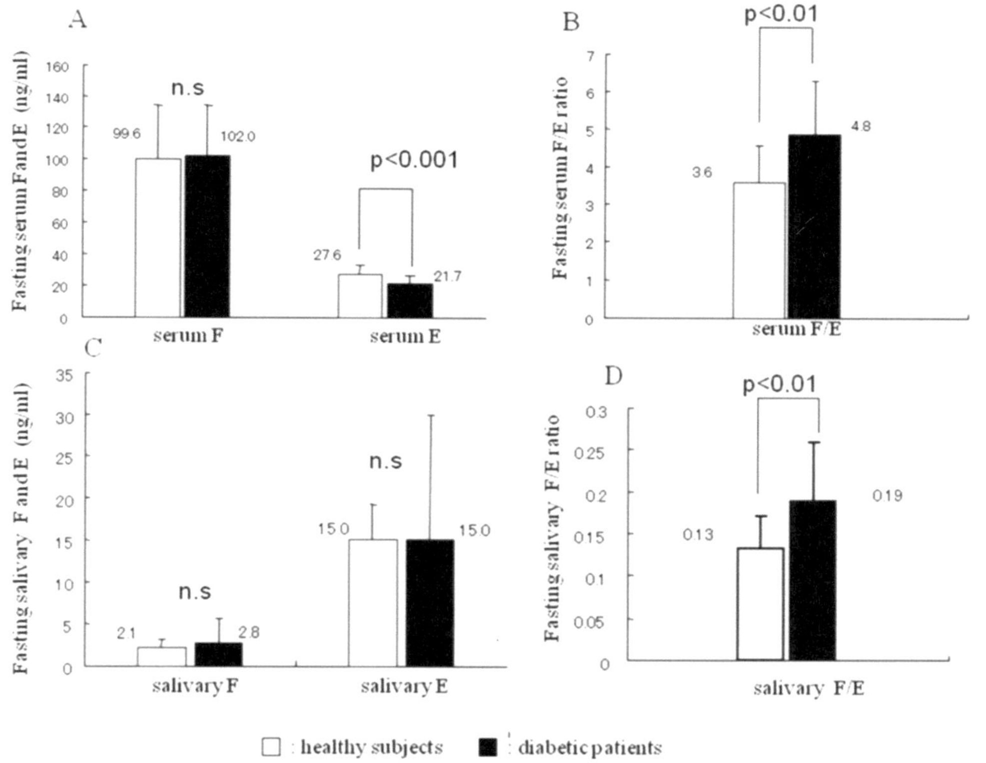

Serum levels of F and E were not different between healthy subjects and diabetic patients (A), and the ratio of F to E was significantly higher in the patient group (B). A similar result was observed for saliva (C, D). Data are expressed as the means±S.D. Statistical significance between healthy and diabetic subjects is described inside the figure.

Fig. 1. Comparison of F, E, and F/E ratios between healthy subjects and diabetic patients in the fasting phase in the morning.

3.2 Relationship between F/E ratio and body weight

As shown in Fig. 1, no significant difference was noted in the blood cortisol (F) level before breakfast between the healthy and patient group, but the cortisone (E) level was lower in the patient group. Accordingly, the ratio of F to E (F/E) in blood was significantly higher in the patient group (3.6 vs. 4.8, respectively, $p<0.01$).

There was no significant difference in F or E level in saliva before breakfast between the healthy and patient group. Unlike the blood levels, E level was higher than F level in saliva. This is considered to be the influence of 11β-HSD2 expressed in the salivary gland (Tannin et al.,1991). However, the F/E ratio in saliva was significantly higher in the patient group, as in blood (0.13 vs. 0.19, respectively, $p<0.01$).

There was no correlation between the blood F/E ratio before breakfast and body mass index (BMI) in healthy subjects (Fig.2A), while there was a strong positive correlation between the blood F/E ratio and BMI in the patient group (Fig.2B). This correlation also remained significant after correction with age, HbA1c and blood glucose level before breakfast. Furthermore, a similar result was observed in salivary samples. The salivary F/E ratio tended to show a positive correlation with BMI in diabetic patients, but not in healthy subjects (Fig.2C, D).

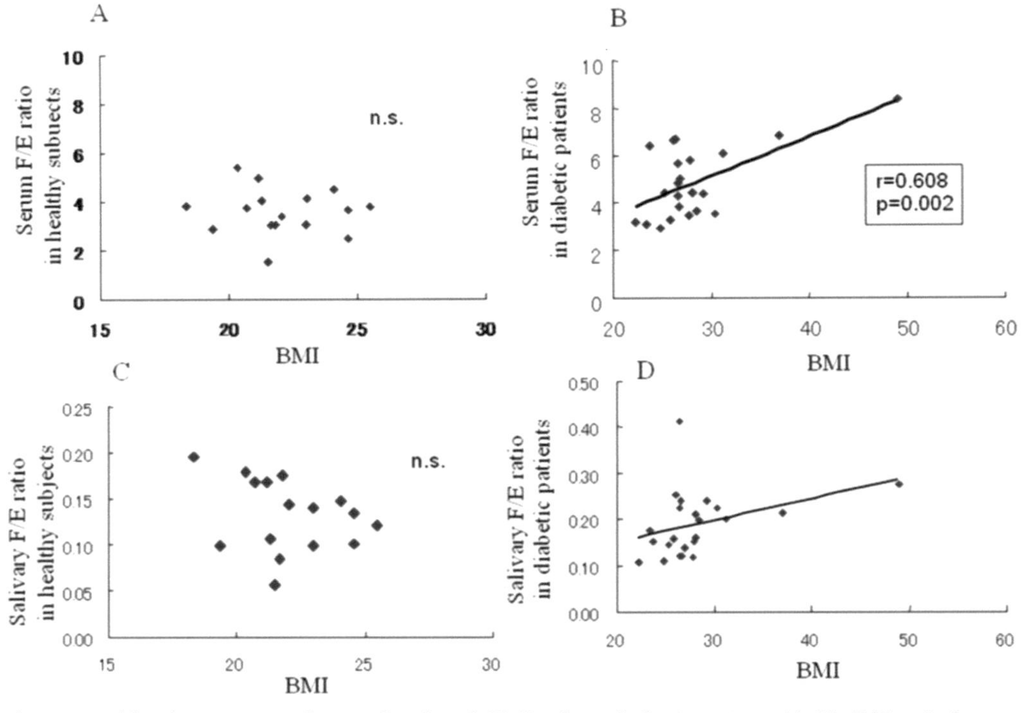

F/E ratio in blood was positively correlated with BMI only in diabetic patients (A, B). F/E ratio from salivary samples also showed a similar tendency, although the correlation was not statistically significant in diabetic patients (C, D).

Fig. 2. Correlation between fasting F/E ratio and BMI.

Fig. 3 shows the relationship between the fasting blood F/E ratio and fat volume assessed by abdominal CT in the patient group. The F/E ratio was positively correlated with the subcutaneous fat area, but was not correlated with the area of visceral fat. Furthermore, the fasting blood and salivary F/E ratio was strongly correlated with serum leptin level ($r=0.652$, $p<.0.01$ for blood, $r=0.469$, $p<.0.05$ for saliva), but was not correlated with the plasma concentration of high molecular weight adiponectin or the severity of insulin resistance measured by glucose clamping (data not shown).

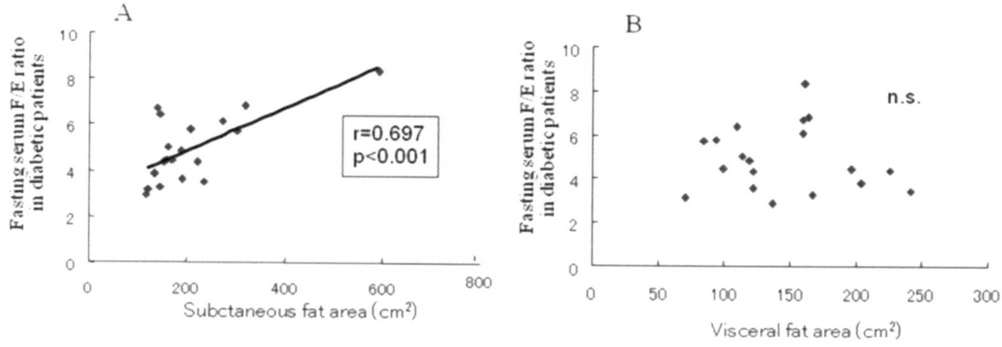

Fasting blood F/E ratio positively correlated with subcutaneous fat area (A), but no correlation was found between F/E ratio and visceral fat area (B).

Fig. 3. Relationship between fasting blood F/E ratio and body fat area assessed by CT scan.

3.3 Relationship between salivary cortisol and insulin sensitivity

Blood and saliva were collected at 4-time points: before breakfast and 2 hours after each meal in the patient group. Fig. 4 shows the diurnal variation of F after assessing the level before breakfast as 1.0. The F level significantly decreased with time and the variation was larger in saliva than in blood. The within-day variation of the F/E ratio was smaller than that of the F level.

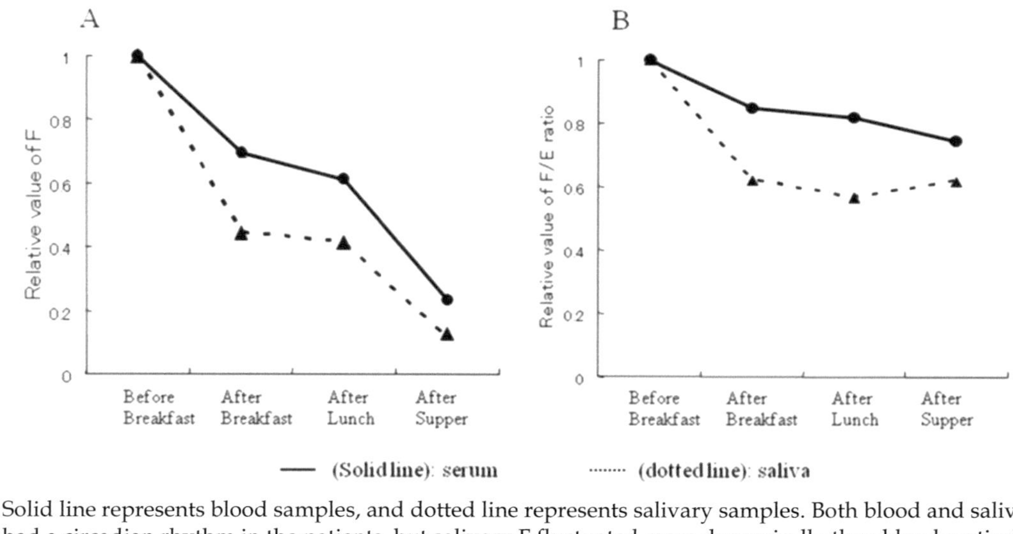

Solid line represents blood samples, and dotted line represents salivary samples. Both blood and saliva had a circadian rhythm in the patients, but salivary F fluctuated more dynamically than blood cortisol within a day.

Fig. 4. Circadian rhythm of F (A) and F/E ratio (B) in diabetic patients.

The salivary F level after breakfast was strongly correlated with the severity of insulin resistance measured by the glucose clamp (Fig. 5). This relationship with insulin resistance was not significantly noted in blood F.

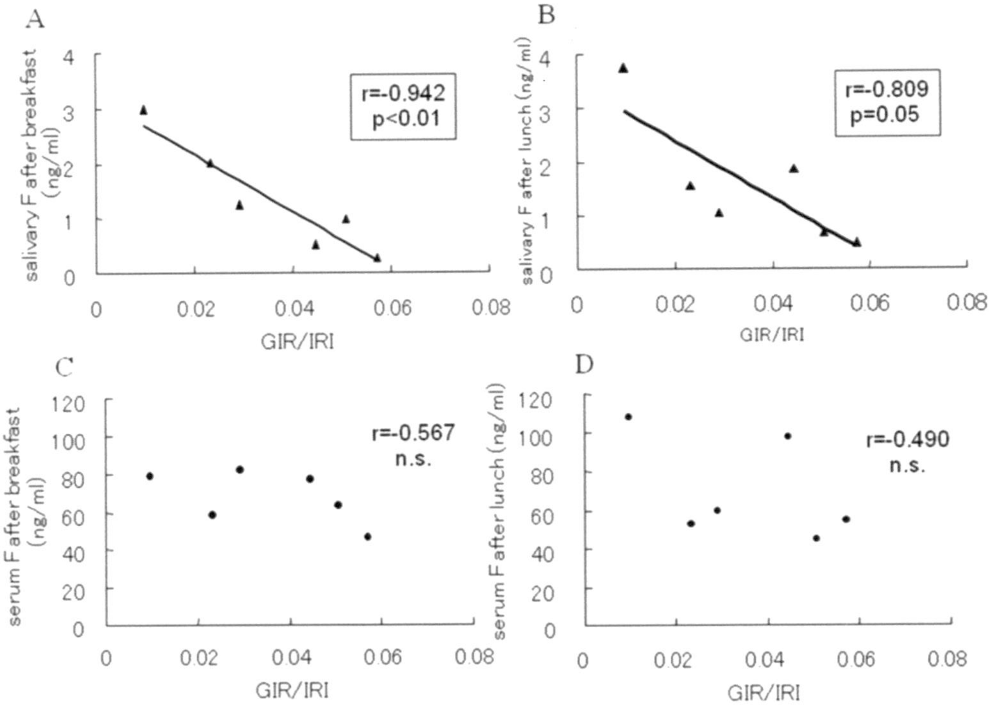

Salivary F after breakfast showed the strongest negative correlation with GIR/IRI (A, B), while serum F(C, D) does not show significant correlation with insulin sensitivity.

Fig. 5. Relationship between insulin sensitivity (GIR/IRI) and F.

4. Discussion

The present study clearly demonstrated that obese patients with type 2 diabetes had a higher fasting F/E ratio in blood and saliva in the morning, comparing with healthy control subjects. Consistent with our results, an elevated blood F/E ratio in patients with type 2 diabetes has been reported (Valsamakis et al.,2004, Homma et al.,2001, Sinha & Caro 1998). Moreover, this is the first report demonstrating a significant increase in the F/E ratio in obese diabetic patients in saliva as well as in blood. Thus, it is suggested that overweight seems to induce much more F formation rather than E production via some mechanism(s) of changing steroidogenic enzymes, including 11β-HSD1 and 2.

Our data also showed a positive relationship between the fasting F/E ratio and BMI, between the fasting F/E ratio and total fat volume, and between the fasting F/E ratio and leptin, in diabetic obese patients. It is, therefore, suggested that the fasting F/E ratio may reflect the severity of adiposity accumulated to both of subcutaneous and visceral areas in obese diabetics, since circulating leptin levels are reported to be the best predictor of total body fat mass (Sinha & Caro,1998). Thus it can be postulated that increased fat mass may lead to increased F production, at least partly mediated by 11β-HSD1 in adipose tissue, resulting in an elevated F/E ratio after overnight fasting. It was also reported that the expression of 11β-HSD1 is increased in adipose tissue in simple obesity (Rask et al.,2002, Paulmyer-Lacroi et al.,2002, Lindsay et al.,2003), suggesting that the ratio of F to E is a biomarker for assessing the adiposity in obese patients.

Oltmanns et al. (Oltmanns et al.,2006) recently reported that the level of salivary F of which sample was taken between breakfast and lunch was significantly related to metabolic findings in type 2 diabetes, such as fasting and postprandial blood glucose, urinary glucose, and glycosylated hemoglobin, although insulin sensitivity was not directly assessed in their study. Our data demonstrated that a circadian rhythm of F was apparently observed both in blood and saliva, and salivary F 2 hours after breakfast was shown to significantly correlate with insulin sensitivity assessed by euglycemic glucose clamping in obese patients with type 2 diabetes. Salivary F has been reported to have a circadian rhythm, highest in the morning, with lunch followed by a peak (Rosmond et al.,1998), suggesting that the salivary level of F usually decreases before lunch under normal conditions. Thus, it is suggested from our data that the level of salivary F before lunch, reflecting insulin sensitivity, may be up-regulated by food intake after breakfast despite of decreasing ACTH level by diurnal rhythm, since eating was reported to stimulate F secretion and women with abdominal obesity have also been reported to have a greater rise of F in response to food than those with peripheral obesity in simple obesity (Pasquali et al.,1998, Duclos et al.,2005, Korbonits et al.,1996). It had been recently reported that U-shaped associations were apparent between diurnal slope in salivary F and both BMI and waist circumference (Kumari et al.,2010), and also that 6 wk of supplementation with fish oil significantly increased lean mass and decreased fat mass, which were significantly correlated with a reduction in salivary F following fish oil treatment (Noreen et al.,2010).

Moreover, we should consider why salivary F could reflect insulin resistance in diabetic patients, while blood F could not. First, F measured in blood was the total of the free form and protein-bound form, while F in saliva reflected the biologically active blood unbound F level (Vining et al.,1983). The level of blood F can be altered by the concentration of blood F binding globulin (CBG), and CBG levels are shown to correlate negatively with BMI, waist-to-hip ratio, and HOMA (Fernandez-Real et al.,2002). Hence, salivary F is supposed to indicate the level of 'real' F activity in vivo, and thus correlates strongly with insulin resistance. Second, as shown in Fig. 4, salivary F fluctuates more dynamically than blood F within a day. None of our patients were diagnosed as overt or subclinical Cushing syndrome, and their levels of F were within the normal range. However, even a small increase in blood F within the normal range may contribute to abnormal glucose metabolism in metabolic syndrome and type 2 diabetes (Khani & Tayek,2001), and salivary F seems to be more sensitive than blood F to detect subtle changes in the metabolic state.

On the other hand, our results demonstrated that there is not significantly positive correlation between salivary F after breakfast and visceral fat mass. Visceral fat volume is known to be one of the most important factors to determine insulin resistance (Bergman et al.,2007), but our data suggest that F has a significant influence on insulin resistance, and intimately related to total fat volume. Furthermore, many factors including levels of glucose and insulin are supposed to modulate F metabolism after meals. Therefore, measuring salivary F after breakfast in obese diabetic patients may be a useful and noninvasive simple method to predict overall insulin sensitivity and severity of adiposity in such patients.

In conclusion, we tried to investigate the role of blood and salivary F and E in the regulatory mechanisms of obesity in obese men with type 2 diabetes. They had a higher fasting F/E ratio in both blood and saliva than that in healthy controls. Moreover, the fasting F/E ratio showed a significant correlation with total fat volume, suggesting that the fasting ratio of F to E in saliva and blood seems to directly reflect the adiposity in type 2 diabetic patients with obesity. Our data also demonstrated that salivary F after breakfast is suggested to be one of the most useful markers of insulin sensitivity in these patients. On the other hand, our study was conducted with a cross-sectional design, which does not allow us to assume any direct causality of F to insulin resistance. The role of F metabolism in adipogenesis and insulin resistance in type 2 diabetes will require further investigation with a prospective design.

5. Acknowledgment

This work was partly supported by Health and Labour Sciences Research Grants for Research on Intractable Diseases from Japanese Government.

6. References

Arnaldi G., Mancini T., Polenta B. & Boscaro M. (2004) Cardiovascular risk in Cushing's syndrome. *Pituitary* 7:253-6.

Atanasov A.G., Odermatt A. 2007 Readjusting the glucocorticoid balance: an opportunity for modulators of 11β-hydroxysteroid dehydrogenase type 1 activity? *Endocr Metab Immune Disord Drug Targets*.7:125-40.

Bergman R.N., Finegood D.T. & Ader M. (1985) Assessment of insulin sensitivity in vivo. *Endocr Rev.* 6:45-86.

Bergman R.N., Kim S.P., Hsu I.R., Catalano K.J., Chiu J.D., Kabir M., Richey J.M. & Ader M. (2007) Abdominal obesity: role in the pathophysiology of metabolic disease and cardiovascular risk. *Am J Med* 120: S3-8; discussion S29-32

Bolufer P., Gandia A & Antonio P. (1989) Salivary corticosteroids in the study of adrenal function. *Clin Chem Acta*, 183: 217-225

Chen Y.M, Cintron N.M & Whitson P.A. (1985) Long-term storage of salivary cortisol samples at room temperature. *Clin Chem* 38: 304

Chiodini I, Adda G, Scillitani A, Coletti F, Morelli V, Di Lembo S, Epaminonda P, Masserini B, Beck-Peccoz P, Orsi E, Ambrosi B & Arosio M (2007) Cortisol secretion in patients with type 2 diabetes. *Diabetes Care* 30: 83-88

Draper N & Stewart P.M. (2005) 11β-hydroxysteroid dehydrogenase and the pre-receptor regulation of corticosteroid hormone action. *J Endocrinol* 186: 251-271

Duclos M. Pareira P.M., Barat P., Gatta B. & Roger P. (2005) Increased cortisol bioavailability, abdominal obesity, and the metabolic syndrome in obese women. *Obesity Research* 13: 1157-1166

Edwards CR, Stewart PM, Burt D, Brett L, McIntyre MA, Sutanto WS, de Kloet ER & Monder C. (1988) Localization of 11β-hydroxysteroid dehydrogenase: tissue specific protector of the mineralocorticoid receptor. *Lancet* 2(8618): 986-989

Fernandez-Real JM, Pugeat M, Grasa M, Broch M, Vendrell J, Brun J & Ricart W. (2002) Serum corticosteroid-binding globulin concentration and insulin resistance syndrome: a population study. *J Clin Endocrinol Metab* 87: 4686-90

Godoy-Matos A.F., Vieira A.R & Meirelles R.M. (2006) The potential role of increased adrenal volume in the pathophysiology of obesity-related type 2 diabetes. *J Endocrinol Invest* 29:159-63

Homma M, Tanaka A, Hino K, Takamura H, Hirano T, Oka K, Kanazawa M, Miwa T, Notoya Y, Niitsuma T & Hayashi T. (2001) Assessing systemic 11β-hydroxysteroid dehydrogenase with serum cortisone/cortisol ratios in healthy subjects and patients with diabetes mellitus and chronic renal failure. *Metabolism* 50: 801-804

Khani S, Tayek J.A. 2001 Cortisol increases gluconeogenesis in humans: its role in the metabolic syndrome. *Clinical Science* 101: 739-747

Korbonits M, Trainer PJ, Nelson ML, Howse I, Kopelman PG, Besser GM, Grossman AB & Svec F. (1996) Differential stimulation of cortisol and dehydroepiandrosterone levels by food in obese and normal subjects: relation to body fat distribution. *Clin Endocrinol.* 45: 699-706.

Kumari M, Chandola T, Brunner E & Kivimaki M. (2010) A nonlinear relationship of generalized and central obesity with diurnal cortisol secretion in the Whitehall II study. *J Clin Endocrinol Metab.* 95:4415-23.

Lindsay R.S., Wake D.J., Nair S., Bunt J., Livingstone D.E.W., Permana P.A., Tataranni P.A. & Walke B.R. (2003) Subcutaneous adipose 11β-hydroxysteroid dehydrogenase type 1 activity and messenger ribonucleic acid levels are associated with adiposity and insulinemia in Pima Indians and Caucasians. *J Clin Endocrinol Metab* 87: 2701-2705

Masuzaki H, Paterson J, Shinyama H, Morton NM, Mullins JJ, Seckl JR & Flier JS. (2004) A transgenic model of visceral obesity and the metabolic syndrome. *Science* 294: 2166-2170

Morton NM, Paterson JM, Masuzaki H, Holmes MC, Staels B, Fievet C, Walker BR, Flier JS, Mullins JJ & Seckl JR. (2004) Novel adipose tissue-mediated resistance to diet-induced visceral obesity in 11β-hydroxysteroid dehydrogenase type 1 deficient mice. *Diabetes* 53: 931-938

Nishikawa T, Iizuka T, Omura M, Kuramoto N, Miki T, Ito H & Chiba S. (1996) Effect of mazindol on body weight and insulin sensitivity in severely obese patients after a very-low-calorie diet therapy. *Endocr J.* 43:671-7.

Noreen EE, Sass MJ, Crowe ML, Pabon VA, Brandauer J & Averill LK. (2010) Effects of supplemental fish oil on resting metabolic rate, body composition, and salivary cortisol in healthy adults *Journal of the International Society of Sports Nutrition* 2010, 7:31

Oltmanns KM, Dodt B, Schultes B, Raspe HH, Schweiger U, Born J, Fehm HL & Peters A. (2006) Cortisol correlates with metabolic disturbances in a population study of type 2 diabetic patients. *Eur J Endocrinol* 154: 325-311

Pasquali R, Biscotti D, Spinucci G, Vicennati V, Genazzani AD, Sgarbi L & Casimirri F. (1998) Pulsatile secretion of ACTH and cortisol in premenopausal women: effect of obesity and body fat distribution. *Clin Endocrinol.*48: 603-12,

Pasquali R, Vicennati V, Cacciari M & Pagotto U. (2006) The hypothalamic-pituitary-adrenal axis activity in obesity and the metabolic syndrome. *Ann N Y Acad Sci.*1083:111-28.

Paulmyer-Lacroi O, Boullu S, Oliver C, Alessi MC & Grino M (2002) Expression of the mRNA coding for 11β-hydroxysteroid dehydrogenase type 1 in adipose tissue from obese patients: an *in situ* hybridization study. *J Clin Endocrinol Metab* 87: 2701-2705

Rask E., Olsson T., Soderberg S., Andrew R., Livingstone D.E., Johnson O. &Walker B.R. (2001) Tissue-specific disregulation of cortisol metabolism in human obesity. *J Clin Endocrinol Metab* 86: 1418-1421

Rask E, Walker BR, Söderberg S, Livingstone DE Eliasson M, Johnson O, Andrew R & Olsson T. (2002) Tissue-specific changes in peripheral cortisol metabolism in obese women: Increased adipose 11β-hydroxysteroid dehydrogenage type 1 activity. *J Clin Endocrinol Metab* 87: 3330-3336

Rosmond R., Dallman M.F. & Bjorntorp P. (1998) Stress-related cortisol secretion in men: relationships with abdominal obesity and endocrine, metabolic and hemodynamic abnormalities. *J Clin Endocrinol Metab* 83: 1853-1859

Sinha, M.K. & Caro, J.F. (1998) Clinical aspects of leptin. *Vitam Horm.* 54: 1-30

Stewart PM, Boulton A, Kumar S, Clark PM & Shackleton CH. (1999) Cortisol metabolism in human obesity: impaired cortisone-cortisol conversion in subjects with central adiposity. *J Clin Endocrinol Metab* 84: 1022-1027

Tannin G.M, Agarwal A.K., Monder C, New M.I. & White, P.C. (1991) The human gene for 11β-hydroxysteroid dehydrogenase. Structure, tissue distribution, and chromosomal localization. *J Biol Chem* 266: 16653-16658

Valsamakis G, Anwar A, Tomlinson JW, Shackleton CH, McTernan PG, Chetty R, Wood PJ, Banerjee AK, Holder G, Barnett AH, Stewart PM & Kumar S. (2004) 11β-hydroxysteroid dehydrogenase type 1 activity in lean and obese males with type 2 diabetes mellitus. *J Clin Endocrinol Metab.* 89:4755-61

Vining RF, McGinley RA, Maksvytis JJ & Ho KY. (1983) Salivary cortisol: a better measure of adrenal cortical function than serum cortisol. *Ann Clin Biochem* 20:329-335

Walker B.R. & Andrew R. (2006) Tissue production of cortisol by 11β-hydroxysteroid dehydrogenase type 1 and metabolic disease. *Ann.N.Y.Acad.Science* 1083:165-184

8

Music and Steroids – Music Facilitates Steroid–Induced Synaptic Plasticity

Hajime Fukui and Kumiko Toyoshima
Nara University of Education
Japan

1. Introduction

Music and medicine have always been closely related. This remains true even in hunter-gatherer cultures that are thought to reflect primitive human forms, as clarified by cultural anthropological and ethno-musicological studies (Lee & Daly, 2005; Merriam & Merriam, 1964). Interestingly, music has also been used for the treatment of neuropsychiatric disorders in hunter-gatherer cultures (Lee & Daly, 2005; Merriam & Merriam, 1964). However, in westernized societies, no established music therapy exists for neuropsychiatric disorders such as stress disorders, mood disorders (depression), and dementia. Experience has shown that music has certain therapeutic effects on neuropsychiatric disorders (both functional and organic disorders), and music therapy is currently being used in the United States and Europe in clinical and welfare settings. However, the mechanisms of action underlying music therapy remain unknown.

Various studies have examined the effects of listening to music on the brain (Bermudez & Zatorre, 2005; Nan et al., 2008). The study by Rauscher et al. on the "Mozart effect" is one of the most famous studies and has had both positive and negative impacts on music therapy (Rauscher et al., 1993). However, many subsequent studies have questioned the reliability of those results, and Chabris et al. published a study disproving the Mozart effect (Chabris, 1999). However, the fact that music affects the human body and mind was not disproved. In fact, more scientific studies on music have been conducted in recent years, mainly in the field of neuroscience, and the level of interest among researchers is increasing (Zatorre, 2003; Zatorre & McGill, 2005). Results of past studies have clarified that music influences and affects cerebral nerves in humans from fetuses to adults (Abbott, 2002).

The most significant finding has been that music enhances synaptic changes in the brain. In other words, studies comparing musicians and non-musicians and music learners and non-learners have clarified that music brings about cerebral plasticity. Music affects neuronal learning and readjustment (response of brain cells to sound and music stimuli, and changes in cell counts), and this effect lasts for a long period (Abbott, 2002). For example, even when neurodegenerative diseases such as Alzheimer's disease cause memory loss, patients can still remember music from the past, and listening to music can facilitate the recovery of other memories. This type of memory recovery is accompanied by the reconfiguration of existing neuron networks, which may allow access to long-term memory. However, most studies have been based on brain imaging modalities such as positron emission tomography (PET) or functional magnetic resonance imaging (fMRI). The effects of music at a cellular level have not been clarified, and the mechanisms of action for the effects of music on the brain have not been elucidated.

The effects of steroids on changes in the brain have been documented in many animal species. For instance, vocal communication is a common characteristic among many vertebrates, and steroid hormones are implicated in the formation of neural mechanisms of vocal behavior in fish, amphibians, birds, and mammals (including primates) (Bass, 2008). The most fully known relationship between steroids and cerebral plasticity is vocal (singing) behavior in birds. The development of vocal behavior in singing birds involves complicated processes including neurons and muscles, and steroid hormones (testosterone and 17β-estradiol) are involved during many steps, such as neuron organization, neuron survival, and neural song-system formation (Fusani & Gahr, 2006; Nottebohm, 1981).

In humans, steroid hormones are associated with spatial perception and cognition. The relationship between testosterone and cognitive abilities is negative in men and positive in women (Gouchie & Kimura, 1991; Grimshaw et al., 1995a; Grimshaw et al., 1995b; Kimura & Hampson, 1994; O'Connor et al., 2001; Silverman et al., 1999). In women, the equilibrium of testosterone and 17β-estradiol associated with the menstrual cycle alters cognitive abilities (Silverman et al., 1999; Silverman & Phillips, 1993). Furthermore, in women, age-related decreases in 17β-estradiol are thought to be involved in cognitive dysfunction, memory disorder, learning disorder, depression, and other mood disorders. Numerous studies have also examined the relationship between 17β-estradiol and Alzheimer's disease accompanied by marked cognitive dysfunction (Gillies & McArthur, 2011; Wharton et al., 2001). The level of 17β-estradiol is lower for Alzheimer patients than for healthy individuals, and this decrease in estrogen level may lead to the progression of Alzheimer's disease and facilitate amyloid beta accumulation, one of the causes of memory disorders. Furthermore, testosterone administration to elderly men reportedly improves cognitive function (Gruenewald & Matsumoto, 2003).

The correlation between musical ability and spatial cognition is well recognized (Cupchik, 2001; Hassler, 1992; Hassler & Birbaumer, 1984). Many studies have investigated the relation between musical ability and spatial perception and cognition in humans. The assumption that some correlation exists between musical ability and steroid hormones also appears reasonable. In fact, Hassler discovered that the relationship between testosterone and musical ability (music composition) corresponded to that between testosterone and other forms of spatial perception and cognition (Hassler, 1991, 1992).

Furthermore, the relationship between music and steroid hormones is not confined to musical ability. Many studies in the field of behavioral endocrinology and neuroendocrinology have documented that musical stimulation (listening) affects various biochemical substances (Hassler et al., 1992; Kreutz et al., 2004; VanderArk & Ely, 1993).

2. Music and human physiology

The fact that music has an effect on the human body, particularly on stress and easing pain or anxiety, has been generally known since the Greeks (Aristoteles). Music influences the endocrine system to keep the body normal, as shown by many studies (e.g., Gardner et al., 1960; Logan & Roberts, 1984; Maslar, 1986; Standley, 1986; Hodges, 1996). Musical behavior is believed to invigorate several parts of the nervous system, as auditory information passes through the limbic and paralimbic systems including the thalamus, the hypothalamus, and amygdala, to the neocortex, and influences the pituitary gland; as a result, various physiological effects are induced. Much research has been done regarding the physiologic effects of music, with results showing increases or decreases in respiration, heart rate, blood pressure, skin temperature, GSR (galvanic skin response), and electroencephalogram findings (Hodges, 1996). However, because of problems with experimental methods, results are inconsistent. Unfortunately, there is still no unified concept regarding the physiological effects of music, although the fact that music causes physiological effects in the human body is well accepted. Enormous advances have been made in recent years toward an understanding of the brain structures involved in music. Using the brain imaging techniques of PET, fMRI, and magnetoencephalography, the brain structures and activity related to music were clarified (Koelsch, 2010; Zatorre, 2003). Interestingly, these structures (limbic and paralimbic structures) are involved in the initiation, generation, detection, maintenance, regulation, and termination of emotions that have survival value for the individual and the species (Koelsch, 2010). Needless to say, emotions are deeply affected by steroids (Garcia-Segura, 2009).

3. Effects of steroids on auditory and musical behavior

Recently, endocrinologic research on human behavior has progressed. Evidence to date suggests that hormones not only have organizational effects but also affect cognition, perception, and other behaviors. Because the endocrine and nervous systems do not function in isolation but as an integrated whole, many aspects of neuronal functioning are affected by hormones (gonadal steroids). However, we still lack data regarding the effect of music on hormones. In addition, although knowledge regarding endocrinologic function and music has begun to accumulate, results are contradictory. Some studies indicate that music influences humans endocrinologically and other studies indicate that hormones influence musical behavior. Below we will review the substances that have been examined thus far and explore the physiological function of music.

Many reports support the correlation between hormones and hearing or vocal behaviors. The fact that testosterone influences growth of the larynx is well known. It is believed that testosterone also influences the auditory sense and the vocal organ (Kelley & Brenowitz, 1992; Marler et al., 1988; Silver, 1992). Reports also indicate that the utterance of song birds is influenced by testosterone (Nottebohm, 1972; Marler et al., 1988) and point to the existence of similarities between the vocal tract of song birds and humans (Bridgeman, 1988). The fact that the auditory sense of the human females undergoes cyclical changes affected hormones has been reported (Wynn, 1971). Moreover the female voice is also influenced by 17β-estradiol (Abitbol et al., 1989). The hypothesis that the perception of sound is influenced by hormones is based on the idea that hormones influence dorsal division and reticular formation in the auditory pathways.

Testosterone influences the development of the neural pathways of the brain and stimulates cerebral lateralization (Geschwind & Galaburda, 1985). As Lovejoy said, this provides males with right brain superiority, which results in making him proficient in spatial ability, such as securing food and adapting to the environment (Lovejoy, 1981). Other reports also show that spatial ability is influenced by sex hormones; for example, men with lower testosterone levels performed better than men with higher testosterone levels whereas women with higher testosterone levels performed better than women with lower testosterone levels on spacial ability tests (Gouchie & Kimura, 1991; Hampson & Kimura, 1992; Nyborg, 1983). Further a relation between spatial ability and musical ability has been reported (Hassler et al., 1985), and listening to music has been shown to improve spatial ability (IQ) (Rauscher et al., 1993).

4. Musical behavior and steroids

4.1 Cortisol

Psychological and physiological stress affects testosterone and cortisol levels in both sexes. Generally, cortisol levels increase significantly in the presence of stress. It has been reported that music eases stress responses psychologically, physiologically, and endocrinologically. It is well known that listening to music reduces uneasiness (Gerdner & Swanson, 1993; Kaminski & Hall, 1996), depression, and fatigue (Field et al., 1997; Hanser & Thompson, 1994), changes mood (Cadigan et al., 2001; Gfeller & Lansing, 1991; McCraty et al., 1998; Sousou, 1997), and suppresses pain (Allen et al., 2001; Browning, 2000; Maslar, 1986). However, some reports that compare listening to music with other relaxation methods show no differences in alleviation of anxiety, depression, and fatigue (Field et al., 1997; Hanser & Thompson, 1994) or reduction of heart rate (Guzzetta, 1989; Scheufele, 2000). In addition, some authors have reported that there is differences in psychological and physiological responses among different genres of music (classical, hard rock, "favorite music," "relaxation music") (Allen & Blascovich, 1994) and others have reported no such differences (Burns, 1999).

Most of these studies have been on the stress-reducing effects of listening to music, and listening to music has been reported to cause a reduction in the cortisol levels. Cortisol is involved in many vital functions such as glucose metabolism and immune function, but in cases of chronic stress, it has been known to induce symptoms such as hypertension and impaired cognitive function (Lundberg, 2005). In addition, increasing cortisol levels with age may lead to a decline in memory or progression of Alzheimer's disease (Huang et al., 2009). Thus, the reduction of cortisol through the passive activity of listening to music may be useful for the treatment and prevention of diseases and disabilities.

Listening to music for short periods could lower cortisol regardless of the subject' s mental state (Field et al., 1998; Möckel et al., 1994), and music has been shown to significantly lower (Escher et al., 1993; Miluk Kolasa et al., 1994; Rider et al., 1985) or suppress cortisol levels (Schneider et al., 2001) even during surgery. Other papers reported that not only listening to music but also playing music (percussion instruments) lowered cortisol levels (Bittman et al., 2001; Burns et al., 2001). In addition, studies have shown that cortisol responses differed by music experience, such as (Vander Ark & Ely, 1992, 1993) and the subject's preference (Gerra et al., 1998). However, so far results are contradictory and there is no consensus regarding the relation between cortisol and music category or preference. However, judging from published research results, listening to one's favorite music decreases cortisol levels (Fukui, 1996).

4.2 Testosterone

Contrary to cortisol, several investigations have been conducted on the relationship between music and testosterone.

Testosterone has been shown to influence musical ability (Hassler, 1991), and its effects produce discrepancies between the sexes (Schumacher & Balthazart, 1986). Hassler hypothesized the existence of an optimal testosterone level in proportion to musical ability. Reports also discuss the existence of a correlation between hormone levels (testosterone) and musical ability in puberty (Durden-Smith & Simone, 1983; Hassler, 1987; Hassler and Birbaumer 1987). Another report indicates that during puberty, children show poor results in music tests because of low testosterone levels at this stage (Serafine, 1988). Moreover, there is a report that composition has a seasonality that might be influenced by the circannual rhythm of testosterone (Fukui, 1995). In addition, most composers are male, and composers tends to show a low level of testosterone compared with control (Hassler et al., 1990). Further reports show that musicians have a tendency to demonstrate relatively low levels of sex-role stereotyping (Kemper, 1990), which again, may be related to testosterone levels. The point is that testosterone influences musical ability.

Regarding musical ability and testosterone, there is a high positive correlation between spatial cognitive ability and musical ability (talent) (Rauscher et al., 1993). A high correlation is also found between spatial cognitive ability and testosterone (Nyborg, 1983). Furthermore, these correlations differ between males and females. Hassler reported that male composers had relatively low testosterone levels, and that testosterone values increased as musical ability increased in female composers (Hassler, 1991).

On the other hand, only one report is available on sex-related differences in testosterone responses associated with music playing or listening. Fukui examined testosterone level changes between before and after listening to a wide variety of music, including favorite music, pop, jazz, and classical, in male and female students, and showed sex-related differences (Fukui, 2001). Specifically, testosterone values decreased in males and increased in females after listening to music, regardless of genre. Interestingly, the sex-related difference in testosterone levels while listening to music were the same as sex-related differences in stress responses. Grape et al. compared between patients with irritable bowel syndrome who took part in singing in a choir with those who took part in a group discussion and found that testosterone levels decreased in the singing group (Grape et al., 2010).

So far, there is no research investigating music and estrogen.

5. Hypothesis and the study

We propose that listening to music facilitates the regeneration and repair of cerebral nerves by adjusting the secretion of steroid hormones in both directions (increase and decrease), ultimately leading to cerebral plasticity. Music affects levels of cortisol, testosterone, and 17β-estradiol, and we believe that music also affects the receptor genes related to these substances and related proteins.

5.1 Methods

Subjects were recruited from healthy elderly women aged 60 or older who were participating in a 90 min. singing group (choir) as part of disease prevention and health-promoting activities hosted by the local government. The session was taught by a music therapist. Inclusion criteria were as follows: attended all four sessions (once a month); healthy; and not taking any medications such as steroids that could affect endocrinologic factors. A total of 50 volunteers (8 males and 42 females) were enrolled, however because of missing value, male's data was not possible to use. Finally, 42 female volunteers were enrolled. Mean age was 72.9 years (range: 64-83 years).

After obtaining informed consent, subjects participated in four choral sessions, once a month for 4 consecutive months. The sessions took place at a facility owned by the local government. The flow of the experiment was as follows: first, health status and medication were checked. Then a saliva sample was collected before and after each session (about 90 min). Saliva samples were stored at -20ºC in the freezer immediately after collection, and cortisol, testosterone, and 17ß-estradiol levels were measured by enzyme immunoassay. Intra- and inter-assay coefficients of variation ranged between 3.35–3.65% and 3.75–6.41% for cortisol, 2.5–6.7% and 7.9–8.6% for testosterone, and 6.3–8.1% and 6.0–8.9% for 17β-estradiol.

The musical preference of subjects was ascertained before the study, and several pieces of music were selected for the session. The contents of all four sessions were the same.

To assess depression and anxiety as psychological states, the Japanese version of the Profile of Mood States (POMS) as executed before and after the session (Yokoyama & Araki, 1994). The POMS is a highly reliable test that is often used in studies on mood states and the test we used were revised for use by the elderly in terms of terminology and style. In the present study, of the six subscales of POMS ("tension/anxiety" (TA), "depression/dejection" (DD), "anger/hostility," "vitality," "fatigue," and "confusion," the DD and TA subscales were used.

Cognitive tests were carried out at the same time as the POMS. Tests performed were as follows: 1) Digit Symbol-Coding (WAIS: Wechsler Adult Intelligence Scale III) memory task (Silverman and Eals' Object Location Memory Task), and 3) mental rotations test (Vandenberg and Kuse Mental Rotations test "3-dimensional").

5.2 Results

Cortisol, testosterone, and 17ß-estradiol levels for subjects were biphasic, and subjects were divided into two groups (high and low) with respect to pre-session median values. Mean hormone levels prior to the choral session were 0.2243 μg/dL for cortisol, 66.0579 pg/mL for testosterone, and 6.1332 pg/mL for 17β-estradiol.

Analysis of variance (ANOVA) was conducted on changes in cortisol, testosterone, and 17β-estradiol levels before and after each session, between the high and low groups, and between each session.

In terms of cortisol levels, the main effect of cortisol changes before and after the choral session was significant ($F(1,122)=28.16$, $p=0.0000$). In addition, the main effect between the high and low groups ($F(1,122)=35.05$, $p=0.0000$) was significant. Cortisol significantly decreased after each session in both the high and low groups (Fig. 1).

The main effect of testosterone changes before and after the choral session ($F(1,284)=4.26$, $p=0.0399$), the main effect between the high and low groups ($F(1,284)=289.99$, $p=0.0000$), and the interaction between testosterone changes and the high and low groups ($F(1,244)=15.04$, $p=0.0001$) were significant. In the high group, testosterone levels significantly decreased after the choral session; in contrast, in the low group, testosterone levels increased significantly after the session (Fig. 2).

The main effect of 17β-estradiol changes ($F(1,244)=23.23$, $p=0.0000$), the main effect between the high and low group ($F(1,244)=193.72$, $p=0.0000$), and the interaction between 17β-estradiol changes and the high and low groups ($F(1,244)=58.27$, $p=0.0000$) were significant. In the high group, 17β-estradiol levels significantly decreased after the choral session. Conversely, in the low group, 17β-estradiol levels significantly increased after the session (Fig. 3).

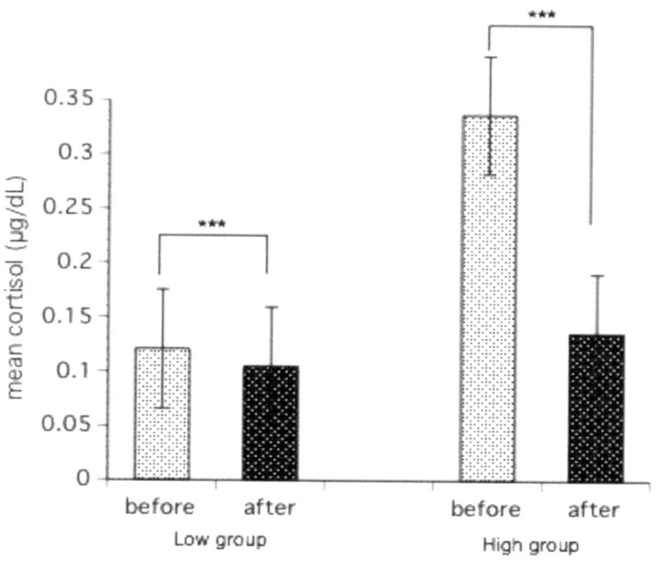

The main effect of cortisol changes before and after the choral session was significant (F (1,122)=28.16, p=0.0000). In addition, the main effect between the high and low groups (F (1,122)=35.05, p=0.0000) was significant. Cortisol decreased after each session in both the high and low groups.

Fig. 1. Cortisol levels of 42 female subjects

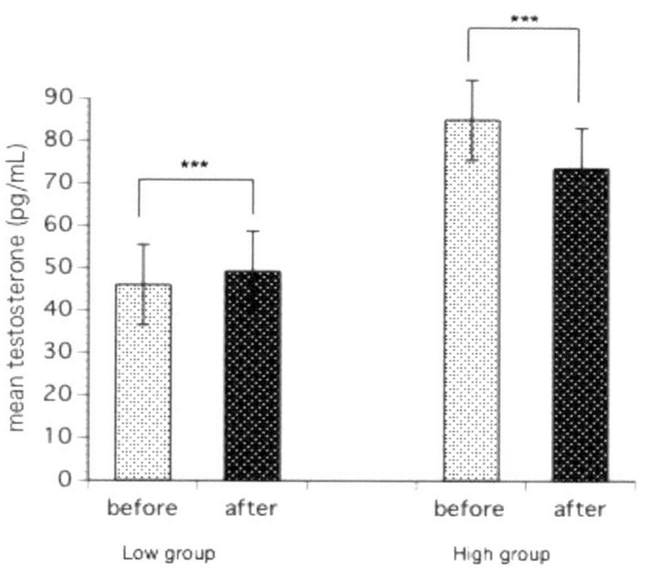

The main effect of testosterone changes before and after the choral session (F (1,284)=4.26, p=0.0399), the main effect between the high and low groups (F (1,284)=289.99, p=0.0000), and the interaction between testosterone changes and the high and low groups (F (1,244)=15.04, p=0.0001) were significant. In the high group, testosterone levels decreased after the choral session; in contrast, in the low group, testosterone levels increased after the session.

Fig. 2. Testosterone levels of 42 female subjects

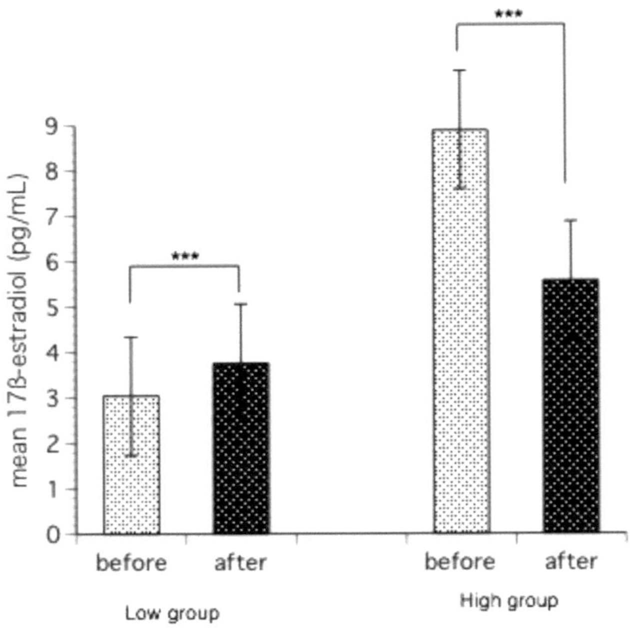

The main effect of 17β-estradiol changes (F (1,244)=23.23, p=0.0000), the main effect between the high and low group (F (1,244)=193.72, p=0.0000), and the interaction between 17β-estradiol changes and the high and low groups (F (1,244)=58.27, p=0.0000) were significant. In the high group, 17β-estradiol levels decreased after the choral session. Conversely, in the low group, 17β-estradiol levels increased after the session.

Fig. 3. 17ß-estradiol levels of 42 female subjects

ANOVA was conducted on changes in cortisol, testosterone, and 17β-estradiol levels before and after each session, between the high and low groups, and between each session. No significant difference was found in any factor of the TA scores. The main effect of the DD scores was significant for cortisol (F (1,122)=4.02, p=0.0473), testosterone (F (1,117)=3.70, p=0.05), and 17β-estradiol (F (1,119)=4.25, p=0.0414). The scores of high and low groups significantly decreased after the session.
ANOVA was conducted on changes in cortisol, testosterone, and 17β-estradiol levels before and after each session, between the high and low groups, and between each session. No significant difference was found in any factor of the Digit Symbol-Coding. For the memory task, only the main effect of high and low groups for 17ß-estradiol was significant (F (1,120)=10.85, p=0.0013). The main effect of the mental rotations test was significant for cortisol (F (1,123)=9.16, p=0.0030), testosterone (F (1,116)=8.48, p=0.0043), and 17β-estradiol (F (1,120)=9.03, p=0.0032). The scores of high and low groups significantly increased after the session (Fig. 4, 5, 6).

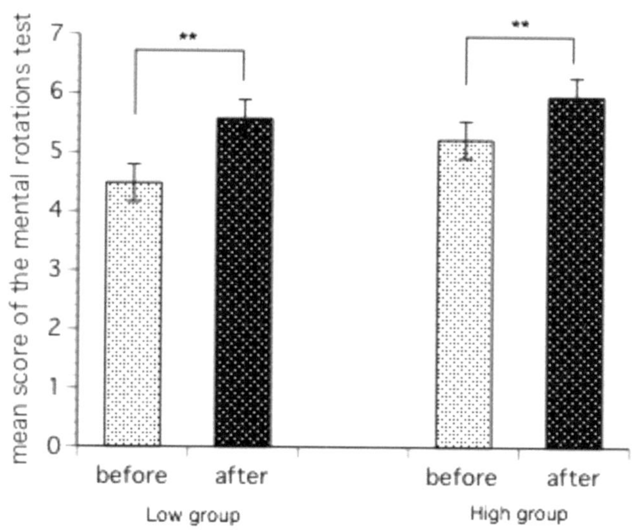

The main effect of the mental rotations test was significant for cortisol (F (1,123)=9.16, p=0.0030). The scores of high and low groups increased after the session.

Fig. 4. Mean score of the mental rotations test in cortisol levels

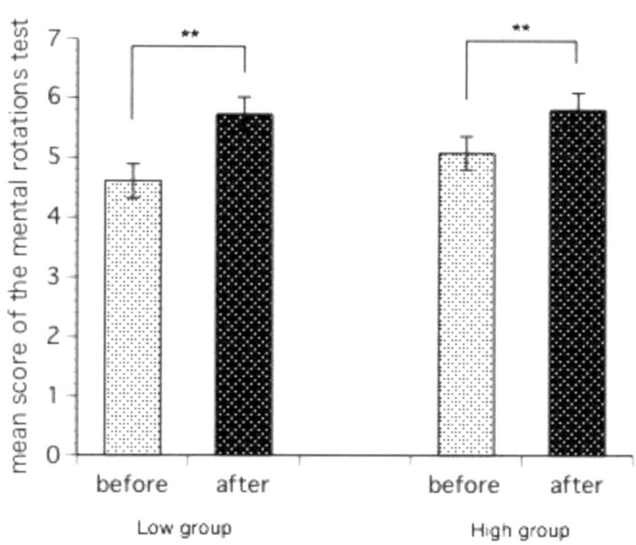

The main effect of the mental rotations test was significant for testosterone (F (1,116)=8.48, p=0.0043). The scores of high and low groups increased after the session.

Fig. 5. Mean score of the mental rotations test in testosterone levels

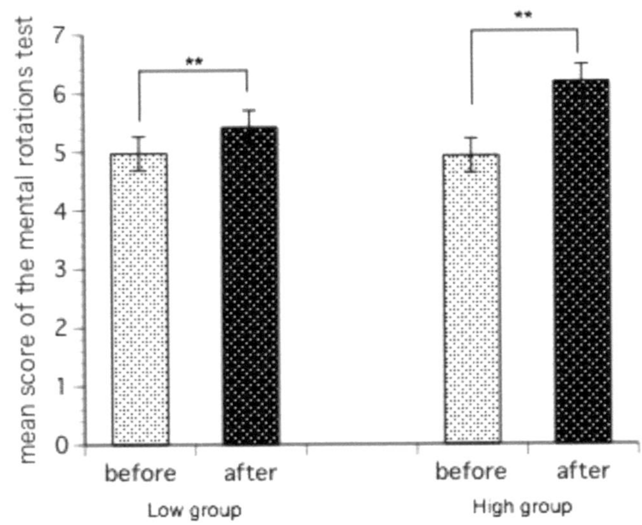

The main effect of the mental rotations test was significant for 17β-estradiol ($F(1,120)=9.03$, $p=0.0032$). The scores of high and low groups increased after the session.

Fig. 6. Mean score of the mental rotations test in 17ß-estradiol levels

6. Discussion

Coristol, testosterone, and 17β-estradiol were affected by musical behavior (chorus). Cortisol levels decreased after each choral session, whereas changes in testosterone and 17β-estradiol levels were dependent on the subject's baseline hormone level. After all sessions, testosterone and 17β-estradiol levels increased in the low groups and decreased in the high groups.

Anxiety and depression score (POMS) decreased after all sessions. The interesting finding was a result of the cognitive test (mental rotations test). The score increased regardless of the initial hormone level. Mental rotation involves spatial ability and is localized to the right hemisphere and is associated with intelligence (Hertzog & Rypma, 1991); Johnson, 1990; Jones & Anuza, 1982). It has been documented that music training improves verbal, mathematical, and visuo-spatial performance in children and adults (Brochard, 2004; Ho et al., 2003). However, no study has investigated music and mental rotation beside the "Mozart effects," especially in elderly people (Cacciafesta, et al., 2010). Our study is the first report to show that music improved mental rotation ability in elderly women.

Results of this study clarified that musical activities affect steroid secretion in elderly women and are likely to alleviate psychological states such as anxiety and tension. Furthermore, levels of steroids changed in both directions, increasing in subjects with low hormone levels and decreasing in subjects with high hormone levels. Thus, the hypothesis that listening to music affects the steroid hormone cascade and facilitates neurogenesis, regeneration, and repair of neuron appears highly plausible.

This study has several limitations, including the fact that only data obtained from a small number of elderly women were analyzed. However, the finding that musical behavior (chorus in this study) altered steroid levels agrees with results of previous studies that have documented strong correlations between steroids and spatial perception and cognition and the effects of listening to music on steroid secretion.

At this point, the effects of music on steroids are unclear, but music appears to be involved with steroid production via the pathway from the auditory system to the auditory area, particularly the neural pathway (emotion circuits) mediated by the cerebral limbic system (hypothalamic-pituitary-adrenal axis and amygdaloid complex). In recent years, the possible involvement of nerve damage in neuropsychiatric disorders has been suggested, and musical activities may enable the protection, repair, and even regeneration of human cerebral nerves.

Music is noninvasive, and its existence is universal and mundane. Thus, if music can be used in medical care, the application of such a safe and inexpensive therapeutic option is limitless.

7. Acknowledgment

This work was supported by Nissei Foundation.

8. References

Abbott, A. (2002). Music, maestro, please. *Nature*, Vol.416, (March 2002), pp. 12-14, ISSN 0028-0836

Abitbol, J., Brux, J., Millot, G., Masson, M.F., Mimoun, O.L., Pau, H. & Abitol, B. (1989). Does a Hormonal Vocal Cord Cycle Exist in Women? Study of Vocal Premenstrual Syndrome in Voice Performers by Videostroboscopy-Glottography and Cytology on 38 Women. *Journal of Voice*, Vol.3, (June 1989), pp. 157-162, ISSN 08921997

Allen, K. & Blascovich, J. (1994). Effects of music on cardiovascular reactivity among surgeons. *JAMA : the journal of the American Medical Association*, Vol.272, No.11, (September 1994), pp. 882–884, ISSN 0098-7484

Allen, K., Golden, L.H., Izzo, J.L., Ching, M.I., Forrest, A., Niles, C.R., Niswander, P.R. & Barlow, J.C. (2001). Normalization of hypertensive responses during ambulatory sur- gical stress by perioperative music. *Psychosomatic medicine*, VOl.63, No.3, (May 2001), pp. 487–492, ISSN 0033-3174

Bass, A.H. (2008). Steroid-dependent plasticity of vocal motor systems: novel insights from teleost fish. *Brain research reviews*, Vol.57, No.2, (March 2008), pp. 299-308, ISSN 0165-0173

Bermudez, P. & Zatorre, R.J. (2005). Differences in gray matter between musicians and nonmusicians. *Annals of the New York Academy of Sciences*, Vol.1060, (December 2005). pp.395–399, ISSN 0077-8923

Bittman, B.B., Berk, L.S., Felten, D.L., Westengard, J., Simonton, O.C., Pappas, J. & Ninehouser, M. (2001). Composite effects of group drumming music therapy on modulation of neuroendocrine-immune parameters in normal subjects. *Alternative therapies in health and medicine*, Vol.7, No.1, (January 2001), pp. 38–47, ISSN 1078-6791

Bridgeman, B. (1988). *The biology of behavior and mind.* NY: John Wiley & Sons Inc, ISBN 9780471876212, NY.

Brochard, R., Dufour, A. & Despres, O. (2004). Effect of musical expertise on visuospatial abilities: Evidence from reaction times and mental imagery. *Brain and Cognition*, Vol.54, No.2, (March 2004), pp. 103-109, ISSN 0278-2626

Browning, C.A. (2000). Using music during childbirth. *Birth*, Vol.27, No.4, (December 2000), pp. 272–276, ISSN 0730-7659

Burns, J., Labbe, E., Williams, K.M. & McCall, J. (1999). Perceived and physiolog- ical indicators of relaxation: as different as Mozart and Alice in chains. *Applied psychophysiology and biofeedback*, Vol.24, No.3, (September 1999), pp. 197–202, ISSN 1090-0586

Burns, S.J., Harbuz, M.S., Hucklebridge, F. & Bunt, L. (2001). A pilot study into the therapeutic effects of music therapy at a cancer help center. *Alternative therapies in health and medicine*, Vol.7, No.1, (January 2001), pp. 48–56, ISSN 1078-6791

Cacciafesta, M., Ettorre, E., Amici, A., Cicconetti, P., Martinelli, V., Linguanti, A., Baratta, A., Verrusio, W. & Marigliano, V. (2010). New frontiers of cognitive rehabilitation in geriatric age: the Mozart Effect (ME). *Archives of Gerontology and Geriatrics*, Vol.51, No.3, (November 2010), pp. e79-e82, ISSN 0167-4943

Cadigan, M.E., Caruso, N.A., Haldeman, S.M., McNamara, M.E., Noyes, D.A., Spadafora, M.A. & Carroll, D.L. (2001). The effects of music on cardiac patients on bed rest. *Progress in cardiovascular nursing*, Vol.16, No.1, (Winter 2001), pp. 5–13, ISSN 0889-7204

Chabris, C.F. (1999). Prelude or requiem for the 'Mozart effect'? *Nature*, Vol.400, (August 1999), pp. 826–827, ISSN 0028-0836

Cupchik, G.C., Phillips, K. & Hill, D.S. (2001). Shared processes in spatial rotation and musical permutation. *Brain and cognition*, Vol.46, No.3, (August 2001), pp. 373-382, ISSN 0278-2626

Durden-Smith, J. & Simone, D. (1983). *Sex and the Brain*, Arbor House Pub Co, ISBN 9780877954842, New York

Escher, J., Hoehmann, U., Anthenien, L., Dayer, E., Bosshard, C. & Gaillard, R.C. (1993). Music during gastroscopy. *Schweizerische medizinische Wochenschrift*, Vol.123, No.26, (July 1993), pp. 1354–1358, ISSN 0036-7672

Field, T., Martinez, A., Nawrocki, T., Pickens, J., Fox, N.A. & Schanberg, S. (1998). Music shifts frontal EEG in depressed adolescents. *Adolescence*, Vol.33, No.129, (Spring 1998), pp. 109–116, ISSN 0001-8449

Field, T., Quintino, O., Henteleff, O., Wells-Keife, L. & Delvecchio-Feinberg, G. (1997). Job stress reduction therapies. *Alternative therapies in health and medicine*, Vol.3, No.4, (July 1997), pp. 54–56, ISSN 1078-6791

Fukui H. (1996). Behavioral endocrinological study of music and testosterone. *The Annual of Music Psycholog & Therapy*, Vol.25, (1996), pp. 14–21, ISSN 1345-5591

Fukui H. (2001). Music and testosterone. A new hypothesis for the origin and function of music. *Annals of the New York Academy of Sciences*, Vol.930, (June 2001), pp. 448–451, ISSN 0077-8923

Fukui, H. (1995). Seasonality of Composition. *Journal of Music Perception and Cognition*, Vol.1, (December 1995), pp. 17-24, ISSN 1342-856X

Fusani, L. & Gahr, M. (2006). Hormonal influence on song structure and organization: the role of estrogen. *Neuroscience*, Vol.138, No.3, (November 2005), pp. 939-946, ISSN 0306 4522

Garcia-Segura, L.M. (2009). *Hormones and Brain Plasticity*, Oxford University Press, ISBN 9780195326611, New York, USA

Gardner, W.J., Licklider, J.C.R. & Weisz, A.Z. (1960). Suppression of Pain by Sound. *Science*, Vol.132, (July 1960), pp. 32-33 ISSN 0036-8075

Gerdner, L.A. & Swanson, E.A. (1993). Effects of individualized music on con- fused and agitated elderly patients. *Archives of psychiatric nursing*, Vol.7, No.5, (October 1993), pp. 284–291, ISSN 0883-9417

Gerra, G., Zaimovic, A., Giucastro, G., Folli, F., Maestri, D., Tessoni, A., Avanzini, P., Caccavari, R., Bernasconi, S. & Brambilla, F. (1998). Neurotransmitter-hormonal responses to psychological stress in peripubertal subjects: relationship to aggressive behavior. *Life Sciences*, Vol.62, No.7. (January 1998), pp. 615–627, ISSN 0024-3205

Geschwind, N., & Galaburda, A.M. (1985). Cerebral lateralization: Biological mechanisms, associations, and pathology: I. A hypothesis and a program for research. *Archives of Neurology*, Vol.42, (May 1985), pp. 428–459, ISSN 0003-9942

Gfeller, K. & Lansing, C.R. (1991). Melodic, rhythmic, and timbral perception of adult cochlear implant users. *Journal of speech and hearing research*, Vol.34, No.4, (August 1991), pp. 916–920, ISSN 0022-4685

Gillies, G.E. & McArthur, S. (2011). Estrogen actions in the brain and the basis for differential action in men and women: a case for sex-specific medicines. *Pharmacological Reviews*, Vol. 62, No.2, (June 2010), pp.155-198, ISSN 0031-6997

Gouchie, C. & Kimura, D. (1991). The relationship between testoster- one levels and cognitive ability patterns. *Psychoneuroendocrinology*, Vol.16, No.4, (January 1992), pp. 323-334, ISSN 0306-4530

Grape, C., Wikström, B.M., Ekman, R., Hasson, D. & Theorell, T. (2010). Comparison between choir singing and group discussion in irritable bowel syndrome patients over one year: saliva testosterone increases in new choir singers. *Psychotherapy and psychosomatics*, Vol.79, No.3, (October 2009), pp. 196-198, ISSN 0033-3190

Grimshaw, G.M., Bryden, M.P. & Finegan, J.A. (1995). Relations between prenatal testosterone and cerebral lateralization in children. *Neuropsychology*, Vol.9, no.1, (January 1995), pp. 68-79, ISSN 0894-4105

Grimshaw, G.M., Sitarenios, G. & Finegan, J.A. (1995). Mental rotation at 7 years: relations with prenatal testosterone levels and spatial play experiences. *Brain and cognition*, Vol.29, No.1, (October 1995), pp. 85-100, ISSN 0278-2626

Gruenewald, D.A. & Matsumoto, A.M. (2003). Testosterone supplementation therapy for older men: potential benefits and risks. *Journal of the American Geriatrics Society*, Vol.51, No.1, (January 2003), pp. 101-115, ISSN 0002-8614

Guzzetta, C.E. (1989). Effects of relaxation and music therapy on patients in a coronary care unit with presumptive acute myocardial infarction. *Heart & lung : the journal of critical care*, Vol.18, No.6, (November 1989), pp. 609–616, ISSN 0147-9563

Hampson, E. & Kimura, D. (1992). Sex Differences and Hormonal Influences on Cognitive Function in Humans. *In Behavioral Endocrinology*, Becker, J., Breedlove, S.M. & Crews, D., (Ed.), pp. 357-397, MIT Press, ISBN 978-0262023429, Cambridge, MA

Hanser, S.B. & Thompson, L.W. (1994). Effects of a music therapy strategy on depressed older adults. *Journal of gerontology*, Vol.49, No.6, (November 1994), pp. 265–269, ISSN 0022-1422

Hassler, M. (1991). Testosterone and Musical Talent. *Expermental Crinical Endocrinology*, Vol.98, No.2, (1991), pp. 89-98, ISSN 0232-7384

Hassler, M. (1991). Testosterone and artistic talents. *The International journal of neuroscience*, Vol.56, No.1-4, (January 1991), pp. 25-38, ISSN 0020-7454

Hassler, M. (1992). Creative musical behavior and sex hormones: musical talent and spatial ability in the two sexes. *Psychoneuroendocrinology*, Vol.17, No.1, (March 1992), pp. 55-70, ISSN 0306-4530

Hassler, M. & Birbaumer, N. (1984). Musical talent and spatial ability. *Archiv für Psychologie*, Vol.136, No.3, (1984), pp. 235-248, ISSN 0066-6475

Hassler, M., Birbaumer, N. & Feil, A. (1985). Musical Talent and Visual-Spatial Abilities: A longitudinal Study. *Pschology of Music*, Vol.13, No.2, (October 1985), pp. 99-113, ISSN 0305-7356

Hassler, M., Birbaumer, N. & Feil, A. (1987). Musical Talent and Visual-spatial Ability: Onset of Puberty. *Psychology of Music*, Vol.15, (October 1987), pp. 141-151, ISSN 0305-7356

Hassler, M., Gupta, D. & Wollmann, H. (1992). Testosterone, estradiol, ACTH and musical, spatial and verbal performance. *The International journal of neuroscience*, Vol.65, No.1-4, (July 1992), pp. 45-60, ISSN 0020-7454

Hassler, M., Nieschlag, E. & Motte, D. (1990). Creative Musical Talent, Cognitive Functioning, and Gender: Psychological Aspects. *Music Perception*, Vol.8, No.1, (Fall 1990), pp. 35-48, ISSN 0730-7829

Hertzog, C. & Rypma, B. (1991). Age differences in components of mental rotation task performance. *Bulletin of the Psychonomic Society*, Vol.29, No.3, (1991), pp. 209-212, ISSN 0090-5054

Ho, Y.C., Cheung, M.C. & Chan, A.S. (2003). Music Training Improves Verbal but Not Visual Memory: Cross-Sectional and Longitudinal Explorations in Children. *Neuropsychology*, Vol.17, No.3, (July 2003), pp. 439–450, ISSN 0894-4105

Hodges, D.A. (Ed.). (1996). *Handbook of Music Psychology*, MMB Music,ISBN 978-0964880306, St. Louis, Missouri

Huang, C.W., Lui, C.C., Chang, W.N., Lu, C.H., Wang, Y.L. & Chang, C.C. (2009). Elevated basal cortisol level predicts lower hippocampal volume and cognitive decline in Alzheimer's disease. *Journal of clinical neuroscience : official journal of the Neurosurgical Society of Australasia*, Vol.16, No.10, (October 2009), pp. 1283-1286, ISSN 0967-5868

Johnson, A.M. (1990). Speed of mental rotation as a function of problem solving strategies. *Perceptual and motor skills*, Vol.71, (December 1990), pp. 803-806, ISSN 0031-5125

Jones, B. & Anuza, T. (1982). Effects of sex, handeness, stimulus and visual field on "mental rotation". *Cortex*, Vol.18, (December 1982), pp. 501-514, ISSN 0010-9452

Kaminski, J. & Hall, W. (1996). The effect of soothing music on neonatal be- havioral states in the hospital newborn nursery. *Neonatal network : NN*, Vol.15, No.1, (February 1996), pp. 45–54. ISSN 0730-0832

Kelley, D.B. & Brenowitz, E. (1992). Hormonal Influences on Courtship Behavior, In: *Behavioral Endocrinology*, Becker, J., Breedlove, S.M. & Crews, D., (Ed.), pp. 187-216, MIT Press, ISBN 978-0262023429, Cambridge, MA

Kemper, T.D. (1990). *Social Structure and Testosterone: Explorations in the Socio-Bio-Social Chain*, Rutgers University Press, ISBN 978-0813515519, London, England

Kimura, D. & Hampson, E. (1994). Cognitive pattern in men and women is influenced by fluctuations in sex hormones. *Current Directions in Psychological Science*, Vol.3, (April 1994), pp. 57-61, ISSN 0963-7214

Koelsch, S. (2010). Towards a neural basis of music-evoked emotions. *Trends in cognitive sciences*, Vol.14, No.3, (March 2010), pp. 131-137, ISSN 1364-6613

Kreutz, G., Bongard, S., Rohrmann, S., Hodapp, V. & Grebe, D. (2004). Effects of choir singing or listening on secretory immuno- globulin A, cortisol, and emotional state. *Journal of behavioral medicine*, Vol.27, No.6, (December 2004), pp. 623-635, ISSN 0160-7715

Lee, R.B. & Daly, R. (Eds.). (2005). *The Cambridge Encyclopedia of Hunters and Gatherers*, Cambridge University Press, ISBN 978-0521609197, Cambridge

Logan, T.G. & Roberts, A.R. (1984). The effects of different types of relaxation music on tension level. *Journal of Music Therapy*, Vol.21, No.4, (October 1984), pp. 177-183, ISSN 0022-2917

Lovejoy, C.O. (1981). The Origin of Man. *Science*, Vol.211, No.4480, (January 1981), pp. 341-350, ISSN 0036-8075

Lundberg, U. (2005). Stress hormones in health and illness: the roles of work and gender. *Psychoneuroendocrinology*, Vol.30, No.10, (November 2005), pp. 1017-1021, ISSN 0306-4530

Marler, P., Peters, S., Ball, G.F., Dufty, A.M.Jr. & Wingfield, J.C. (1988). The role of sex steroids in the acquisition and production of birdsong. *Nature*, Vol.336, (December 1988), pp. 770-772, ISSN 0028-0836

Maslar, P.M. (1986). The effect of music on the reduction of pain: a review of the literature. *The Arts in Psychotherapy*, Vol.13, (Fall 1986), pp. 215–219, ISSN 0197-4556

McCraty, R., Barrios-Choplin, B., Atkinson, M. & Tomasino, D. (1998). The effects of different types of music on mood, tension, and mental clarity. *Alternative therapies in health and medicine*, Vol.4, No.1, (January 1998), pp. 75–84, ISSN 1078-6791

Merriam, A.P. & Merriam, V. (1964). *The Anthropology of Music*, Northwestern University Press, ISBN 978-0810106079, Evanston, Illinois

Miluk Kolasa, B., Obminski, Z., Stupnicki, R. & Golec, L. (1994). Effects of music treatment on salivary cortisol in patients exposed to pre-surgical stress. *Experimental and clinical endocrinology*, Vol.102, No.2, (1994), pp. 118–120, ISSN 0232-7384

Möckel, M., Rocker, L., Stork, T., Vollert, J., Danne ,O., Eichstadt, H., Müller, R. & Hochrein, H. (1994). Immediate physiological responses of healthy volunteers to different types of music: cardiocascular, hormonal and mental changes. *European journal of applied physiology and occupational physiology*, Vol.68, (March 1994), pp. 451–459, ISSN 0301-5548

Nan, Y., Knösche, T.R., Zysset, S. & Friederici, A.D. (2008). Cross-cultural music phrase processing: an fMRI study. *HUMAN BRAIN MAPPING*, Vol.29, No.3, (March 2008), pp. 312–328, ISSN 1065-9471

Nottebohm, F. (1972). The origin of vocal learning. *The American Naturalist*, Vol.106, No.947, (January 1972), pp. 116-140, ISSN 0003-0147

Nottebohm, F.A. (1981). A brain for all seasons: cyclical anatomical changes in song control nuclei of the canary brain. *Science*, Vol.214, No.4527, (December 1981), pp. 1368–1370, ISSN 0036-8075

Nyborg, H. (1983). Spatial ability in men and women: Review and new theory. *Advances in Behaviour Research and Therapy*, Vol.5, (1983), pp. 89-140, ISSN 0146-6402

O'Connor, D.B., Archer, J., Hair, W.M. & Wu, F.C. (2001). Activational effects of testosterone on cognitive function in men. *Neuropsychologia*, Vol.39, No.13, (September 2001), pp. 1385-1394, ISSN 0028-3932

Rauscher, F.H., Shaw, G.L. & Ky, K.N. (1993). Music and spatial task performance. *Nature*, Vol.365, (October 1993), pp. 611, ISSN 0028-0836

Rider, M.S., Floyd, J.W. & Kirkpatrick, J. (1985). The effect of music relaxation on adrenal corticosteroids and the re-entrainment of circadian rhythms. *Journal of music therapy*, Vol.22, No.1, (Spring 1985), pp. 46–58, ISSN 0022-2917

Scheufele, P.M. (2000). Effects of progressive relaxation and classical music on measurements of attention, relaxation, and stress responses. *Journal of behavioral medicine*, Vol.23, No.2, (April 2000), pp. 207–228, ISSN 0160-7715

Schneider, N., Schedlowski, M., Schurmeyer, T.H. & Becker, H. (2001). Stress reduction through music in patients undergoing cerebral angiography. *Neuroradiology*, Vol.43, No.6, (June 2001), pp. 472–476, ISSN 0028-3940

Schumacher, M. & Balthazart, J. (1986). Testosterone-Induced Brain Aromatase Is Sexually Dimorphic. *Brain Research*, Vol.370, (April 1986), pp. 285-293, ISSN 0006-8993

Serafine, M.L. (1988). *Music as Cognition: The development of thought in sound*, Columbia University Press, ISBN 0231057423, New York

Silver, R. 1992. Environmental Factors Influencing Hormone Secretion. *In Behavioral Endocrinology*, Becker, J., Breedlove, S.M. & Crews, D., (Ed.), pp. 401-422, MIT Press, ISBN 978-0262023429, Cambridge, MA

Silverman, I. & Phillips, K. (1993). Effects of estrogen changes during the menstrual cycle on spatial performance. *Ethology and Sociobiology*, Vol.14, (July 1993), pp. 257-270, ISSN 0162-3095

Silverman, I., Kastuk, D., Choi, J. & Phillips, K. (1999). Testosterone levels and spatial ability in men. *Psychoneuroendocrinology*, Vol.24, No.8, (November 1999), pp. 813-822, ISSN 0306-4530

Sousou, S.D. (1997). Effects of melody and lyrics on mood and memory. *Perceptual and motor skills*, Vol.85, No.1, (August 1997), pp. 31–40, ISSN 0031-5125

Standley, J.M. (1986). Music Research in Medical/Dental Treatment: Meta-Analysis and Clinical Applications. *Journal of music therapy*, Vol.23, No.2, (Summer 1986), pp. 56-122, ISSN 0022-2917

Vander Ark, S.D. & Ely, D. (1992). Biochemical and galvanic skin response to music stimuli by college students in biology and music. *Perceptual and motor skills*, Vol.74, (June 1992), pp. 1079–1090, ISSN 0031-5125

Vander Ark, S.D. & Ely, D. (1993). Cortisol biochemical and galvanic skin responses to music stimuli of different preference values by college students in biology and music. *Perceptual and motor skills*, Vol.77, (August 1993), pp. 227–234, ISSN 0031-5125

Wharton, W., Baker, L.D., Gleason, C.E., Dowling, M., Barnet, J.H., Johnson, S., Carlsson, C., Craft, S. & Asthana, S. (2011). Short-term Hormone Therapy with Transdermal Estradiol Improves Cognition for Postmenopausal Women with Alzheimer's Disease: Results of a Randomized Controlled Trial. *Journal of Alzheimer's disease*, (June 21. 2001) [Epub ahead of print], ISSN 1387-2877

Wynn, V.T. (1971). "Absolute" Pitch-a Bimensual Rhythm, *Nature*, Vol.230, (April 1971), pp. 337, ISSN 0028-0836

Yokoyama, K. & Araki, S. (1994). *The Profile of Mood States (POMS) Japanese Version*, Kaneko shobo, ,Tokyo, Japan

Zatorre, R.J. (2003). Music and the brain. *ANNALS- NEW YORK ACADEMY OF SCIENCES, Annals of the New York Academy of Sciences*, Vol.999, (November 2003), pp. 4-14, ISSN 0077-8923

Zatorre, R. & McGill, J. (2005). Music, the food of neuroscience? *Nature*, Vol.434, (March 2005), pp. 312-315, ISSN 0028-0836